Achieving Competencies for Nursing Practice

A handbook for student nurses

Achieving Competencies for Nursing Practice

A handbook for student nurses

Edited by Sheila Reading and Brian Webster

Mc Graw Hill Education

Open University Press

Open University Press
McGraw-Hill Education
McGraw-Hill House
Shoppenhangers Road
Maidenhead
Berkshire
England
SL6 2QL

email: enquiries@openup.co.uk
world wide web: www.openup.co.uk

and Two Penn Plaza, New York, NY 10121-2289, USA

First published 2013

A catalogue record of this book is available from the British Library

ISBN-13: 978-0-335-24674-8
ISBN-10: 0-335-24674-5
eISBN: 978-0-335-24675-5

Library of Congress Cataloging-in-Publication Data
CIP data applied for

Typeset by Aptara, Inc.

Praise for this book

"What we have in this textbook is a user friendly but rigorous presentation of the main competencies for professional nursing practice. Its easy style and 'readability' is one of its most pleasing features and the case studies, information boxes and key learning points give structure to the book as well as helping to engage readers. The short chapters are interesting and authoritative and can be read on a 'stand-alone' basis, allowing readers to 'dip in and out'.

This book has arrived at an opportune time. The public and the nursing profession has been shocked by the findings of the Francis Review of the Mid Staffordshire NHS Foundation Trust. Research informed competencies were never more necessary. To provide patient care without expertise in the competencies required would be like starting a new journey without a map. This book is one of the best maps of the competency terrain that I have come across.

I recommend with enthusiasm this book to would-be readers. It is a solid and significant contribution to the on-going development of best nursing practice. It should be on the recommended reading list of any nurse who plans, delivers and evaluates patient care."

Professor Hugh P. McKenna CBE, PhD, B.Sc(Hons), RMN, RGN, RNT, DipN(Lond), AdvDipEd, FFN RCSI, FEANS, FRCN, FAAN, Pro Vice Chancellor, Research and Innovation, University of Ulster, UK

"[This book] clearly fills an important niche in the market. It frames the notions of competence, and addresses the NMC standards for pre-registration nursing clearly for students, mentors and educators in ways that are easy to understand, and encourages students to consider the implications behind the words they encounter and what these mean for them in their own practice. The expertise held by the range of authors ensures the book presents informed detail relating to nursing domains and competencies, and enhances the relevance of interpretation and examples through the four fields of nursing and both core and field specific concepts. To date, I would consider this the 'must-have' book on achieving competence for any nursing student in all four countries of the United Kingdom."

Melanie Jasper, Professor of Nursing and Head of the College of Human and Health Sciences, Swansea University, UK

Contents

List of tables

List of figures

The editors and contributors

The editors

Sheila Reading is an adult nurse who has worked in a variety of clinical, research and education roles including primary care contexts in the NHS and the university sector. She is currently a principal teaching fellow in the Faculty of Health Sciences, University of Southampton. She has wide-ranging experience of planning, developing and leading on a large number of undergraduate and postgraduate programmes and teaches on several professional courses, study days and workshops. Her education and research interests are broad but have a particular focus on exploring the student experience of undergraduate project supervision. She is interested in supporting student learning about the importance of research and evidence related to implementing sound clinical practice and how it can best be used by practitioners to enhance the quality of patient care.

Brian Webster is professor of nursing and Assistant Dean at the Faculty of Health, Life & Social Sciences at Edinburgh Napier University. He is both a mental health nurse and an adult nurse and has worked in a wide range of clinical settings including substance misuse, forensic psychiatry, emergency medicine, oncology and gastroenterology. A nurse for over 30 years, Brian also chairs the Scottish Heads of Academic Nursing & Allied Health Professions which is the voice of nursing education and research in Scotland, as well as being an executive member of the Council of Deans of Health UK. His research focus is on alcohol use and misuse especially among higher education students.

The contributors

Mary Addo is a lecturer in mental health nursing at the Robert Gordon University, Aberdeen. She has a range of clinical experience in mental health which is grounded in effective communication and interpersonal relationships with clients in order to empower them to improve the quality of care. She is an active researcher in mental health and has a distinctive passion for communication skills as a pivotal part of all nursing care.

Heather Bain is a lecturer at the Robert Gordon University, Aberdeen. She is currently the course leader of the masters awards portfolio at the School of Nursing and Midwifery and has a wealth of experience in district nursing. She has written several books and journal papers on this subject and has developed and implemented several prescribing courses for non-medical prescribers.

Mary-Jane Baker is a lecturer in adult nursing in the Faculty of Health Sciences, University of Southampton. She has extensive experience of nursing and her role as a student academic tutor and practice academic coordinator has enabled her to continue to work closely with clinical practitioners at all levels and in different settings. The NMC domain of nursing practice and decision-making encapsulates one of her particular areas of expertise in promoting students' development of critical thinking and application of knowledge and skills to practice. Mary-Jane is keen to encourage, support and guide students to make sense of decision-making within the various complex settings of contemporary clinical practice.

Debbie Banks is a senior lecturer and teaching fellow at the Robert Gordon University. She is an experienced mental health nurse and has worked in a wide range of clinical settings. She has written and created many undergraduate programmes during her time as an academic and has also implemented several creative pedagogical initiatives as part of the student experience in nursing. Her passion for listening to service users and incorporating their views and experience into student learning is a pivotal part of her role.

Owen Barr is professor of nursing and head of the School of Nursing at the University of Ulster. He is dual registered in learning disabilities and adult nursing. Owen was a member of the NMC Generic Writing Group who developed the draft competency statements and contributed to the development of the *Standards for Pre-registration Nurse Education*. He views professional values as core in the development of a student nurse's identity and behaviour, and in the promotion of a competent and confident registered nurse who will integrate the NMC Standards and guidance documents into their daily work to deliver a professional and competent service.

Pauline Black is a lecturer in nursing at the School of Nursing at the University of Ulster. Her clinical background is in acute and critical care nursing. She was a member of the team involved in developing the new undergraduate pre-registration nursing curriculum at Ulster and has a keen interest in developing methods to support effective learning for students. Pauline has a particular interest in the impact of effective teamwork in acute care, developed during her experience and research in the intensive care unit, Belfast City Hospital.

Jackie Bridges is a senior lecturer in the Faculty of Health Sciences, University of Southampton. Her expertise is in the care of the older person, particularly in acute hospital settings. Her clinical work with older people and a well-established research programme in this area have enabled her to pursue an interest in the nursing contribution to health care, including the factors that influence how nurses make decisions.

Alison Brown is a senior lecturer in practice learning at the Robert Gordon University. She has worked in a variety of settings including cancer care and sees communication as a pivotal aspect of both nursing practice and education. Her current role and partnership working with practitioners in a range of clinical settings allows her to remain up to date with the importance of communication as a fundamental and pivotal aspect of quality care for all nurses.

Jean Cowie is a lecturer at the Robert Gordon University. She has a wide-ranging clinical background including accident & emergency nursing as well as being a qualified and practising health visitor. She has played an active role in supporting the Erasmus Programme within the pre-registration nursing programme at the university as well as running the health visiting pathway in the post-registration portfolio.

Debbie Goode is a lecturer in nursing at the University of Ulster School of Nursing with a clinical background in intensive care. She is the course director for the BSc (Hons) Nursing Adult Course. Her interest in leadership and management began during her BA (Hons) in business studies. This interest was developed further as a team leader in the regional intensive care unit.

Kate Goodhand is a senior lecturer in clinical skills and a teaching fellow at the Robert Gordon University. She is an experienced nurse and academic who is well experienced in developing students learning through simulated practice and using feedback to improve their performance. In addition she has the role of a learning enhancement coordinator, responsible for embedding new and creative approaches to learning, teaching and assessment to enhance the student experience.

Chris McLean is a lecturer in adult nursing in the Faculty of Health Sciences at the University of Southampton and held the role of field lead for adult nursing in the undergraduate nursing programme between 2010 and 2012. He played a central role in the development of the 'values-based' curriculum, one of the first validated undergraduate programmes in England. He has a particular interest in the philosophy of care, particularly in relation to concepts of virtue and character in nursing practice. His doctoral research explored aspects of how nurses think and talk about patients.

 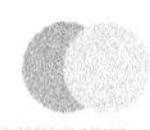

Yvonne Middlewick is a lecturer in the Faculty of Health Sciences at the University of Southampton and her current role is the mental health field lead for undergraduate programmes. Yvonne is a dual registered nurse, adult and mental health. She has a keen interest in how nurses can influence teams and organizations to enhance patient care, strongly believing that this should begin early in nurse education. The NMC *Standards* fully support this and her interest is to focus on leadership, management and team working, helping students to see how these influence their development as a nurse in preparing for an exciting and challenging career.

Avril Milne is a senior lecturer at the Robert Gordon University. She has established several Erasmus links within the pre-registration nursing programme as well as pioneering international exchanges for students in the USA. She is currently the head of pre-registration programmes at the School of Nursing and Midwifery as well as developing a research profile in cultural competence in nursing.

Elosie Monger is the faculty lead for clinical skills in the Faculty of Health Sciences at the University of Southampton. She has been actively involved in developing the practice and research of simulation in the undergraduate nursing and midwifery curricula in the faculty since 2002. Her doctoral research has developed a novel technique for the analysis of video-captured behaviour in simulated practice to elicit the factors which contribute to mentors' assessment of student nurse competence.

Delia Pogson has worked as a senior lecturer in the Faculty of Health Sciences, University of Southampton and is a registered nurse in learning disabilities. Her interest is in the complexities faced when working for people with learning disabilities and the communication challenges that they may experience. She recognizes that staff working with people with learning disabilities sometimes also experience difficulties in understanding people and hence she views the development of students' communication skills as fundamental to achieving the NMC competencies and fulfilling their role of working with people.

Mark Rawlinson is a lecturer and pathway lead for community nursing in the Faculty of Health Sciences, University of Southampton. He passionately believes that every nurse has the capability to improve the quality of care to patients, families and carers, and considers that this can be demonstrated not only through care and compassion, but also through the ability to lead. As a nurse with 25 years' experience in community nursing, Mark notes that it is apparent that the direction set by the NMC endorses this view.

Beth Sepion is currently a lecturer in children's nursing in the Faculty of Health Sciences at the University of Southampton, following on from a well-established clinical career in children's cancer nursing. Beth has particular interest in the use of experiential learning strategies such as sculpting and forum theatre to facilitate child field students' development of effective communication skills. She has significant experience of communication skills training in children's palliative and end-of-life care. Her motivation as a lecturer is the desire to develop child field practitioners who can facilitate compassionate and sensitive conversations with children and their families encountering end-of-life situations.

Steve Smith Is a lecturer in mental health nursing and an enterprise fellow at the School of Nursing and Midwifery, Robert Gordon University. He is a leading solution-focused therapist and heads one of the few training courses in solution focused brief therapy in the UK. Steve has a range of skills in developing tailor-made education for practitioners in this area as well as progressing research to improve the patient experience.

Cathy Sullivan is a lecturer at the Faculty of Health Sciences, University of Southampton. She has a professional background in adult nursing and mental health practice. She is keenly interested in learning in practice and believes that a practice experience is not just the place where students put 'theory into practice' but is most essentially the time where the principles of practice are learned, as well as giving students an opportunity to build on the knowledge and skills already gained. She considers this learning to be crucial, as it is where each student will learn the culture and skills of nursing that will ensure they offer high quality care for all service users and their families.

Ruth Taylor is Professor of nursing and Deputy Dean at Anglia Ruskin University. Ruth's expertise is in education relating to clinical leadership, and she has a keen focus on the enhancement of care through the development of students who have a commitment to achieving high standards.

Kay Townsend is a lecturer in cancer care in the Faculty of Health Sciences at the University of Southampton. Coming to this role from a well-established clinical career in cancer nursing, Kay has a particular interest in the educational use of narratives and in critical companionship. She has significant experience of communication skills training in palliative and end-of-life care. Her teaching is driven by the need to develop practitioners who can have sensitive and compassionate conversations with people who are faced with end-of-life situations.

Alison Trenerry is the education, quality and learning environment lead at University Hospital Southampton NHS Foundation Trust. Her role focuses on enhancing the learning experience in the clinical practice setting for students and on the support of mentors and educators who work closely with students who over three years are developing their competencies for registration. She is an experienced nurse with a clinical background in cardio-thoracic nursing.

Foreword

It is a significant honour to be asked to write the foreword for this important new book. I was closely involved with the process of developing the Nursing and Midwifery Council (NMC) *Standards for Pre-registration Nursing Education* over a period of about five years, latterly as the chair of the NMC's Stakeholder Advisory Group. I believe, and said at the time of their launch, that the *Standards* provide a flexible professional framework, delivering on the NMC's core responsibility for protection of the public, and also offering significant opportunities for innovation in programme development and delivery. It will be for education providers and clinical practice, working together, to make the most of the opportunity offered. I believe that this book will make a significant contribution to delivering that for student nurses.

It is also the right book at the right time. Criticisms of the quality of health care and, by extension, criticisms of nursing, have become commonplace in the past few years. While I am certain that most nurses are able to demonstrate the care, compassion and technical expertise that service users and carers should reasonably expect, it is clear that this is not always achieved by all. I am also convinced that nursing education is not fundamentally flawed, and this belief is regularly reinforced through contact with student nurses who seem well able to demonstrate the best of the caring attributes I would look for in a registered nurse.

The context of nursing practice has, however, become increasingly complex and nursing education has a responsibility to ensure future graduate nurses are well equipped for contemporary nursing practice. The nurse of the future will practise in an increasingly differentiated context. He or she will often be expected to work autonomously, crossing what had previously seemed impenetrable professional and institutional boundaries, leading and managing teams, and being accountable for the care delivered. There is no reason to believe that those realities will change or that the role of the nurse in the delivery of care will become less complex.

There are core issues that confront all nurses whatever their specific field of practice. Health care should be safe, personalized and effective. Nurses should demonstrate the skills, values and knowledge to provide skilful, intelligent and compassionate care wherever they work. These issues are reflected in the four domains of the NMC competency framework that sets out the standards for competence, and the individual competencies, to be successfully achieved for registration as a nurse.

It is a significant strength of this book that it uses those domains to organize the chapters, but it is not constrained by this. I like the domains: professional values; communication and interpersonal skills; nursing practice and decision-making; and leadership, management and team working. There could have been other legitimate ways of dividing up what nursing is, what nurses do and how nurses and nursing relate to others, but this seems to ring true as encapsulating the important conceptual and practical issues for nurses. It is also a strength that the authors have chosen to address all four fields of practice of nursing in a single volume. Past distinctions in terms of the service user population or the location of practice are becoming meaningless, and the NMC's concept of generic and specific competences is intended to address this. The thematic, domains-based approach of this book means that students, and their teachers, will find great value in each chapter whatever their destination field of practice.

One of the most significant changes to the NMC *Standards* was to establish that the newly-qualified nurse would be a graduate at the point of registration. Looking back, this was probably one of the least contentious of the developments. There have been nurses with degrees for many years, many more nurses 'top-up' to a degree post-qualification, and there has been a widespread belief that the increasing complexity of the nursing role would be best served by graduate preparation. While 'graduateness' implies a level of education and expertise within the subject area, it also implies a set of general and transferable attributes that will help prepare the graduate for a future that is largely unknowable. I believe that it is in the strengthening of these attributes and abilities (to be reflective; to weigh evidence; to articulate clear professional values; to demonstrate resilience; to communicate effectively in challenging situations; to demonstrate personal and professional accountability) that the strengths of the new preregistration nursing programmes will lie. Universities and their partners in practice will develop programmes that reflect their local needs and priorities, and this book can support that process.

While it is clearly aimed at students, this book will be of great value to educators, mentors and to nurses in practice who want to refresh their thinking and practice. Sheila and Brian have assembled a remarkable group of contributors, whose breadth and depth of experience, insight and passion for excellence in nursing education and practice are reflected in each chapter. It is my view that this book is a 'must read' for all student nurses.

Iain McIntosh
Dean, Faculty of Health, Life & Social Sciences,
Edinburgh Napier University

Introduction

In an environment of increasing public expectations and demands this book specifically highlights the nature and importance of the Nursing and Midwifery Council (NMC) competencies which apply to all nurse education programmes in the UK. The NMC safeguards the health and well-being of the public by maintaining a register of qualified nurses and midwives. To be accepted onto the register student nurses need to demonstrate that they have achieved the knowledge, skills, attitudes and technical abilities to be qualified graduates who are fit for practice in a range of roles. In addition, the education providers are required to confirm that students who have met all course requirements are in both good health and of good character. The successful delivery of quality patient care relies on the demonstration of competencies by nurses at all stages of their education and developing career.

The NMC competency framework

The NMC competency framework has laid out the standards for competence and the related competencies that every nursing student must acquire under the following four domains:

- professional values;
- communication and interpersonal skills;
- nursing practice and decision-making;
- leadership, management and team working.

These four domains are at the heart of professional health care and in this book are explored in a way that will encourage you as a student to consider, on your own and with others, including peers, clients/patients, practice educators, academic staff and other health care professionals, how the competencies support the provision of effective care in practice.

We believe that the competencies, which are integral to all nursing programmes, require some interpretation, discussion and analysis by you as a student nurse who will be experiencing theoretical learning in a university setting and undertaking practice in a diverse range of clinical environments.

About this book

This book is for all student nurses on pre-registration degree programmes in nursing across the UK. It supports the development of graduate thinking and the demonstration of graduate attributes by the individual student in clinical practice. The primary aim of the book is to offer a text for student nurses, whatever their chosen field of practice, to explore the relevance and meaning of the NMC competencies to their personal learning throughout the duration of their course. There are chapters that relate to all four fields of practice – child, adult, mental health and learning disabilities. Each field of nursing is acknowledged and addressed as every student requires an insight into all fields of nursing practice. The book also provides a basis for exploring other fields of care and identifying areas of best practice for the student to adopt. Furthermore, it addresses the radical move to specific *generic* and *field* competencies – that is, competencies required by all nurses, irrespective of their chosen field of study as well as specific competencies to their chosen field of study. The book also supports the rich opportunities in shared learning required by all nurses to develop their graduate thinking. We believe that it will also be helpful for academics, educators, mentors and the many other practitioners that support students in diverse settings as part of their preparation for their roles as first-year, second-year, third-year or even fourth-year students (Scotland) and finally as graduate practitioners.

The chapters have been written by expert and experienced nurses in their fields who explore the competencies from a variety of perspectives. The chapters are divided into sections according to the domain which they address, but inevitably there will be some overlap as the reality is that as part of holistic health care competencies are not discrete or separate from each other. Each chapter provides a specific focus and offers examples to enable a creative understanding of how the competencies may be demonstrated in the different contexts where practice occurs with individuals, groups or communities. The intention is to provoke ideas to support your understanding and help you to reflect on how the competencies underpin professional health care practice and can best be achieved. Due to the fact that competencies can be measured and assessed both in theory, practice and simulated settings and at different progression points, the book is a valuable resource for you to use with others and to revisit throughout your entire programme. In fact an important and pivotal part of a graduate nursing programme is to ensure that previous concepts, knowledge and skills learned at the start of university education are revisited, built upon and analysed further as in order to develop the professional application of these as a nurse.

This book aims to offer a rich and wide-ranging exploration of existing theoretical and knowledge bases relating to the competencies, which will challenge you to ask questions and think about situations you may experience in practice. It will also challenge you to reflect on your own underpinning values and belief systems and analyse how these may differ from others with whom you work or those you may care for (Chapters 2 and 3). It is intended to be used to foster an approach which promotes an honest and open exploration of different understandings of competence and to promote in-depth exploration, questioning and analysis of different attitudes and beliefs which underpin communication styles (Chapters 4, 5 and 6) and actions used by clients/patients and other professionals within your chosen field of practice. We make no apology for the emphasis on seeking or using knowledge/evidence (Chapter 1) to help solve problems in practice and make clinical decisions (Chapters 7 and 8) which support patients and clients in improving, maintaining or recovering health. As graduate nurses you will work in teams, managing complex situations and lead others – therefore, it is important to begin to learn how to achieve these competencies at an early stage of your programme and constantly develop your expertise as leaders in various health care settings (Chapters 9, 10 and 11).

As simulation is increasingly used to support health care professional learning and provides an opportunity to learn, practise and perfect your knowledge, clinical skills and competencies, this book includes a chapter to support your achievement of competencies in this way (Chapter 12).

It will be important for you to assess what has been achieved and what further personal development you may require. The use of personal development portfolios, learning contracts and working with mentors and others in practice are addressed in relation to achieving the competencies and demonstrating excellence in practice (Chapter 13).

Our view is that it is important that all health care students are encouraged to think about health care beyond the UK context and indeed, as some have an opportunity to undertake an elective placement outside the UK, the text acknowledges the importance of recognizing the global health care setting and the richness and benefits that working in a different global health care setting can provide to your own knowledge, skills and confidence (Chapter 14).

Using this book

This book will provide you the reader with a guide, or handbook, which, rather than being a text to read from cover to cover, can be used to dip in and out of as you progress through your programme of learning and encounter new situations in practice.

The book will also be a valuable tool to you for use in the practice setting to encourage dialogue with clients/patients, and for mentors and others who are pivotal in assessing practice achievements.

We envisage that you will use this book as a tool for promoting peer and group discussion both in practice and in the university context, possibly during seminars or action learning groups. In particular it would be useful for sharing experiences and learning from practice, and for identifying further theoretical knowledge that may be required. The text can be used to encourage your learning through reflection on critical incidents when elements of your clinical practice may have been very successful or possibly when you need future adaptation for specific situations.

Reflecting on current and future contexts of health care provision, case studies are included to illustrate how you might demonstrate competencies in specific settings with a particular individual, client group, community or society. The book focuses on illustrating specific concepts and themes to provoke wider thinking through a series of activities and some suggested further reading.

The chapter topics are not intended to be prescriptive but rather to be illustrative. The hope is that this will promote and develop the attributes of a graduate nurse. We think it is important to encourage you as students to add your own voices to the interpretation of the competencies in order to make them meaningful for yourselves. The activities in each chapter will help you to think about the underlying principles, literature, research and other evidence that informs understanding.

A note on terminology

It is important to note that throughout the book, rather than attempt to apply one term consistently across all chapters, the words 'patient', 'clients', 'service user' and 'individual' are used as the chapter contributors felt best, in recognition of the variations observed and applied within different health care contexts.

In conclusion

We hope you will find this a helpful and constructive book as you develop your graduate thinking, analysis of evidence and application of your knowledge and skills to the quality care that you learn to provide to patients. It is our intention in writing this book that your development as professionals will ultimately lead you to provide a high standard of evidence-based care to the patients you care for. We wish you well.

Sheila Reading and Brian Webster

1

The importance of evidence-based professional nursing practice

Sheila Reading and Brian Webster

Chapter contents

Introduction

The concept of evidence-based practice underpins contemporary health care. Throughout your programme of nursing study you will develop the skills to demonstrate the application of evidence-based nursing practice. You will learn to think critically about the theoretical literature, research and other evidence informing your understanding to help you achieve the Nursing and Midwifery Council (NMC) competencies (2010) which are arranged within the following four domains.

- professional values;
- communication and interpersonal skills;
- nursing practice and decision-making;
- leadership, management and team working.

Throughout this book you are provided with examples of how to integrate existing evidence into your practice to illustrate and support your learning. For all aspects of nursing, there is a wealth of diverse evidence to draw on and you will become familiar with accessing and using various sources of knowledge concerning values, ethics and compassionate care; communication studies, interactional research and theory; approaches to decision-making and leadership; and management research.

Evidence-based practice is a fundamental aspect of all you do as a nurse and this chapter will support your learning and achievement of the competencies within the NMC *Standards for Pre-registration Nursing Education* (NMC 2010) by facilitating you to:

- understand what is meant by evidence-based practice;
- appreciate the diverse types of evidence that can be used to inform practice;
- explain the importance of evidence-based practice;
- develop the knowledge and skills you need to demonstrate evidence-based practice;
- critically consider the limitations and challenges of evidence-based practice.

This chapter specifically addresses the following NMC standards but evidence-based information underpins all the standards.

Domain 1: Professional values – generic standard for competence

9 All nurses must appreciate the value of evidence in practice, be able to understand and appraise research, apply relevant theory and research findings to their work, and identify areas for further investigation.

Domain 3: Nursing practice and decision-making

1 All nurses must use up-to-date knowledge and evidence to assess, plan, deliver and evaluate care, communicate findings, influence change and promote health and best practice. They must make person-centred, evidence-based judgements and decisions, in partnership with others involved in the care process, to ensure high quality care. They must be able to recognise when the complexity of clinical decisions requires specialist knowledge and expertise, and consult or refer accordingly.

What is evidence-based practice?

Evidence-based practice first came to the fore during the 1970s and one of the most quoted definitions is:

> the conscientious, explicit and judicious use of current best evidence in making decisions about the care of individual patients. The practice of evidence based medicine means integrating individual clinical expertise with the best available external clinical evidence from systematic research.
>
> (Sackett *et al.* 1996: 71)

This definition captures a broad overview of the key considerations of how evidence should be used to inform practice. Often it appears that the main focus is on being able to critique research and apply it to practice, but read the definition carefully again and you will recognize that much more is being indicated.

1 The words **conscientious**, **explicit** and **judicious**

These words convey how each health care practitioner embracing an evidence-based approach to care should conduct themselves. Conscientious means being *thorough*, *meticulous* and *painstaking*. Explicit means being *open*, *clear* and *precise* and judicious indicates the need to be *cautious*, *shrewd*, *prudent* and *well-judged*.

2 When using '**best evidence**'

What counts as best evidence has been contested and remains controversial (Rycroft-Malone *et al.* 2004). Therefore a consideration of the value of a range of evidence available should be made.

3 The **care of individual patients**

Transferring evidence to the real world of practice which involves caring for individual patients is challenging and complex. While research-based knowledge provides theories and clear-cut solutions it is often difficult to use in practice where there are uncertainties and multiple variables which are unable to be controlled for (Schön 1983; Mantzoukas 2007). In addition, every nurse and patient and their interaction is unique and subjective (Kitson 2002; Rolfe and Gardner 2005).

4 Integrating **individual clinical expertise** with **the best available external clinical evidence**

Kitson (2002: 181) has highlighted that in nursing:

> EBP [evidence-based practice] should embrace ways of being able to demonstrate the effectiveness of expert knowledge on individual and collective patient decisions; the impact of existing research and outcomes and the ability to integrate patient experience into decisions about outcome.

Sackett *et al.* (2000: 1) describe the value of tailoring care and using professional experience and clinical judgement as:

> the ability to use our clinical skills and past experience to rapidly identify each patient's unique health state and diagnosis, their individual risks and benefits of potential interventions, and their personal values and expectations.

The rationale for basing practice on the best available evidence is to ensure that nursing practice is informed, appropriate, transparent and safe. Underpinning this is a question concerning what counts as evidence.

Activity 1.1

- Think about the types of evidence that might underpin how you assess a person's need for pain relief.
- List all the possible sources of this knowledge you might draw on.

Allcock and Day (2012) provide information which enables nurses to adopt an evidence-based approach when caring for people with pain. Their chapter focuses on how best to assess pain and use evidence to manage, relieve and evaluate pain. Various sources of evidence are provided:

- prevalence of pain;
- the science/theories of pain;
- the human, social and financial burden of pain;
- pain assessment tools (using validated tools);
- accessing evidence to pain management;
- using evidence to manage pain (pharmacological and non-pharmacological).

In reality there are many different types of evidence which inform nursing and add to its knowledge base. Did you manage to consider the following after completing **Activity 1.1**?

- randomized controlled trials (RCTs);
- systematic reviews – the Cochrane Collaboration (www.cochrane.org) is one source and academic journals also produce such reviews (e.g. the *International Journal of Nursing Studies*, www.journalofnursingstudies.com);
- clinical guidelines such as those produced by the National Institute for Health and Clinical Excellence (NICE) for England and Wales and the Scottish Intercollegiate Guidelines Network (SIGN: www.sign.ac.uk);
- controlled trials;
- case control;
- cohort studies;
- case studies;
- descriptive studies/reports;
- qualitative studies.

However, it is pivotal to your practice as a nurse to understand that evidence is not *solely* derived from research. There are other non-research sources of evidence such as:

- evidence from theory (e.g. theories about the grieving process, parent and child bonding, etc.);
- psychosocial, cultural and pharmacological knowledge that can inform patient care and clinical practice by offering evidence regarding

possible non-concordance with drug treatment (e.g. unpleasant side-effects, personal belief systems);
- evidence of experts, experienced professional opinions, professional consensus and respected authorities;
- audit data;
- quality/performance data;
- evidence from patients and carers (e.g. patient feedback);
- evaluation data;
- guidelines;
- knowledge of the organization and the culture;
- clinical expertise/professional experience;
- professional networks;
- policy documents, national and local.

While research-based information is a key element informing the provision of quality care and meeting patient needs, audit data, patient surveys, patient and carer stories, laboratory tests and other results also help build up a picture of best care.

Activity 1.2

You may hear people say things that justify why they have chosen to do something in a particular way in practice. Below is a list of phrases/expressions you may have heard used in the clinical practice environment. Do you think any of these has a role in helping us develop evidence-based practice? If so, why? If not, why not?

- 'In my opinion this is what should be done.'
- 'In my experience this seems to work.'
- 'I have always done it this way.'
- 'Traditionally, we do it this way.'
- 'Well it's not clear what is best so let's give this a try.'

Justify your responses and discuss with colleagues.

There are many texts for nursing which provide a balance of evidence for practice (e.g. Newell and Gournay 2000; Bullock *et al.* 2012). Bullock *et al.*'s book for adult nurses demonstrates how evidence can be used to benefit the patient with common health conditions or with specific health needs, and improve the patient experience of care.

Knowledge that informs nursing practice is not always based on studies of clinical effectiveness such as systematic reviews and RCTs. In reality, relatively little health care is based on evidence which indicates precisely what effective care is and there is often no suitable guidance for practice. However, it can never be acceptable to ignore evidence that already exists and carry out patient care if we are unable to justify and explain why we are doing it. Where there really is no published evidence, it is acceptable to base practice on what we know works and be ready to defend this position based on confirmed expert knowledge, experience and patient viewpoints. This provides an opportunity to then monitor and evaluate the results of that care and make proposals for further research.

Kitson (2002: 185) has argued for a broadening of the concept of using evidence in health care which acknowledges the importance of patient-focused care:

> Nursing's theoretical and practice base requires a broad interpretation of the term evidence. Definitions of evidence need to be understood in the context of establishing effective therapeutic relationships with clients and by balancing evidence from patients, clinical experience and research in order to arrive at the best clinical decision for care . . . This does not mean that nursing science cannot draw from studies of effectiveness but it may be that as a discipline, it still needs to do a lot more describing, refining and classifying of basic constructs and concepts before it can put great reliance on the evidence that emerges from intervention studies alone. Researchers within nursing need to be equipped with the full range of methodological

 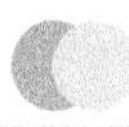

approaches, and not create a hierarchy that sets one approach above another.

We would suggest that rather than focus on a debate as to what counts as best evidence, nurses must become competent in asking practice-based questions, accessing and synthesizing the full range of available information to answer the question, improve their clinical practice and enhance patient care.

> **Key learning**
>
> - There is a range of types of evidence that you will be required to understand to inform your practice.
> - Evidence from a range of sources, including audit documents, patient surveys, clinical guidelines and policy documents plays a pivotal role in informing your practice as a nurse.

The importance of evidence-based practice within the current context of nursing

Nursing is never a static practice and during the last decade there has been a significant increase in the skill set and knowledge base expected of the qualified nurse. Nursing has become a more diverse and complex profession across the four fields of practice and the opportunities to develop and grow in a chosen field are now greater than they have ever been. In the UK nurses can now aspire to become a:

- staff nurse (community or hospital based);
- GP practice nurse;
- public health nurse;
- school nurse;
- occupational health nurse;
- sister/ward manager;
- clinical nurse specialist;
- nurse practitioner/advanced practice nurse;
- practice education facilitator;
- lecturer/practitioner;
- nurse consultant/consultant practitioner;
- research nurse.

It is clear from the list above, which is not exhaustive, that a range of roles are available for you once you have qualified. What is certain is that these roles require graduate-prepared nurses, with clear skills of problem-solving, leadership, critical analysis and an ability to gather, interpret and apply the best possible evidence to care and support the patients they are looking after. Many roles will require further education and preparation, often to masters level and some to doctoral level, and this development gives recognition to the important autonomous and patient-focused approach that nurses can bring to patient care and management.

> **Activity 1.3**
>
> - In choosing to become a nurse what skills and attributes do you think you bring to this profession?
> - How might these support you in the delivery of evidence-based clinical care?

There are many skills and attributes to support you in being an evidence-based practitioner including:

- being ready to question care and practice;
- wanting to understand more about what you do and why you do it;
- the desire to be knowledgeable, well informed and aware of the latest policies, guidelines and research;
- the desire to provide the best high quality care based on clear evidence;
- the ability to challenge, and be challenged, about aspects of your practice;
- a readiness to change your own practice to improve patient or health outcomes;
- wanting to be a consumer of research and possibly even generate some research-based knowledge.

Your role in promoting evidence-based practice

When you graduate and register as a qualified nurse you will be in a position to lead others in delivering high quality evidence-based care within a complex and changing health care environment. Increasingly people, are able to access the extensive health information available to them and are well informed about their own health care needs (Kitson 2002). It is essential that your clinical practice is supported by the best available evidence in order to ensure that what you do actually improves individual, and population, health outcomes. This means that you will need to remain up to date with the latest and best evidence to keep yourself informed and be able to draw on the many sources of knowledge to ensure quality care.

During your nursing programme you will become familiar with academics presenting you with research-based information and giving you a sound understanding of other types of evidence, including the science and theory underpinning a range of health care initiatives. As a student nurse you will learn to access, judge and use evidence to present clear reasons for the care you deliver, both in written assignments and in clinical placements. However, as evidence is constantly being added to, you will need to maintain and adapt your knowledge and skills of searching for evidence, synthesizing and using it to inform your practice once registered as a professional nurse with the NMC.

RCN competences: finding and using information

One helpful tool for nurses has been produced by the Royal College of Nursing (RCN 2011) which introduced a strategy and document called *'Finding, Using and Managing Information: Nursing, Midwifery Health and Social Care Information Literacy Competences* to support the enhancement of skills in accessing information from the various sources available in health care practice and delivery of patient care. The intention was to enable nurses to find and analyse evidence for use in the provision of safe and effective clinical practice. Online resources have been provided with the intention of supporting graduate student nurses in achieving competencies for practice. The aim is to assist nurses in evaluating evidence derived from professional standards and benchmarks.

Using evidence for decision-making and problem-solving in practice

Many sources of evidence are used in the decision-making process for nursing practice (see Chapters 7 and 8) and it is important to emphasize again that evidence is not the only dimension informing how you deliver care. It is now clear that your knowledge and the clinical care given to patients is informed by a variety of sources and adapted to suit your patient preferences (related to their values: see Chapter 2) in light of your experience and developing expertise.

During your time at university, whether attending lectures or action learning groups, reading articles and books, or undertaking online learning, you will engage in activities that encourage you to identify problems, think critically, generate knowledge or information and ultimately solve problems. Modules of study will include both theory and practice and encourage you to apply one to the other, or to integrate knowledge from theory and practice (see **Figure 1.1**). The same will be true of your practice experience. Fundamental to this is the application of your theoretical knowledge to your developing clinical practice and care of patients, whether that be at a hospital, in a home or some other area where you have contact with patients. In practice you will assess specific individual needs by looking at care plans and observing patients for a range of signs and symptoms to add to the evidence needed to identify and solve their particular problems.

Some of the skills you will develop as a student nurse will focus on how to best make use of the wide range of knowledge available to you and

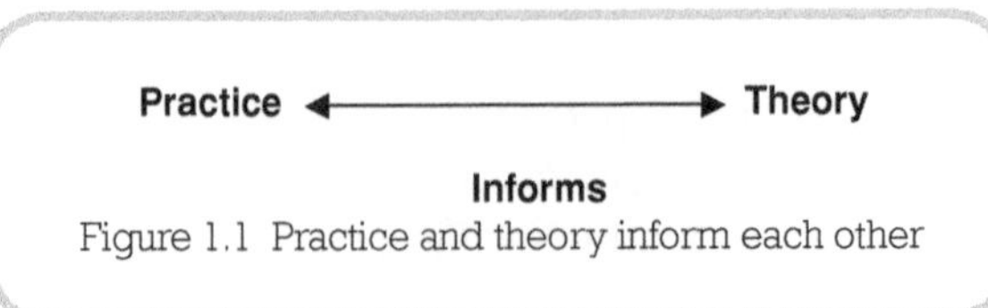

Figure 1.1 Practice and theory inform each other

 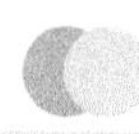

apply this to your care of patients. These skills will be developed as an integral part of your education as a student nurse and will continue to grow, be shaped by and enhanced in your role as a qualified practitioner. This is part of your journey as a lifelong learner, a professional who is willing, able and open to change, gathering new information and using this to inform your clinical practice. We believe that learning how to use evidence and the knowledge and skills required to do this is a developing attribute of the graduate nurse.

Knowledge and skills needed to use evidence in practice

The evidence-based practice process

The process of using evidence to best inform your clinical practice usually starts with *you* asking a question regarding an aspect of care you require an answer to. It is necessary to translate the question into one that will help you focus your ideas and guide your search for evidence from a range of sources. The following evidence-based practice process is usually adopted.

1. Develop a well-framed practice-based question.
2. Search systematically for evidence to address the question.
3. Search and select the best available evidence to answer your question.
4. Appraise that evidence, synthesize and summarize: translate into recommendations or guidelines.
5. Apply the evidence in practice, taking account of patient preference and local organizational context.
6. Evaluate the result of the use of that evidence.
7. Disseminate the evidence to others.

Creating evidence

It is possible that you may choose to undertake some research yourself either as part of a research module or for an honours component within your degree, or indeed at a later stage in your professional career. Whenever you do this the aim will be to generate new evidence that will add to the existing knowledge base of nursing-focused and patient-centred findings. Many nurses actively engage in research to build the knowledge base underpinning practice. Some follow a career in research or combine clinical practice with research and practice development. As the profession of nursing builds and strengthens its research and evidence base it is important to understand that as a nurse you can be active in generating evidence, translating evidence and using that evidence to inform your own practice and therefore provide the best possible care to your patients.

Using evidence in practice

We take here hygiene needs as an example. All of us attach great importance to our personal care and hygiene needs, and it is only when the usual facilities for showering, brushing teeth and washing our hair are removed that we are reminded of the impact this has on our feelings of comfort, self-esteem and general well-being. During periods of illness many people require nursing interventions to meet their hygiene needs and of course the very young and the very old will require specific interventions as part of their daily care.

Activity 1.4

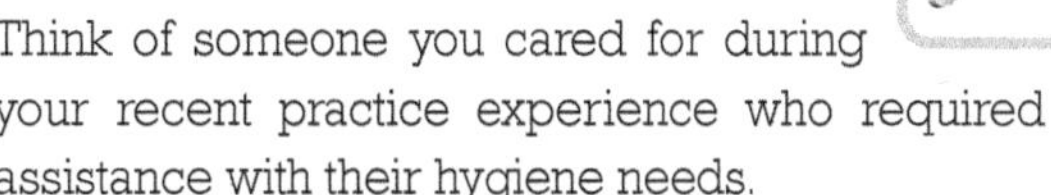

Think of someone you cared for during your recent practice experience who required assistance with their hygiene needs.

- What evidence did you draw on and use to inform your care to best meet that person's hygiene needs?
- What resources/evidence/guidelines did you use to ensure best clinical practice?
- Were you aware of that person's view of being assisted with their personal hygiene?
- Did you assess their specific hygiene needs and personal preferences, rather than adopt routine and ritualized care?
- Reflect on what other evidence/information/knowledge you would like to have in the future to improve this aspect of care.

You may want to discuss your answers to **Activity 1.4** with peers, your tutor, your mentor or even with some patients you have cared for. This is likely to reveal areas where you need to learn more about what evidence exists to help you improve patient care in this area.

Some people will require specifically adapted nursing interventions to support their hygiene needs. For example:

- people who are unconscious, semi-conscious or sedated;
- people with certain mental health problems;
- people with physical disabilities;
- people with learning disabilities;
- people receiving end-of-life care;
- babies and young children.

You should consider how evidence of best practice might need to be adapted for these patient groups.

Using audit data

In relation to hygiene needs, evidence gathered by the Healthcare Commission (2007) (now known as the Care Quality Commission – CQC) indicated that 30 per cent of complaints by patients about hospital care related to poor attention to dignity, privacy and basic personal care. This audit data provides evidence of areas where improvement is needed.

Using benchmarks, clinical guidelines and protocols to inform practice

Rather than expecting every nurse to access and search for evidence related to improving this aspect of care, quality benchmarks for hygiene care have been produced and published in *Essence of Care* (DH 2010). In this document quality indicators to support best practice are provided and include:

- assessing individual preferences and agreeing personal care needs for individuals for their skin, teeth, nails, eyes, ears and nose;
- documenting, communicating and evaluating the hygiene care provided;
- ensuring the evidence base that underpins care is reviewed and kept up to date.

This example highlights just one area where the generation of audit data, guidelines and benchmark standards is valuable for ensuring health care professionals are enabled to use evidence in practice that there are improvements in patient care as a result. Clinical guidelines help you make decisions about what is effective in clinical practice. Summaries of evidence do exist and these are helpful as they combine evidence from various sources which inform care. In mental health nursing, the quantity and quality of evidence is increasing and numerous guidelines inform the organization of clinical practice (Newell and Gournay 2000).

Other evidence gathered from patients, such as NHS surveys (see www.nhssurveys.org) also help to inform best practice. But, as always, there is a need to be cautious and to carefully and critically consider the value of these types of evidence for your own context and local practice. Guidelines can become outdated and need regular reviewing.

RCN information literacy competences

The RCN suggests that when seeking evidence for practice you use the following framework.

1. Identify why information is needed (question practice and recognize gaps in evidence).
2. Identify what information is needed (what type of evidence is needed to address a practice topic?).
3. Carry out a search to find information (identify and select best evidence available).
4. Evaluate how the information meets the identified need (judging the quality and relevance of the evidence).
5. Use information and knowledge inclusively, legally and ethically.
6. Manage information.
7. Create new information or knowledge, draw conclusions and make recommendations for practice.

This framework will support health care professionals to ensure care is informed by best evidence,

 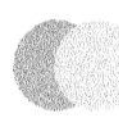

which inevitably will have an impact on the patients you look after.

Critically assessing evidence

We take here the Mental Health Network (MHN) as an example. In 2011 the MHN NHS Confederation produced a fact sheet on mental health statistics and resources. This kind of evidence is drawn from several sources and helps to set in context key information when deciding on NHS service provision, budgets and investment in new services for people with mental health problems.

One example taken from the fact sheet is:

> There are currently 750,000 people in the UK with dementia, which is expected to grow to over one million by 2021. The cost to the UK economy currently stands at £20 billion per annum and is projected to rise to £27 billion per annum by 2018.

It is essential to first understand how this information was generated and critically analyse what the figures actually mean. For example, prevalence figures such as this vary as they do not always measure the same thing. This can be for a number of reasons. For example, in practice, psychiatric diagnosis can be difficult and different health care professionals may diagnose dementia differently. As a result figures of prevalence and incidence may be distorted. A further problem that arises is that data may be collected on the number of people who are cared for by mental health professionals. It has to be recognized that many individuals may never be in contact with health care services and as a result the 'facts' may not be entirely accurate.

Statistics appear to be convincing but should not be treated as facts. It is important to explore how statistical figures were arrived at and examine the reliability and validity of the data in question. The following questions could be asked:

- What was the sample size?
- How representative is the sample of the population?
- Are there any methodological weaknesses in how data was collected?

Key learning !

- Always approach evidence with a critical stance which looks for both strengths and weaknesses in the research which may impact on the findings.
- All studies have strengths and weaknesses in spite of attempts to ensure rigour.

Using different types of evidence to answer practice questions

Statistics derived from surveys and other quantitative studies only represent part of the clinical practice scenario. For example, we may know how many people in the population have depression, but what may be equally important is to understand the experiences and perspectives of those who have this condition in order to respond effectively and meet their needs. Such information is usually provided by both quantitative and qualitative evidence addressing questions such as:

- Why do people suffer from depression?
- Are some people more at risk of becoming depressed than others?
- How can we maintain personal well-being in order to try and prevent or avoid depression (consider social, economic and employment factors, and how stress relates to these)?
- How does depression impact on the person and their family?
- How long might it last for any individual?

Challenges and limitations of evidence-based practice

It can be a challenge to know what to do in a situation when there is no evidence, conflicting evidence or a lack of consensus across the evidence. Indeed, in nursing the evidence for effectiveness in clinical practice and improving patient outcomes is still limited (Randell *et al.* 2007).

A lack of research undertaken

A systematic review by Griffiths *et al.* (2009) concluded that the body of evidence informing learning disability nursing remains small and underdeveloped, and consists mainly of small-scale evaluations which can offer some guidance for service development. Importantly this review highlighted that more research is needed and learning disability health care requires more focus, funding and resources to develop the evidence base for practice and care.

In addition the review helped identify areas where particular research is required as a priority. For example, the need to identify strategies for improving the experience of general health care for people with behavioural problems, as this was identified as being particularly problematic. As a nurse it is important to be aware that in some areas the evidence informing practice is limited or simply just not available (French 2002), and to recognize this as an opportunity to identify areas for future research that will support the growth of evidence-based practice.

A lack of clarity on how to proceed

It is not unusual that the interpretation of research evidence leads to conflicting or contradictory ideas about how evidence may be used. You will be aware of reports in the media on a weekly basis regarding research that seems to indicate conflicting findings. This can cause confusion for people who receive health care as well as for professionals attempting to provide it. Even rigorous research does not always provide a clear answer on what to do in practice.

To give an example of this, a systematic review and meta-analysis is now explored (see below).

The reality of clinical practice is that people experience health problems in a range of diverse ways and respond to treatment in similar ways. The nature of nursing itself is complex and subtle. 'Gold standard' research seldom offers absolute certainty and is rapidly superseded by new research that is constantly being produced (Rycroft-Malone *et al.* 2004). Despite the difficulties encountered in finding and using evidence, it is important not to

Example of a systemic review identifying a lack of evidence to inform nursing practice

Clark, C.E., Smith, L.F.P., Taylor, R.S. and Campbell, J.L. (2010) Nurse led interventions to improve control of blood pressure in people with hypertension: systematic review and meta-analysis, *British Medical Journal*, 341: c3995.

Background

A major cause of cardiovascular morbidity is essential hypertension, a public health problem which is increasing with the ageing population. A Cochrane review (by Fahey *et al.* 2005) indicated that an organized system of regular review along with anti-hypertensive drug therapy significantly reduced blood pressure in those with hypertension above target level.

Clarke *et al.* considered that perhaps the primary care setting could offer a nurse-led intervention which would effectively deliver best monitoring and treatment of people with hypertension. Evidence from previous studies indicated that nurse-led care was associated with greater observance of protocols and guidelines as well as increased patient satisfaction – possibly all at a lower cost. However, the evidence was conflicting. Clarke *et al.* undertook a systematic review of RCTs of interventions by nurses, nurse prescribers and nurse practitioners which aimed to improve blood pressure. However, they had to conclude that there was little evidence that could be applied to a UK setting that indicated any benefit of nurse involvement in hypertension within the NHS.

This example highlights the complexity of applying evidence to practice. The study provided no clear answer; instead it highlighted the need for more research and that in itself is an important research outcome.

 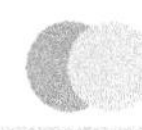

surrender to the problem but rather remain hopeful and tackle 'sub-problems' and look for answers which can enhance care. This is part of the complexity of nursing and demonstrates the need for the nurse graduate to continue to apply the skills of problem-solving, critical thinking and analysis.

Where there is insufficient, conflicting or inconclusive evidence it is important to look for the most robust quality of evidence available. Hierarchies of evidence tend to put systematic reviews and RCTs at the top. However, central to your role as a nurse is the need to use your own knowledge, judgement and interrogation of a range of evidence available to inform the best outcome for patient care. Rather than have a debate about which evidence is best for nursing, remember that *all* evidence informs practice and interventions are not the be-all and end-all. McKenna *et al.* (1999) propose that a lack of research does not prevent evidence-based decisions from being made.

The informed and knowledgeable practitioner

We cannot emphasize enough the importance of being an informed and knowledgeable practitioner who can use their clinical expertise and that of other health care professionals to make careful, judicious use of current best evidence when caring for individual patients. Your clinical expertise will provide you with knowledge of the context of care, local resources, the patient, their family and carers. In addition it is now not unusual that users of health care services are involved in the decision-making process regarding their care (see Chapters 7 and 8). Rolfe (2006) provides wise advice in suggesting that there are different approaches to using evidence in practice. Pivotal to this is the consideration of what evidence-based practice really means to your own practice as a professional.

Evidence-based practice is a continuous process and as a student you will learn much about the importance of evidence for your practice. As nursing research increases and new technologies and approaches to care are developed, it becomes clear that competence in evidence-based practice will require a commitment to lifelong learning. The dynamic nature of knowledge which is constantly being added to and revised will require you to maintain an interest in the latest evidence once you graduate and qualify in your chosen field. It is a professional requirement that you continue to build on your knowledge and, importantly, remain curious about practice issues which present challenges (Yoder-Wise 2008). This curiosity will enable you to remain open to new evidence, which will in turn enrich your personal practice and patient care and set the foundation for your continuing professional development (CPD).

The NMC field standard competence for adult Mental Health, Learning Disabilities and Children's nurses (2010) highlights this:

Domain 1 Professional value

7 All nurses must be responsible and accountable for keeping their knowledge and skills up to date through continuing professional development. They must aim to improve their performance and enhance the safety and quality of care through evaluation, supervision and appraisal.

8 All nurses must practise independently, recognising the limits of their competence and knowledge. They must reflect on these limits and seek advice from, or refer to, other professionals where necessary.

Reflection in and on your practice

It is important to ensure as a practitioner that the knowledge base you are using is credible and informed. This can be achieved through reflection and made transparent to others for critical analysis. Benner (1984) made an important contribution to the understanding of nursing practice by uncovering and articulating the knowledge embedded in practice experience. Her research identified five levels of competency in clinical nursing practice:

Level 1 novice practitioner
Level 2 advanced beginner
Level 3 competent practitioner
Level 4 proficient practitioner
Level 5 expert practitioner

Activity 1.5

Using Benner's five levels of practice, try to identify individuals you have worked with and begin to make an assessment as to where they stand on the scale. Why did you think that? What skills and attributes of a professional nurse did they demonstrate for you to make that assessment? It will be helpful for you to discuss this with your peers.

Importantly, Benner argues that experience refers to 'the refinement of preconceived notions and theory through encounters with many actual practical experiences that add nuances or shades of difference to theory'. This highlights how formal theory is used to inform practice in the real world. An experienced nurse has a wealth of knowledge on which to draw for interpreting new situations but that knowledge remains difficult to articulate.

Throughout this book there are many references to the place and value of *refection* for practice and to various models of reflection. According to Mantzoukas (2007) reflection makes it possible for us to consider what information is informing our decision-making and in that way we can review the extent to which our practice is based on best evidence rather than habitual practice. Reflection is identified in Chapter 7 as integral to clinical decision-making and can support you in changing your practice.

Conclusion

Evidence informing clinical practice can be drawn from many disciplines such as epidemiology, sociology, psychology and biology. Accessing best evidence, critiquing it, and translating it for use in your particular area of practice presents challenges within daily nursing. The main consideration in promoting evidence-based practice is ensuring that robust and relevant knowledge is generated, synthesized, disseminated and used in practice.

The reality of evidence-based practice is complex and requires skills that are developed, adapted and applied over a period of time. As a graduate nurse we would encourage you to engage with the concept and application of evidence-based practice from the early stages of your career and education, and develop the necessary skills so that it becomes a fundamental part of your everyday working life. This is an important aspect of your role in delivering high quality patient-focused care and a professional requirement as a lifelong learner.

Further reading and resources

Barker, J. (2010) *Evidence-based Practice for Nurses*. London: Sage.

Newell, R. and Burnard, P. (2011) *Research for Evidence-based Practice in Healthcare*. Chichester: Wiley/Blackwell.

RCN (Royal College of Nursing) (2007) *Understanding Benchmarking: RCN Guidance for Nursing Staff Caring for Children and Young People*. London: RCN.

RCN (Royal College of Nursing) (2011) *Finding, Using and Managing Information: Nursing, Midwifery Health and Social Care Information Literacy Competences*. London: RCN. This publication complements the RCN's clinical competence framework, helping nurses and nursing students develop their skills in using information and knowledge and applying this to their practice. The competences are intended to support the individual's and the nursing team's thinking about the information required to inform activities of varying complexity.

Joanna Briggs Institute: www.joannabriggs.edu.au. Supports evidence-based health care by providing a range of resources.

References

Allcock, N. and Day, R. (2012) Managing pain, in I. Bullock, J. Macleod Clark and J. Rycroft-Malone (eds) *Adult Nursing Practice: Using Evidence in Care*. Oxford: Oxford University Press.

 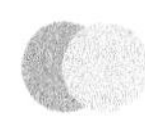

Benner, P. (1984) *From Novice to Expert: Excellence and Power in Clinical Nursing Practice*. Menlo Park, CA: Addison-Wesley.

Bullock, I., Macleod Clark, J. and Rycroft-Malone, J. (eds) (2012) *Adult Nursing Practice: Using Evidence in Care*. Oxford: Oxford University Press.

Clark, C.E., Smith, L.F.P., Taylor, R.S. and Campbell, J.L. (2010) Nurse led interventions to improve control of blood pressure in people with hypertension: systematic review and meta-analysis, *British Medical Journal*, 341: c3995.

DH (Department of Health) (2010) *Essence of Care: Benchmarks for Fundamental Aspects of Care – Personal Hygiene*. London: DH.

Fahey, T., Schroeder, K., Ebrahim, S. and Glynn, L. (2005) Interventions used to improve control of blood pressure in patients with hypertension, *Cochrane Reviews*, CD005182.

French, P. (2002) What is the evidence on evidence-based nursing? An epistemological concern, *Journal of Advanced Nursing*, 47(3): 250–7.

Griffiths, P., Bennett, J. and Smith, E. (2009) The size, extent and nature of the learning disability nursing research base: a systematic scoping review, *International Journal of Nursing Studies*, 46(4): 490–507.

Healthcare Commission (2007) *Caring for Dignity: A National Report on Dignity in Care for Older People While in Hospital*. London: Commission for Healthcare Audit and Inspection, available at www.healthcarecommission.org.uk/_db/_documents/Caring_for_dignity.pdf.

Kitson, A. (2002) Recognising relationships: reflections on evidence based practice, *Nursing Inquiry*, 9(3) 179–86.

Mantzoukas, S. (2007) A review of evidence-based practice, nursing research and reflection: levelling by hierarchy, *Journal of Clinical Nursing*, 17: 214–23.

McKenna, H., Cutcliffe, J. and McKenna, P. (1999) Evidence based practice: demolishing some myths, *Nursing Standard*, 14(16): 39–42.

Newell, R. and Gournay, K. (eds) (2000) *Mental Health Nursing: An Evidence-based Approach*. Edinburgh: Churchill Livingstone Elsevier.

NMC (Nursing and Midwifery Council) (2010) *Standards for Pre-registration Nursing Education*. London: NMC.

Randell, R., Mitchell, N., Dowding, D., Cullum, N. and Thompson, C. (2007) Effects of computerised decision-support systems on nursing performance and patient outcomes: a systematic review, *Journal of Health Services Research and Policy*, 12: 242–9.

RCN (Royal College of Nursing) (2011) *Finding, Using and Managing Information: Nursing, Midwifery, Health and Social Care Information Literacy Competences*. London: RCN.

Rolfe, G. (2006) Evidence-based practice, in M. Jasper (ed.) *Professional Development, Reflection and Decision-Making*. Oxford: Blackwell.

Rolfe, G. and Gardner, L. (2005) Towards a nursing science of the unique: evidence, reflexivity and the study of persons, *Journal of Research in Nursing*, 10: 297–310.

Rycroft-Malone, J., Seers, K., Titchen, A., Harvey, G., Kitson, A. and McCormack, B. (2004) What counts as evidence in evidence-based practice? *Journal of Advanced Nursing*, 47(1): 81–9.

Sackett, D.L., Rosenberg, W.M.C., Muir Gray, J.A., Haynes, R.B. and Richardson, W.S. (1996) *Evidence based* medicine: what it is and what it isn't, *British Medical Journal*, 312: 71–2.

Sackett, D.L., Straus, S.E., Richardson, W.S., Rosenberg, W. and Haynes, R.B. (2000) Evidence based medicine: how to practise and teach EBM, 2nd edn. London: Churchill Livingstone.

Schön, D. (1983) *The Reflective Practitioner*. London: Temple Smith.

Yoder-Wise, P.S. (2008) Lifelong learning in nursing: a drill down of the Macy Foundation Report, *Journal of Continuing Education in Nursing*, 38(3): 99.

SECTION

1

Professional values

Professional values for nursing

2

Owen Barr and Chris McLean

Chapter contents

Introduction

In applying for your nursing programme it is likely you read about and prepared answers to possible interview questions concerning why you wanted to become a nurse and what you thought the qualities of a 'good' nurse were. In preparing for your interview you will have realized that nursing is not only about having the appropriate up-to-date knowledge and skills, but is also about the values you are expected to hold as a student nurse and as a registered nurse (RN). Indeed there is increasing consideration being given to how to establish or at least get an indication of the values of potential student nurses during the recruitment and selection of students for nurse education programmes. The need to pay attention to the values (and previous conduct) of people applying to nursing is due to the centrality of person-centred care and professional conduct that will justify public trust in the profession (NMC 2011). The perceived need for specific attention to the values of applicants has been heightened with reports of poor nursing care in the areas of maintaining privacy, dignity and communication with people as individuals (Parliamentary and Health Service Ombudsman 2009; Patients' Association 2009; Independent Commission on Dignity in Care 2012).

Your programme of nurse education is designed to ensure that you achieve the competencies required by the Nursing and Midwifery Council (NMC) that are necessary for you to register as a nurse, but the introduction to this book has already observed that competence is a complex concept. In all activities, be they in work or recreational contexts, to be competent at something requires possession of certain knowledge, skills and technical abilities. Your programme of nurse education will enable you to develop these important areas, and they are the subject of later chapters in this book. It is clear though that knowledge and technical ability alone are not enough to make a good nurse, and that all aspects of nursing are dependent upon possessing appropriate *professional values and attitudes*. Nursing education programmes must also address these areas and they are the focus of this chapter.

This chapter specifically addresses the following NMC standards.

Domain 1: Professional values – generic standard for competence

All nurses must act first and foremost to care for and safeguard the public. They must practise autonomously and be responsible and accountable for safe, compassionate, person-centred, evidence-based nursing that respects and maintains dignity and human rights. They must show professionalism and integrity and work within recognised professional, ethical and legal frameworks. They must work in partnership with other health and social care professionals and agencies, service users, their carers and families in all settings, including the community, ensuring that decisions about care are shared.

1 All nurses must practise with confidence according to *The code: Standards of conduct, performance and ethics for nurses and midwives* (NMC 2008),* and within other recognised ethical and legal frameworks. They must be able to recognise and address ethical challenges relating to people's choices and decision-making about their care, and act within the law to help them and their families and carers find acceptable solutions.

2 All nurses must practise in a holistic, non-judgmental, caring and sensitive manner that avoids assumptions, supports social inclusion; recognises and respects individual choice; and acknowledges diversity. Where necessary, they must challenge inequality, discrimination and exclusion from access to care.

3 All nurses must support and promote the health, wellbeing, rights and dignity of people, groups, communities and populations. These include people whose lives are affected by ill health, disability, ageing, death and dying. Nurses must understand how these activities influence public health.

4 All nurses must work in partnership with service users, carers, families, groups, communities and organisations. They must manage risk, and promote health and wellbeing while aiming to empower choices that promote self-care and safety.

8 All nurses must practise independently, recognising the limits of their competence and knowledge. They must reflect on these limits and seek advice from, or refer to, other professionals where necessary.

The NMC and professional standards

Within the UK the NMC is responsible for the regulation of nurses and midwives in so far as 'to safeguard the health and wellbeing of the public, as required by the Nursing and Midwifery Order 2001' (NMC 2010a: 4). To ensure this is achieved the NMC maintains a register of nurses and midwives (which all practising nurses and midwives must be on), and sets standards of education, training and conduct. The NMC also publish mandatory guidance and advice as well as reviewing the professional practice to ensure that nurses and midwives keep their skills and knowledge up to date, and uphold the standards of their professional code (NMC 2008).

The NMC stipulates that nursing practice and nurse education are underpinned by *values*. The public need to be assured that RNs and midwives, along with students of these courses, will 'act with professionalism and integrity', and practise in ways that are 'compassionate' and 'respectful, and which maintain dignity (NMC 2010a: 5). In order to ensure that these values are achieved the NMC publishes

* Relates to the *Standards* in place at the time of the publication of the NMC (2010a) *Standards for Pre-registration Nursing Education*. It is important to be aware that the standards for education will also relate to the most recent NMC standards for conduct and therefore student nurses must remain up to date with any revision of standards by regularly reading the nursing press and also visiting to the NMC website at www.nmc-uk.org.

and regularly updates standards for professional conduct which RNs and midwives are required to meet (NMC 2008). The NMC also publishes guidance on the expected professional conduct of students of nursing and midwifery (NMC 2011). It is important that RNs and student nurses keep up to date with the latest versions of these documents.

Thinking about values

Values underpin nursing practice and your programme of nurse education. We have begun to examine how these values underpin the standards of behaviour that are expected of you are as a practitioner and as a student. In order to examine the nature of these professional values it is important to explore the nature of values themselves.

In order to gain registration with the NMC on completing your programme, you are required to make a statement that you are of 'good character' (NMC 2010b). This requirement appears to suggest that in order to be a nurse you need to be a particular kind of person (apparently a good one!). It can therefore be challenging to realize that nurse education explicitly sets out to develop your personal values. After all, 'our values express who and what we are' (Mohr *et al.* 2001). They are personal values and are normally considered to be just that – *personal.* You may believe that it is important to simply respect, rather than seek to change, the values of others, and may be inclined to question whether it is legitimate for nurse educators to try to change *your* values. By engaging with the ideas and activities presented in this chapter you will begin to appreciate why this is necessary. This will mean examining the nature of values, what characterizes *professional* values, and the importance of specific values which characterize nursing as a profession.

Before beginning to consider the nature of professional values, it is important to consider what a *value* actually is. We have noted that it is natural when we first think about values to consider that our values (perhaps like our beliefs) are personal. In order to illustrate the nature of values themselves it is therefore appropriate to begin by considering your own personal values in **Activity 2.1** below.

This activity makes it clear that our values represent general and broad goals about what we consider a good life to be. Our values relate to what we consider to be a good life, but this does not mean that they are self-centred or egocentric. Very often our own idea of what constitutes a good life is intimately linked with our relationships with others. By identifying our values in this way, it becomes clear that we would expect these values to hold in other situations. We would anticipate that the 'fictional' person who wrote the list in **Table 2.1** would also value 'security', 'family and relationships', 'human dignity' and so on in other ways. Values can therefore be seen as 'desirable trans-situational goals' (Schwartz 1994), or as ongoing beliefs or attitudes that certain behaviours or states are desirable and preferred (Rokeach 1973 cited in Rassin 2008).

Activity 2.1

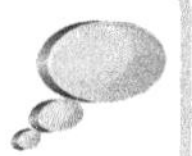

Imagine for a moment that you have just been given a million pounds, legitimately yours to spend as you wish. Now think about each of the three elements of this activity below.

- Spend a few minutes writing a list of the things that you would do with the money, entitled 'A good life for me'. Don't worry too much about exactly how much these things would cost (you can have another million if you need it!) – but create a list of at least five or six items.
- Revisit each of the items you have listed and create another column stating *why* you would want these things.
- Finally, create a third column and ask yourself how these reasons begin to make clear what it is that you value.

Once you have completed this activity you will end up with a similarly formatted list to that shown in **Table 2.1**.

Table 2.1 A good life for me

Item	Because a good life for me involves	Therefore I value
Pay off my mortgage	Being free from debt and having no concerns about where I will live	Security
Take my parents on the holiday of a lifetime	Spending time with family and thanking them for what they have given me in the past	Family and relationships
A long weekend with my partner in a luxury spa hotel	Being able to take time out for myself for rest and relaxation	Myself and my own well-being
Donation to Amnesty International	Living in a world in which other people are not subject to torture and inhuman or degrading treatment	Human dignity
Take a university course in philosophy	Thinking deeply and critically about new subjects	Intellectual challenge and accomplishment
A new car	Not being embarrassed in front of my friends by the car I drive	Social status

We started this section by observing that our values are related to character and therefore to the kind of person we are. The above exercise therefore also makes it clear that our values are revealed by what we actually *do*. If someone *were* to win a million pounds and then spent the whole sum on a very expensive car for themselves, we would generally take this to reveal that person's true values regardless of whether they claimed to value 'relationships' or 'human dignity' above all else. The caveat 'above all else' is important here because we all have a range of different values, and we can attach varying importance to them (Schwartz 1994). An individual may acknowledge that they do value social status, but they may nonetheless hope and assert that this is not more important to them than other things that they value, such as relationships. This demonstrates that on occasion the tensions between our personal values can cause conflict.

While understanding that people may have different values is important in nursing, it is also important to recognize that other people may prioritize their values differently. Consider the case study opposite and then attempt **Activity 2.2**.

Case study 2.1: Tomasz Krawiec

Mr Krawiec is an 83-year-old man who has lived alone since he was widowed three years ago after 53 years of marriage. He spent his early career in the Air Force, and is immensely proud that for the first time in his life he is independently taking care of his own domestic needs such as cooking and laundry. His primary means of socializing is to meet friends in the betting shop a few hundred metres down the road, and he bets small amounts on races on most days. He has a history of heart failure for which he is prescribed diuretic tablets, and has also recently been diagnosed as having early dementia.

A community nurse has visited Mr Krawiec and expressed some concern that he is not looking after himself. She reports that he is not taking his medication in the mornings because it makes him want to go to the toilet while he is at the betting shop. She also feels that he is evasive or vague when asked how he is managing his medication, and that his flat is cluttered and appears chaotic, with laundry hanging over every item of furniture.

 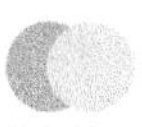

Activity 2.2

From the above information it is reasonable to surmise that there are many things that Mr Krawiec values. Some of these are listed below, and you may wish to add more that you think are relevant to him.

- Safety
- Independence
- Dignity
- Security
- Physical well-being
- Friendships
- Personal cleanliness

Now attempt the following.

- Once you have added any others to this list, try to put the items in the order of priority that you think will be most important to Mr Krawiec.
- Then examine some of the stories and experiences of other people from one or more of the following major reports, all readily available online.
  - *Care and Compassion? Report of the Health Service Ombudsman on Ten Investigations Into NHS Care of Older People* (Parlimentary and Health Service Ombudsman 2009).
  - *Patients Not Numbers, People Not Statistics* (Patients' Association 2009).
  - *The Point of Care: Enabling Compassionate Care in Acute Hospital Settings* (King's Fund 2009).
- Having reflected on some of these experiences, revisit the priorities you attached to the values Mr Krawiec may hold. Have your views changed, and why? What have you learned that will inform your nursing practice?

Your professional conduct as a student nurse

The NMC guidance on students' professional conduct will be reflected in the guidance offered by the institution providing your course, and will be used as criteria to review any allegations of student misconduct. In many ways the expectations in relation to the values held and acted out by student nurses and midwives at all times distinguish them from many other university students who do not have to meet the same expectations.

Activity 2.3

The latest versions of NMC publications are on their website (www.nmc-uk.org). Go to the 'publications' page and download the latest version of *Guidance on Professional Conduct for Nursing and Midwifery Students*. Read through it and note your initial thoughts on the expectations and requirements that the NMC has placed on student nurses and midwives.

Discuss your initial impressions with some of your peers, in particular:

- Whether there are there any points of guidance you feel are central to nursing and must be present?
- Whether there are any points of guidance you feel are not central and should not be required of student nurses and midwives?
- Any areas of guidance that relate to your behaviour as a student on a nursing course and not specifically to the provision of nursing care: what do you think about the need to follow this guidance at all times?
- Any challenges you think you may experience in following the guidance and how you can effectively respond to such challenges.

It is very important to remember that NMC publications are reviewed on an ongoing basis and it is therefore essential that you ensure you are always following the latest published guidance. The guidance discussed in this book was correct and up to date at the time of writing.

Key learning

- Being knowledgeable and skilled as a nurse is not enough; appropriate professional values and attitudes are essential.
- NMC guidance on conduct for student nurses and midwives will be reflected in your university programme.

Variations in the interpretation of values

In a global community the values of nursing in other countries such as the USA are worth examining and comparing with our own in the UK. For example, the American Association of Colleges of Nursing (AACN 2008) identifies the values which student nurses in the USA are expected to aspire to as:

- **altruism:** concern for the welfare and well-being of others;
- **autonomy:** right to self-determination;
- **human dignity:** respect for the inherent worth and uniqueness of individuals and populations;
- **integrity:** acting in accordance with accepted standards of practice; truth-telling;
- **social justice:** upholding moral, legal and humanistic principles; assuring equal treatment and equal access.

Values-based practice

The above activities should have helped you to explore why an understanding of values is of such central importance in nursing practice (or any other health care practice). Values-based practice (Fulford 2004; Fulford *et al.* 2012; McLean *et al.* 2012) is an approach which recognizes that working with people who are receiving health care is dependent upon recognizing and working with their values. Health cannot be narrowly defined, and a holistic understanding of health requires us to recognize that because people have different values they will have different ideas of what constitutes 'health' or a 'good life'. Nurses enable other people to achieve their health-related goals, and this means not only recognizing the values of others, but also that nurses may be involved in helping others to clarify their own values and to work out what 'health' or 'a good life' may be for them.

In order to explore these points, consider the details given about Chloe Arnold in **Case study 2.2**, and then complete **Activity 2.4**.

Case study 2.2: Chloe Arnold

Chloe is 15 years old and attends a local comprehensive school where she is doing well and is predicted to achieve 11 good GCSEs at grades B or above. She hopes to achieve her dream of becoming an architect. Chloe's mother Aileen has been alcohol dependent for a number of years and this was a factor in her divorce six years previously. Chloe therefore lives with her father Andrew, and sees her mother (whose lifestyle is still somewhat chaotic) only occasionally.

Chloe has always been physically healthy and active as a member of the school athletics team, but in the last 18 months her father has noticed that she is running more frequently, eating very little and losing weight. A year ago Chloe was diagnosed as having anorexia nervosa.

Despite support from health services, Chloe has continued to lose weight over recent months, and was yesterday admitted to hospital as her body mass index (BMI) had dropped to a critical level of 13. Sam is a student nurse who meets Chloe on the first day of her hospital admission while she is waiting for a review by the consultant and full medical team.

Sam approaches Chloe and notices that she is sat in bed using a tablet PC to read material on a 'pro-ana' website. Although she turns the screen away, Sam notes the name of the site and decides to investigate it before returning to talk to Chloe again. Sam goes online to look at the website and is particularly struck by the following statements:

Anorexia is a lifestyle not a disease.
Giving in to food shows weakness.
Being thin is more important than being healthy.

Sam also notes that the site recommends that girls who are 'pro ed' (eating disorder) may recognize each other by wearing a red beaded bracelet around their left wrist, and recalls that Chloe is wearing such a bracelet.

(Some content in this case study is taken from: http://proanalifestyle.blogspot.co.uk, accessed 20 August 2012)

Activity 2.4

Consider what you now know about Chloe and take some time to answer the following questions.

- What values do you think she may be expressing in her behaviours? Consider whether you know these are her values or whether they are your presumptions?
- Does Chloe appear to have values which conflict with one another?
- In what ways may Chloe's values conflict with your own?
- How would you say that Chloe was expressing her identity by associating with particular sets of values?

The information about Chloe generates many questions. For example:

- What sort of hospital environment do you think Chloe may be in?
- What environment may be appropriate?
- What field of nursing did you suppose Sam is studying? Children's nursing, mental health nursing, adult nursing or learning disabilities?
- What support from health services may have been available to Chloe prior to her hospital admission?

The above activity may have helped you to begin to understand how meeting the health needs of other people can challenge our own values, but it is also clear that Chloe appears to be establishing who she is in part by adopting the values of the online 'pro-ana' community. Discourse analysts studying websites such as these have observed that they represent communities in which apparent health or appearance concerns are reframed as markers of success. Participants actively (re)produce their identities as people with eating disorders (Riley *et al.* 2009). The quotes from the site mentioned at the end of the case study give a clear indication of the values of this group: that being thin is more valued than being healthy; that resisting food is a sign of strength (and therefore good). In as much as Chloe adopts these values, she is asserting herself as being a member of this group, and this is further reinforced by the fact that she chooses to wear a 'badge' of this identity in the form of the red bracelet.

It can also be seen that Chloe, like anyone else, has a range of conflicting values. An important part of the nurse's role will be in helping Chloe come to understand that the values of the 'pro-ana' group are not consistent with what she otherwise values in relation to being 'healthy' and living a 'good life'.

It is clear that there are several reasons why an understanding of personal values is important in nursing. Firstly, it is important for nurses to have the skills necessary to recognize that other people's values can be different from their own. This means that people will have different ideas of what 'health' means to them. Secondly, nurses need to recognize that people may hold values which conflict with one another. Nurses therefore do not simply help other people to achieve particular values (such as being thin), but set out to work with others in ways which take account of all of their different values so that the individual can 'flourish' (Sellman 2011) or 'thrive' (Aslan and Smith 2012) and live a good life.

Key learning

!

- Your values will be visible to others by what you do and say.
- Meeting the health needs of others requires nurses to recognize and respect other people's values.

Professional values

It was made clear in the discussion about Chloe that adopting particular values can be associated with membership of groups within society. We all know that our personal values are influenced by our family, our culture, our education, our religious upbringing and other social groupings to which we belong, including the professions we work within and the behaviours they expect of us. Acceptance of a set of values is part of being a member of a group. Whether this group is a university swimming club, a set of friends forming a study group or a faith-based organization, it will have goals which reflect some of its values such as physical well-being, academic achievement or celebrating spirituality. Becoming a nurse involves joining a professional group, and therefore means adopting the values of that group. It is important to note that people receiving health care may encounter differing values being embodied by different health professions or between differing fields of nursing practice (see 'Professional values in different fields of practice' on p. 31). Recognizing that these different values may be prioritized and reflected in decisions about care can be a central challenge for the interdisciplinary team.

Professional values underpinning nursing practice

Writers such as Sellman (2011) follow the philosopher Alasdair MacIntyre (1985) in holding that nursing is a 'practice' and a form of cooperative activity which is uniquely defined by having its own standards of excellence, and which seeks to achieve particular goals. It was noted above that nursing has the goal of ensuring that other people 'flourish' or 'thrive', and professional values in nursing are therefore those which help to ensure that the people for whom we care 'flourish'. Nursing practice offers the opportunity to make a difference to people we come into contact with. Central to nursing is the recognition of the privileged nurse–patient relationship, working in partnership, collaboratively with individuals and in teams, and the acceptance of personal accountability for decisions and actions.

Defining precisely what professional values actually entail is not straightforward. It is by no means clear to what degree being 'compassionate' or 'person-centred', or 'respecting human dignity' actually reflects different values or expected behaviours. Within the nursing literature the meaning of terms such as 'care' and 'person-centred' is widely debated, and 'human rights' themselves involve complex ethical and legal questions. The NMC (2010a) makes it clear that professional values are central to the competencies required for registration, and central to *The Code: Standards of Conduct, Performance and Ethics for Nurses and Midwives* (NMC 2008) as well as to *Guidance on Professional Conduct for Nursing and Midwifery Students* (NMC 2011). Nonetheless, these documents do not provide a clear 'list' of what those professional values are. More recently the policy document *Compassion in Practice* (DH 2012c) has attempted to capture the key values and behaviours required of nurses and caregivers into six Cs:

- **Care.** Delivering and enabling people to receive the best possible care.
- **Compassion.** Care given with empathy, thoughtfulness, kindness, respect and dignity.
- **Competence.** Care that is skilled, knowledgeable, based on best evidence and able to deliver excellence for all.

- **Communication.** Recognizes the value of listening to patients' views and involving them in all decisions about their care.
- **Courage.** Speaking up if something is wrong, being an advocate and always doing the right thing.
- **Commitment.** To act in a way that ensures excellent care and being passionate about this.

Absence of value-based care

The importance of holding appropriate professional values becomes clear when we examine what happens when this is not the case. Although *The NHS Constitution* (DH 2009) expresses an ideal of delivering care with care and compassion, reports such as those by the Parliamentary and Health Service Ombudsman (2009, 2011), and the King's Fund (2009) make clear that these ideals are not always realized. If you have examined these reports, or if you use the suggested resources at the end of this chapter, it will become clear that many people experience care that does not respect their dignity or meet their needs so as to help them 'flourish'.

The *National Service Framework for Older People* (DH 2001) identified areas where respect and dignity were not maintained, resulting in what was perceived as ageism and negative patient experiences. Examples of a lack of respect for patients included:

- being made to feel a nuisance;
- being ignored;
- generally being rushed and not being listened to;
- having to eat with fingers rather than helped to eat with a knife and fork.

In the recent case of Winterbourne View Hospital, the abuses revealed there were acknowledged as serious failures in the systems of ensuring quality care. An in-depth review set up in the aftermath of the scandal focused on the lessons to be learned and the actions needed to prevent such failures in future. The findings were published in *Transforming Care: A National Response to Winterbourne View Hospital* (DH 2012a). Specifically highlighted was the need to promote a culture where poor practice can be challenged and individuals enabled to speak out if they see poor care taking place. Hand in hand with this is a need to support an environment where collaboration, partnership working and excellent care are promoted.

Other examples of a person's dignity being violated include being left alone and having the call bell removed, or a patient being refused help to have a shower at night because it does not fit with ward routine or procedures. Sometimes being too busy or short staffed can result in a situation where patient values are ignored, however, everyone has a human right to dignity and it is unethical practice to ignore those rights (Heijkenskjold *et al.* 2010). Nurses can experience ethical conflict when ensuring the rights of individuals are maintained if the organizational culture is such that it overlooks patients' rights. This can be disheartening for individual student nurses, and in such cases it is important to seek support from mentors, managers, personal tutors and the university link staff, and take the courage to speak out or take action.

Complaints received by the Healthcare Commission (2007) cited examples of patients being left in soiled clothing or bedding. In particular the values manifest in the nursing care of older people and people in vulnerable circumstances are perceived by some to be poor (DH 2012b). Poor practice is unacceptable and although it may only be a minority of nurses who behave in such ways, the result is that the values of the profession come under severe scrutiny by the public and the media, who expect the highest professional values to be demonstrated by nurses.

Stretched health care resources, or organizational cultures which clash with nursing's professional values can challenge nurses who seek to deliver value-based care. This not only impacts on people's experience of care, but nurses themselves experience burnout, frustration and disillusionment if they feel themselves to be delivering care that is not consistent with their professional values (King's Fund 2009). Nonetheless, however difficult delivering values-based care may be, the NMC (2010a) makes it clear that a nurse must be 'willing to accept personal and professional accountability for his/her actions'. With this in mind one of the greatest challenges you will face as a student nurse is to always act like the nurse that you want to become.

Competing values

As with personal values, you may well have identified a range of professional values which conflict with one another. For example, it is easy to imagine circumstances in which 'recognizing and respecting individual choice' may conflict with the value placed upon using evidence-based practice. Or, what happens if an individual chooses a treatment option which the evidence suggests is unlikely to have positive outcomes? Similarly, there are challenges involved in managing risk while aiming to empower choices that promote self-care and safety. Consider how to balance the risk of someone falling in the bathroom with the fact that they need to learn to safely care for themselves. While the competences provide guidance on the standards expected, central to the role of a nurse is their individual clinical decision-making as they seek to make decisions to balance competing priorities in the pursuit of the 'provision of care to enable people to improve, maintain or recover health, to cope with health problems, and to achieve the best possible quality of life, whatever their disease or disability until death' (RCN 2003: 5).

In arriving at a decision, student nurses and RNs should be able to explain what factors they considered, how these were weighted against each other with consideration to possible outcomes and why they ultimately made the decision they did and acted accordingly (see Chapters 7 and 8 for further discussion on decision-making).

It can be important to draw on evidence derived from research or clinical guidelines and highlight the benchmarks for care to present the reasons for your practice. *The Essence of Care* (DH 2003) benchmarks for privacy and dignity best practice highlight the need to ensure the following patient outcomes:

- patients always feel they matter;
- patients and carers can access an area that safely offers privacy;
- patients experience care in an environment that takes full account of individual values, beliefs and personal relationships;
- communication between staff and patients takes place in a way that always respects their individuality and rights.

Ethical considerations in nursing practice

The NMC *Code* (2008) obliges nurses to demonstrate sound ethical decision-making skills and, importantly, this is underpinned by law. As a student you will constantly be developing your understanding of legal and ethical issues which influence the maintenance of professional standards. Ethics is concerned with reflecting on values and making decisions. In health care ethics is concerned with 'doing the right thing and with being a certain kind of person' (Gallagher and Hodge 2012). Daily you will be faced with ethical dilemmas and it is important to appreciate that there is not always an easy or 'right' answer. The four moral principles underpinning health care ethics developed by Beauchamp and Childress (2001) are:

- **beneficence:** practising in a way that promotes the good of the person;
- **non-malevolence:** avoiding harming the person;
- **autonomy:** respecting the person's right to make his or her own decisions;
- **justice:** treating the person fairly and equitably.

These principles provide the tools to help you to make choices. However, because we all have different value and belief systems as well as different past experiences, our decisions will not always be aligned with our colleagues or our patients.

You will become increasingly accountable for your actions during your programme as you work towards graduation and explore how related concepts such as respect for individual rights, confidentiality, duty of care and the preservation of dignity are central in providing quality nursing care. However, while standards and codes offer guidance, your decisions will always remain individual ones and will be influenced by the values and ethical stance prioritized by you in any particular context. Making effective decisions will require that you draw on the knowledge developed during your programme related to ethical principles and frameworks, legislation and policies in place within the care environment.

Professional values in different fields of practice

Within the UK there are four 'fields of practice' (previously referred to as 'branches') possible in pre-registration nurse education: mental health, learning disability, children's nursing and adult nursing. To reflect the differing emphasis within these areas of nursing, in addition to the generic competencies already noted, the NMC has also identified 'field specific' competencies within the professional values domain (see Appendix, p. 33). These field specific competences must be incorporated within, and achieved by students undertaking, the related programme. Across the fields of nursing practice there are differing numbers of field specific competences, as a result of the consultation process involved in the development of the *Standards for Pre-registration Nursing Education* (NMC 2010a) and the responses received related to each field of practice. Some fields advocated more detailed competency statements to reflect their priorities while others sought to have broader competency statements. There is also some repetition of field specific competencies across some but not all fields of nursing – for example, the first field specific competency for adult, mental health and learning disability nursing is the same, but is not identified in children's nursing.

This book sets out to help you achieve the competencies for professional nursing practice required by the NMC. These competencies are within four domains, the first of which is that of professional values. Within this domain the NMC expects student nurses to develop competences by the time they have completed their pre-registration nursing education and are applying for entry to the NMC Register.

Now undertake **Activities 2.5 and 2.6** which will help you to identify the values that underpin the NMC overall standard of competence in relation to professional values and the individual competency statements in that domain.

Activity 2.5

Study the generic competencies related to professional values presented on page above, and answer the following three questions for each of them.

- Which competencies do you think reveal values?
- What are the goals that will be achieved if nurses possess these competencies?
- What are the underpinning values of the profession that are being expressed?

Now complete **activity 2.6** which enables you to focus on the specific NMC competencies for your field of nursing.

Activity 2.6

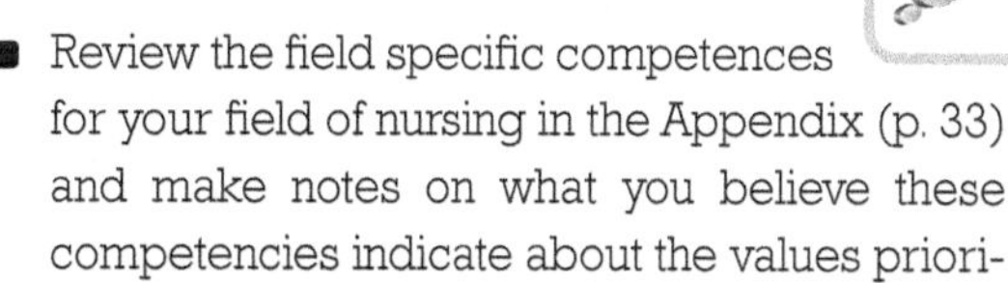

- Review the field specific competences for your field of nursing in the Appendix (p. 33) and make notes on what you believe these competencies indicate about the values prioritized within your field of nursing.
- Now review the field specific competences for the other three fields of nursing and again make notes about what you believe these indicate about the values prioritized within those fields of nursing. Then compare and contrast the similarities and differences with your field of nursing and the possible priorities within the other fields of nursing.

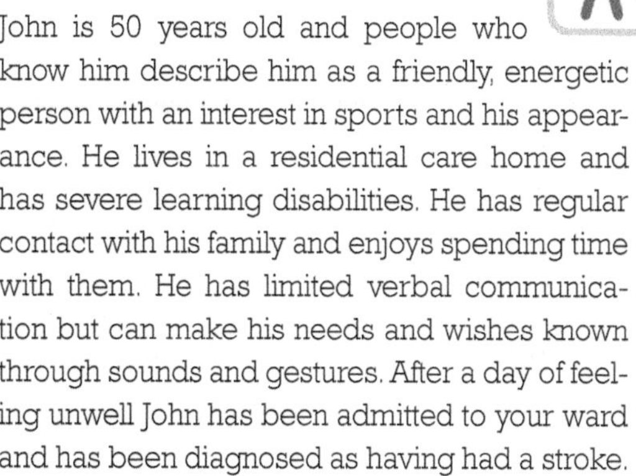

Case study 2.3: John Wetherall

John is 50 years old and people who know him describe him as a friendly, energetic person with an interest in sports and his appearance. He lives in a residential care home and has severe learning disabilities. He has regular contact with his family and enjoys spending time with them. He has limited verbal communication but can make his needs and wishes known through sounds and gestures. After a day of feeling unwell John has been admitted to your ward and has been diagnosed as having had a stroke.

- Make your own notes on how the field specific competences from your course will influence the decisions you make in the provision of care and support for John.
- Discuss your priorities from above with colleagues from another field of nursing and explore how similar values and priorities in relation to John's care provide opportunities for collaboration.
- Discuss how potential areas of differing priority may create challenges in collaborative working and how these could be effectively responded to in order to improve care and support for John.

Review the story of Martin Ryan (Parliamentary and Health Service Ombudsman 2009: 56–61). In this case it was concluded that 'had the care and treatment Mr Ryan received not fallen so far below the relevant standard, it is likely that his death could have been avoided' (p. 60). While health professionals normally seek to provide effective care, harm and indeed death can occur when there is failure to deliver values-based nursing care. It is important that all nurses learn from such examples of poor care if these are to be avoided in the future. What evidence can you see that the values required by your field of practice were applied in Mr Ryan's care and what values appear not to have been applied?

Key learning !

- As a nurse you may at times experience tensions in prioritizing your values in practice.
- Poor standards of care reflect a failure to deliver values-based nursing care.

Conclusion

This chapter has examined the nature of personal and professional values in nursing. It has made clear that people's personal values (including our own) are complex and potentially conflicting. Nurses need to have highly developed skills in order to recognize and work with the values of the people they care for. This ability is a key aspect of nursing decision-making (explored further in Chapters 7 and 8). These values may themselves be seen as the goals which people themselves hold to be important in living a good life and 'flourishing'. The values of the nursing profession relate to our professional goal of ensuring that the people we care for 'flourish'. Nurses value *autonomy* because they recognize that flourishing requires people to have control over their own lives and bodies; nurses value a *respect for dignity* because living a good life requires that we are recognized and treated as unique and valued persons. Above all else, the professional values of nursing require that *nurses prioritize the values of the people they work with.* It is for this reason that the NMC *Code* begins by stating that nurses must 'make the care of people [their] *first* concern' (NMC 2008, emphasis added).

This chapter has helped you to consider the nature of professional values and recognize the values that you wish to embody. However, it is adopting these values and making sure they are reflected in your practice that is central to becoming a nurse. Nursing practice requires nurses to have courage (Day 2007) and to be of 'good character' (NMC 2010b). Becoming a nurse requires you to have the personal integrity to practise in accordance with your professional values at all times (Ekeberg 2011). The NMC (2010a) notes that newly-qualified nurses cannot be expected to have extensive experience or specialist expertise, but makes clear that *all* nurses can be expected to practise with integrity.

Acknowledgements

Our thanks to Chris Gale from the University of Southampton for comments on and improvements to the case study about Chloe.

Appendix

Field specific competence statements

Adult nursing

Adult nurses must also be able at all times to promote the rights, choices and wishes of all adults and, where appropriate, children and young people, paying particular attention to equality, diversity and the needs of an ageing population. They must be able to work in partnership to address people's needs in all healthcare settings.

1.1 **Adult nurses** must understand and apply current legislation to all service users, paying special attention to the protection of vulnerable people, including those with complex needs arising from ageing, cognitive impairment, long-term conditions and those approaching the end of life.

Mental health nursing

Mental health nurses must work with people of all ages using values-based mental health frameworks. They must use different methods of engaging people, and work in a way that promotes positive relationships focused on social inclusion, human rights and recovery, that is, a person's ability to live a self-directed life, with or without symptoms, that they believe is meaningful and satisfying.

1.1 **Mental health nurses** must understand and apply current legislation to all service users, paying special attention to the protection of vulnerable people, including those with complex needs arising from ageing, cognitive impairment, long-term conditions and those approaching the end of life.

2.1 **Mental health nurses** must practise in a way that addresses the potential power imbalances between professionals and people experiencing mental health problems, including situations when compulsory measures are used, by helping people exercise their rights, upholding safeguards and ensuring minimal restrictions on their lives. They must have an in depth understanding of mental health legislation and how it relates to care and treatment of people with mental health problems.

3.1 **Mental health nurses** must promote mental health and wellbeing, while challenging the inequalities and discrimination that may arise from or contribute to mental health problems.

4.1 **Mental health nurses** must work with people in a way that values, respects and explores the meaning of their individual lived experiences of mental health problems, to provide person-centred and recovery-focused practice.

8.1 **Mental health nurses** must have and value an awareness of their own mental health and wellbeing. They must also engage in reflection and supervision to explore the emotional impact on self of working in mental health; how personal values, beliefs and emotions impact on practice, and how their own practice aligns with mental health legislation, policy and values-based frameworks.

Learning disability nursing

Learning disabilities nurses must promote the individuality, independence, rights, choice and social inclusion of people with learning disabilities and highlight their strengths and abilities at all times while encouraging others do the same. They must facilitate the active participation of families and carers.

1.1 **Learning disabilities nurses** must understand and apply current legislation to all service users, paying special attention to the protection of vulnerable people, including those with complex needs arising from ageing, cognitive impairment, long-term conditions and those approaching the end of life.

2.1 **Learning disabilities nurses** must always promote the autonomy, rights and choices of people with learning disabilities and support and involve their families and carers, ensuring that each person's rights are upheld according to policy and the law.

3.1 **Learning disabilities nurses** must use their knowledge and skills to exercise professional advocacy, and recognise when it is appropriate to refer to independent advocacy services to safeguard dignity and human rights.

4.1 **Learning disabilities nurses** must recognise that people with learning disabilities are full and equal citizens, and must promote their health and wellbeing by focusing on and developing their strengths and abilities.

Children's nursing

Children's nurses must understand their role as an advocate for children, young people and their families, and work in partnership with them. They must deliver child- and family-centred care; empower children and young people to express their views and preferences; and maintain and recognise their rights and best interests.

1.1 **Children's nurses** must understand the laws relating to child and parental consent, including giving and refusing consent, withdrawal of treatment and legal capacity.

2.1 **Children's nurses** must recognise that all children and young people have the right to be safe, enjoy life and reach their potential. They must practise in a way that recognises, respects and responds to the individuality of every child and young person.

3.1 **Children's nurses** must act as advocates for the right of all children and young people to lead full and independent lives.

4.1 **Children's nurses** must work in partnership with children, young people and their families to negotiate, plan and deliver child- and family-centred care, education and support. They must recognise the parent's or carer's primary role in achieving and maintaining the child's or young person's health and wellbeing, and offer advice and support on parenting in health and illness.

Further reading and resources

DHSSPS (Department of Health, Social Service and Public Safety) (2008) *Improving the Patient & Client Experience*, available at: www.dhsspsni.gov.uk/improving_the_patient_and_client_experience.pdf.

This document explores how patient and client experience can be positively or adversely impacted upon through the actions or omissions of health and social care professionals. It focuses on the areas of respect, attitude, behaviour, communication, privacy and dignity. It provides practical examples of indicators for how appropriate standards for care can be provided in these areas.

Griffith, R. and Tengnah, C. (2010) *Law and Professional Issues in Nursing*, 2nd edn. Exeter: Learning Matters.

King's Fund (2009) *The Point of Care: Enabling Compassionate Care in Acute Hospital Settings*. London: King's Fund.

Local Government Association/NHS Confederation/Age UK (2012) *Delivering Dignity: Securing Dignity in Care for Older People in Hospitals and Care Homes*, available at: www.nhsconfed.org/documents/dignity.pdf.

Parliamentary and Health Service Ombudsman (2009) *Six Lives: The Provision of Public Services to People with Learning Disabilities, Part 1: Overview and Summary Investigation Reports, Second Report Session 2008–2009*. London: The Stationery Office.

Parliamentary and Health Service Ombudsman (2011) *Care and Compassion? Report of the Health Service Ombudsman on Ten Investigations into NHS Care of Older People*. London: The Stationery Office.

www.nmc-uk.org/Students. The NMC student resource. The NMC provides advice and guidance with a focus on students' conduct during and following their pre-registration nurse education. This is updated regularly.

Listening to the stories of people who use health services can be a powerful way of coming to understand the need for all health care practitioners to embody appropriate professional values. Two useful websites where you can do this are:

www.patientvoices.org.uk. The Patient Voices programme aims to facilitate the telling of some of the unwritten and unspoken stories of ordinary people so that those who devise and implement strategy in health and social

 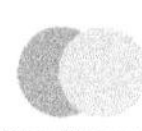

care, as well as the professionals and clinicians directly involved in care, may carry out their duties in a more informed and compassionate manner.

www.tellingstories.nhs.uk. This resource has been developed to promote understanding among all health professionals of the impact genetics has on real life, and its relevance to health care practice. The website draws on stories that cover a range of genetic conditions including single-gene disorders, chromosomal abnormalities and multifactorial conditions such as cancer and heart disease. The section on 'issues raised' is particularly useful.

References

AACN (American Association of Colleges of Nursing) (2008) *The Essentials of Baccalaureate Education*. Washington, DC: AACN.

Aslan, M. and Smith, M. (2012) Promoting health and social inclusion, in S. Tee, J. Brown and D. Carpenter (eds) (2012) *Handbook of Mental Health Nursing*. London: Hodder Arnold.

Beauchamp, T.L. and Childress, J.F.(2001) *Principles of Biomedical Ethics*, 5th edn. Oxford: Oxford University Press.

Day, L. (2007) Courage as a virtue necessary to good nursing practice, *American Journal of Critical Care*, 16(6): 613–16.

DH (Department of Health) (2001) *National Service Framework for Older People*. London: DH.

DH (Department of Health) (2003) *The Essence of Care: Patient Focused Benchmarks for Clinical Governance*. London: DH.

DH (Department of Health) (2009) *The NHS Constitution*. London: DH.

DH (Department of Health) (2012a) *Transforming Care: A National Response to Winterbourne View Hospital, Final Report*. London: DH.

DH (Department of Health) (2012b) *Developing a Culture of Compassionate Care: Creating a New Vision for Nurses, Midwives and Care-givers*. London: DH.

DH (Department of Health) (2012c) *Compassion in Practice: Nursing, Midwifery and Care Staff: Our Vision and Strategy*. London: DH.

Ekeberg, V. (2011) Mature care and the virtue of integrity, *Nursing Philosophy*, 12(2): 128–38.

Fulford, K.W.M. (2004) Ten principles of values based medicine, in J. Radden (ed.) (2004) *The Philosophy of Psychiatry: A Companion*. New York: Oxford University Press.

Fulford, K.W.M., Peile, E. and Carroll, H. (2012) *Essential Values-based Practice: Linking Science with People*. Cambridge: Cambridge University Press.

Gallagher, A. and Hodge, S. (eds) (2012) *Ethics, Law and Professional Issues: A Practice-based Approach for Health Professionals*. Basingstoke: Palgrave Macmillan.

Healthcare Commission (2007) *State of Healthcare 2007: Improvements and Challenges in Services in England and Wales*. London: Healthcare Commission.

Heijkenskjold, K.B., Ekstedt, M. and Lindwall, L. (2010) The patient's dignity from the nurse's perspective, *Nursing Ethics*, 17(3): 313–22.

Independent Commission on Dignity in Care (2012) *Delivering Dignity. Securing Dignity in Care for Older People in Hospitals and Care Homes*. London: Local Government Association/NHS Confederation/Age UK.

King's Fund (2009) *The Point of Care: Enabling Compassionate Care in Acute Hospital Settings*. London: King's Fund.

MacIntyre, A. (1985) *After Virtue: A Study in Moral Theory*, 2nd edn. London: Duckworth.

McLean, C., Fulford, B. and Carpenter, D. (2012) Values based practice, in S. Tee, J. Brown and D. Carpenter (eds) *Handbook of Mental Health Nursing*. London: Hodder Arnold.

Mohr, W., Deatrick, J., Richmond, T. and Mahon, M. (2001) A reflection on values in Turbulent times, *Nursing Outlook*, 49(1): 30–6.

NMC (Nursing and Midwifery Council) (2008) *The Code: Standards of Conduct, Performance and Ethics for Nurses and Midwives*. London: NMC.

NMC (Nursing and Midwifery Council) (2010a) *Standards for Pre-registration Nursing Education*. London: NMC.

NMC (Nursing and Midwifery Council) (2010b) *Good Health and Good Character: Guidance for Approved Higher Education Institutions*. London: NMC.

NMC (Nursing and Midwifery Council) (2011) *Guidance on Professional Conduct for Nursing and Midwifery Students*. London: NMC.

Parliamentary and Health Service Ombudsman (2009) *Six Lives: The Provision of Public Services to People with Learning Disabilities, Part 1: Overview and Summary Investigation Reports, Second Report Session 2008–2009*. London: The Stationery Office.

Parliamentary and Health Service Ombudsman (2011) *Care and Compassion? Report of the Health Service Ombudsman on Ten Investigations into NHS Care of Older People*. London: The Stationery Office.

Patients' Association (2009) *Patients Not Numbers, People Not Statistics*. London: Patients' Association.

Rassin, M. (2008) *The Nature of Human Values*. New York: Free Press.

RCN (Royal College of Nursing) (2003) *Defining Nursing*. London: RCN.

Riley, S., Rodham, K. and Gavin, J. (2009) Doing weight: pro-ana and recovery identities in cyberspace, *Journal of Community & Applied Social Psychology*, 19: 348–59.

Schwartz, S.H. (1994) Are there universal aspects in the structure and contents of human values? *Journal of Social Issues*, 50(4): 19–45.

Sellman, D. (2011) Professional values and nursing, *Medicine, Health Care & Philosophy*, 14(2): 203–8.

Owning your standards of care

3

Ruth Taylor and Debbie Banks

Chapter contents

Introduction

This chapter aims to facilitate your understanding of standards of clinical care and the responsibilities that you have to ensure your own practice achieves the standard expected of you at each stage of your course. It also aims to ensure that you continue to develop your standards of care as you progress through your course and on into professional practice. It builds on the previous chapter and is underpinned by the theories of value-based care. You will be exploring standards in relation to quality through the key concepts of safe, effective and person-centred care and how these relate to you as a developing professional.

Policy and different types of evidence from across the fields of practice including examples of situations where standards have not been achieved will be considered. In addition, carers and former patients bring their voice to the issues that affect good quality care. Finally, we provide you with some practical approaches that will enable you to continually work towards enhancement of your practice, and the achievement of good standards of care. The key message within this chapter is that as a student nurse you have a responsibility to own the standards of care you provide. In this respect, it is clear that all of the Nursing and Midwifery Council (NMC) competencies across the domains are relevant to your learning in this chapter. However, particular attention is paid to Domain 1 (professional values) so that you can contextualize your learning and consider the impact that your actions, approaches to care and attitudes have in the context of owning your own standards of care.

In particular we would draw your attention to the following NMC competencies.

Domain 1: Professional values – generic standard for competence

All nurses must act first and foremost to care for and safeguard the public. They must practise autonomously and be responsible and accountable for safe, compassionate, person-centred, evidence-based nursing that respects and maintains dignity and human rights.

1 All nurses must practise with confidence according to *The Code: Standards of Conduct,*

Performance and Ethics for Nurses and Midwives (NMC 2008), and within other recognised ethical and legal frameworks.

Reflection and owning your standards of care

To commence the chapter, we invite you to consider the role of reflection in relation to the care you provide. It is likely that you will have been introduced to the concepts of reflection and reflective practice as part of your nurse education so far. We offer an overview of reflection and its use for you as a developing professional, but acknowledge that the topic is far-reaching and widely written about. It is an area that you will explore fully as you work your way through your course. What we recommend is that you use this section as a starting point and as a focus for your work within this chapter.

The term reflection is widely described through different theoretical and experiential perspectives. For us, the key focus for reflection is about using a framework to look back on your experiences of practice or your experiences as they are happening, so as to enhance your learning and therefore your competence in practice. This action of reflection should be an ongoing process that takes place every day, and one which develops as you develop as a person and as a professional.

Johns and Freshwater (2005) write eloquently about transforming nursing through reflective practice. Having extensively written about reflective practice, Johns (2010) sets out several key points about the essence of reflection. These mirror our views and are reflected in the statements below.

- Reflection is a way of being rather than doing, it is more than a technique for learning through experience.
- Becoming mindful of self is the central quality of reflective practice.
- Being a reflective nurse is always being mindful in practice.
- The outcome of reflection provides insight and learning that can enable people to become more effective in their personal and professional lives.
- Reflective practice is hard work and requires commitment and practice.

What emerges in Johns' work is the relationship between mindfulness and reflection. He asserts that 'The ultimate expression of reflective practice is mindfulness' (2010: 15). Kabat-Zinn (2004: 4) describes mindfulness as 'paying attention in a particular way: on purpose, in the present moment, and non-judgementally', while Siegel (2010: 26) describes it as a 'particular attitude toward experience – whatever that experience may be [to achieve] awareness of present experience with acceptance'. We will return to the relevance of mindfulness for you later in the chapter.

For the purposes of this chapter we offer a reflective model that should allow you to think more easily about your practice, but recommend that you review the work of Johns who takes a complex and in-depth approach to the development of reflective practice in an attempt to enable us to become all we can be as professionals.

The model by Gibbs (1988) is widely used and comprises a number of specific steps, as follows:

1. Description: what happened?
2. Feelings: what were you thinking and feeling?
3. Evaluation: what was good and bad about the experience?
4. Analysis: what sense can you make of the situation?
5. Conclusion: what else could you have done?
6. Action plan: if it arose again what would you do?
7. Back to Stage 1.

We will be asking you to reflect upon your own experiences of practice later in the chapter and suggest you refer to Gibbs' model to do so.

Activity 3.1

We recommend you keep a log throughout your practice placements, perhaps in your professional development portfolio, of the times you ask patients how their experiences can be improved. You will be able to use the information you gain from these conversations in a number of ways.

- As part of your reflective practice so that you can determine how well the standards of care are enacted in practice settings.
- In group work and other classroom learning activities such as critical incident analysis and enquiry-based learning in order to understand more fully the nature and impact of nursing practice.
- As part of your leadership and management learning at later stages in your course.

Standards of care

The term 'standards' refers to the principles or values that govern a person's decision-making and behaviour. However, the word 'standard' has a variety of meanings, two of which are also relevant to this chapter: one meaning is 'norm' – norms are the customary ways we behave that are accepted by society. A second meaning is 'a level of quality or excellence' to be achieved, which implies that a standard can be used as a benchmark. Kleinman (2006) states that professional standards articulate what is important or desired, and standards what is good or acceptable. Standards of care exist at a micro level in practice at the point of delivery where they impact on the experience of the participants in the care process, through to the macro level of health care as articulated through policy and published statements by a range of professional bodies and stakeholders. A key purpose at the macro level is to make transparent to the public what the government's, professions' and health care providers' intentions are in order to instil public confidence.

The policy context is clearly focused on the achievement of high standards of care within a complex and evolving health care system. The nature and extent of change within health care can be observed through the following (Basford and Kershaw 2008; NMC 2010; Scottish Government 2010):

- patient empowerment;
- co-production;
- scientific and technological advances;
- the importance of outcome as measured by the patient experience and other types of indicators;
- the move towards more stringent professional regulation;
- financial constraints;
- the emergence of more rigorous frameworks for managing risk and promoting safety.

We need to remember that health care is not delivered in isolation, and that increasingly nursing and health care teams are working alongside social care professionals as part of a shift towards delivering integrated care. The challenges associated with working across boundaries are explored in the interprofessional literature (e.g. Taylor and Brannan forthcoming) and can be summarized as:

- the need for flexible approaches to working within and across roles;
- the expansion and evolution of roles and the associated impact on other professions;
- the organizational structures and cultures that impact on team working, leadership and decision-making;
- the professional challenges associated with interprofessional working, including hierarchical issues;
- a collective vision of the meaning of standards and ownership of standards of care.

Despite the emphasis here on interprofessional working, you may feel that some of the challenges noted above apply equally to working towards high standards of care within a team of health professionals. It is imperative that we work towards breaking down the barriers across professions and across health and social care where they exist. When you come to look at cases of care which went wrong later in this chapter, you will see that these boundaries are sometimes the cause of difficulties in ensuring that care is of good quality.

Key learning

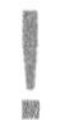

- The standards of care you provide are owned by you.
- Reflection is a pivotal component of enhancing your own standards of care.

In relation to the health care policy context, the three quality ambitions below present a summary of current national policy. You may wish to investigate further and access policy that has specific reference to your own field of practice – the policy documents identified at the end of this chapter are relevant across all fields.

The focus of the NHS Scotland Quality Framework (see resources at end of the chapter) document is to continue to drive up standards of health care across all settings through the enactment of the three quality ambitions:

1. Mutually beneficial partnerships between patients, families and those delivering health care.
2. No avoidable injury or harm for people from the health care that they receive.
3. The most appropriate treatments, interventions, support and services at the right time and in the right way.

Linked into these are the six dimensions of health care quality:

- person-centred;
- safe;
- effective;
- efficient;
- equitable;
- timely.

Policy accentuates standards of care. The way in which we, as a professional group and as individual nurses, enact the policy direction within our practice is crucial. In conjunction with the NMC *Standards* (2010) and *Code* (2008), a clear vision is articulated. Regardless of the fast pace of change, it remains the remit of the nurse to work in partnership to deliver professional, person-centred, safe and effective nursing care that is both evidence-based and values-based (NMC 2010; Scottish Government 2010).

Evidence- and values-based practice, as discussed in Chapters 1 and 2, are crucial components to making care decisions. Evidence-based practice is concerned with how we ensure safety, effective outcomes, efficiency and improvement, and that what we do is best practice. Values-based practice is concerned with how we uphold people's rights, ensure equality, establish meaningful relationships, use communication skilfully, convey compassion and respect, and ensure dignity, so that the patient care experience meets their expectations. The standard of your care is entrenched in how you bring these two elements of care together. As a student nurse, you need to be motivated to learn about both and integrate them into your practice to achieve the level of professionalism that is inherent in the standards of care expected. The NMC has made it clear that our graduate nurses will not only deliver care to certain standards, but will drive up standards of care (NMC 2010). Therefore a priority area for you as a student nurse is to recognize the importance of both theoretical learning and practice learning in influencing the standards of care you deliver and to challenge yourself to engage equally in both.

As a student nurse we would encourage you to bear the following in mind:

- To be clear about your own values so you can explore them in relation to your behaviour and their alignment with the values and principles that relate to professional nursing. You will explore this later in the chapter.

- Within every clinical setting there will be customary ways of doing things that you will observe and perhaps be expected to adopt. You therefore need to be able to make judgements relating to the evidence-base and values associated with practice.
- You will have customary ways of doing things which may or may not reflect the standards expected. As part of your development process you need to be able to accept and discuss feedback and be open to the need for change. This is a key part of your learning process.
- All registered nurses must adhere to codes, practice guidelines, frameworks and procedures. Individual, team and service performance are assessed against these. As a student nurse, your performance will be assessed against the NMC competencies but encompassed within these is the requirement to demonstrate compliance with a range of other standards that are in place within the placement environment.
- The outcome of nursing care is increasingly the subject of measurement to ascertain effectiveness, improve services and the patient experience as well as develop the evidence base. As a student nurse on placement, you will be expected to take every opportunity to become personally effective and enhance the patient experience with the support of your mentors. This aspect of your practice relates to one of the progression assessment points required by the NMC: 'Works more independently, with less direct supervision, in a safe and increasingly confident manner'.

Although published statements make transparent what should be done, it is at the point of delivery that standards of care matter. While much of the care that is provided in practice will be of an appropriate standard, we know that standards are not always as high as they should be. We will now explore the impact of poor standards on practice.

Impact of poor standards

Kleinman's (2006) seminal paper 'Ethical drift: when good people do bad things' highlights some key areas that are worthy of note before we go on to look at examples of poor practice in relation to high profile cases and in day-to-day situations.

- Most nurses enter the profession to care for patients.
- Their values are about maintaining high standards and doing their best for patients.
- Resource constraints are often cited as the main reason nurses feel they work in ways that interfere with or compromise the values they hold.
- Collaboration where managers and clinicians share the same or similar values heightens morale in difficult times.
- Where different agendas are perceived, an 'ethos' gap can occur where professional values and priorities for managers and clinicians conflict.
- In some cases of patient care, deviation from a person's ethical foundation and values can be blatant and represent a major issue or incident.
- In other cases a gradual erosion of ethical standards and care occurs which can go unnoticed as minor deviations are justified as acceptable in that situation.
- Gradual ethical drift can escalate until care is significantly below standard but is not recognized, continues to be rationalized as reasonable in the light of other demands and is usually characterized by a lack of awareness. One concession to self-interest over values makes it easier to continue to act in this way and leads on to others.

As you progress through this section and are introduced to examples of poor practice, you might find it useful to look back at the points Kleinman makes as a way of understanding some of the dynamics of the cases presented.

There are many examples where standards of care have fallen far short of what is required. If you listen to the news regularly you will hear repeated media coverage of problems associated with the care of patients across many settings. In the most serious of cases there are publicly available documents that enable students and professionals to reflect on incidents of poor care and to learn from these. It is not happy reading, but as professionals we have a responsibility to seek out learning from these situations and to make sure that we strive to improve in all aspects of our practice. So, taking ownership of our standards of care involves a proactive approach to learning from difficult situations. Leadership in practice is key within all this – from leadership at a strategic level by the director of nursing for example, to leadership at an individual level at the point of interaction with the patient or family.

Clinical governance

Clinical governance is a set of measures that works towards ensuring that standards of care are appropriate. Recent policy, as discussed earlier, emphasizes the need for patient-centred, safe and effective care and all are relevant to the notion of clinical governance. In terms of nursing practice, we as a group of professionals are responsible for ensuring that our practice is at a high level in all these areas. The challenges associated with this aspiration are rehearsed in the media – resourcing in service, education of nurses, culture in practice, among others (if you look at the BBC website you are very likely to come across topical news items relating to standards of care and, in particular, the public perception of the standards of nursing care – see www.bbc.co.uk/news/health).

In addition, nurse leaders have highlighted concerns about standards of care in certain situations (McSherry *et al.* 2012). The authors counterbalance the concerns by emphasizing that not all care is bad and that the core attributes of nursing (dignity and respect, caring and compassion) can be demonstrated at organizational, team and individual levels. However, not to do anything to change practice in the light of learning from situations in which care was poor is to ignore the responsibilities that each individual has to continuously improve care. We have provided some examples of where care has gone wrong in **Box 3.1**. Take the time to reflect on these cases. Although they relate to specific fields of practice they are relevant for all students to consider in order to enhance their own practice-focused learning and their understanding of organizational cultures and responsibilities.

From these examples you can probably see that there are many aspects of customary practice that went wrong, with ethical drift as a feature. Mason (2002) asserts that part of our professional development is to question and change habitual ways of responding which are often developed to cope with specific situations in practice. As a student going into your practice placements you are a new pair of eyes and can ask relevant questions regarding practice – staff will usually be pleased to discuss critical questions relating to the ways in which care is delivered.

Having looked at incidents of poor practice that have become well known nationally and led to significant changes to policy and practice, we will now look at aspects of poor practice that may occur on a day-to-day basis, that go unreported, and have the potential to escalate. To set the context, take time to think about **Activity 3.1** and how what we are asking you to do within this activity has the potential to impact positively on your awareness of the patient experience. As you will see, the types of practice that have a real impact on the patient experience are often things that are within our control as individuals.

The examples given in **Box 3.2** are based on a range of stories found on the patient opinion website at www.patientopinion.org.uk. They are used to illustrate how poor practice is often about the very things we see as fundamental to good standards of care.

Take some time to think about the key point made earlier about owning your standards of care and the ideas that Kleinman (2006) discusses about why nurses might lose sight of their values and standards. Then undertake **Activity 3.2**.

Box 3.1 Inquiries into poor care

CHILDREN AND YOUNG PEOPLE

***The Victoria Climbié Inquiry Report* (House of Commons Health Committee 2003)**

Victoria Climbié died of multiple injuries inflicted on her by her great aunt and her great aunt's partner over a period of months. They were convicted of her murder. Victoria's story is a harrowing one – and very powerfully written in this document. You will see from the report that there is a vast amount of learning for health and social services. While the problems associated with the case related to a systemic failure of services to provide what was required, specific issues relating to health care included: problems with history-taking, note-keeping, handover of care and monitoring of outcome, among others. Reflection on our responsibilities as individual practitioners and as a profession in relation to any provision of care is vital if we are to learn from tragedies such as this one.

ADULT

***Report of the Mid Staffordshire NHS Foundation Trust Public Inquiry* (Francis 2013)**

The Mid Staffordshire Inquiry was set up following concerns with mortality rates and the standard of care. This far-reaching report documents numerous examples of where care fell far short of what should be expected. When you read the report you will see that there were failings in many areas including continence, bladder and bowel care, safety, personal and oral hygiene, nutrition and hydration, pressure area care, and cleanliness and infection control. These are just some of the areas, and as you can see, they have far-reaching effects on all aspects of the patient journey and standards of care.

MENTAL HEALTH AND ADULT

***Starved of Care: Summary Investigation Report into the Care and Treatment of Mrs V* (MWC 2011)**

Mrs V was a woman with dementia who died in hospital in December 2008. The Scottish Mental Welfare Commission (MWC) decided to investigate because there were concerns that her treatment had not been as good as it should have been. The MWC findings show that Mrs V was treated poorly. Her problems were complex but not uncommon.

LEARNING DISABILITY

***Review of Compliance: Castlebeck Care (Teesdale) Ltd* (CQC 2011)**

This review of services revealed a number of concerns including (but not restricted to):

- poor and outdated practices in the care of patients across a variety of settings;
- inconsistent practice in safeguarding;
- problems with staff supervision;
- inadequate quality assurance mechanisms nationally.

OLDER ADULT

***Care and Compassion? Report of the Health Service Ombudsman on Ten Investigations into NHS Care of Older People* (Parliamentary and Health Service Ombudsman 2011)**

This report provides evidence relating to 10 complaints against NHS Trusts and GP practices. The particular cases are explored and the key message from the ombudsman is that people did not receive the care that they expected and that the patient experiences did not relate to the core values and principles of the NHS. What the ombudsman presents is a picture of an NHS that is failing in its care for older people.

Box 3.2 Illustration of poor practice

'Excellent surgical team let down badly by some'

'Sadly some of the staff on ward let the hospital down badly. They were lazy and treated people with lack of respect and dignity. This was my first time in hospital and I was horrified by what I witnessed on this ward. I had an accident and could not clean myself, the nurse threw a box of wet wipes at me and said, "You have get used to it, clean yourself up." Food left for people to eat on tray when they could not feed [themselves]. Urine left on bathroom floor for long periods, patients walking into it without slippers.'

https://www.patientopinion.org.uk/opinions/58021

'Concerned about poor communication and patient care'

'I was horrified to witness some nurses treating other patients . . . with very little patience and occasionally outright hostility. I soon became the object of the same treatment when I expressed my concern over the fact that I was left waiting up to four hours each time I asked for pain relief.'

https://www.patientopinion.org.uk/opinions/63357

'Very, very bad'

'The nurse[s] and ward sister[s] never remembered a patient's name. I saw no "basic care" given to patients that needed it and some of these patients asked for help, it was not given. Staff told me they were too busy when I said I was in pain. I was left without water and I could not get out of bed . . . All night staff were rude and gave the impression they didn't want to be there. Patients didn't want to ask for anything because of the staff's attitude.'

https://www.patientopinion.org.uk/opinions/51668

'Compassion is sometimes lacking'

'Upon arrival at A&E it was reported that I was just having a panic attack . . . I was then told to sit in a small waiting area to be triaged. When the nurse came to triage me I was talked to with disdain and was asked the circumstance of my being in A&E. I did my best to explain about being unwell and a passer-by calling 999 on my behalf. The nurse stated that I was obviously just anxious and I was asked, "What made you think this is an emergency?" I attempted to explain the situation again but I was dismissed to wait for a Dr. . . . When the same nurse came to carry out some of the tests I . . . happened to ask what I do. I replied, honestly, that I am currently awaiting treatment for a brain tumour . . . From that moment, the attitude of the nurse changed dramatically. On discharge and recalling the nurse's question to me about why I thought my situation that day was an emergency I stopped and apologised for having wasted both the nurse's and the Dr's time. I really will never forget the response which was "Oh, it's fine, I didn't realise you actually had something wrong with you."'

https://www.patientopinion.org.uk/opinions/54848

'Elderly patient care'

'My grandmother was admitted with a broken leg . . . on two days she was left for hours without water at her bedside . . . I asked that she be given extra pillows from the nurses and while assured she would get some she was never given any extra pillows to make her more comfortable . . . As her leg was broken, she was in a lot of pain and need[ed] regular painkillers. One night she rang for the nurse and it took the nurse 30 minutes to come to her bedside. She informed the nurse that she was in a lot of pain and asked if she could be given more painkillers. The nurse said she was not sure what she could be given and said she would have to ask a more senior colleague. However, the nurse did not come back to her bedside and she was left in pain until her next round of painkillers was due. She was also distressed that it would take a nurse sometimes an hour to come to her bedside when she rang the buzzer for help to go to the bathroom. This was very stressful for her as the delay in time meant she was worried she would have an accident . . . Furthermore, some staff members complained to her and other staff loudly in front of patients that they were not being paid enough and their pensions were not good enough. Noise during the night was another issue, as some nursing staff appeared to make no attempts to keep the noise down as they often talked to each other loudly during the night.'

https://www.patientopinion.org.uk/opinions/59553

> **Activity 3.2**
>
> For each of the examples above, make notes about:
>
> - What you think was happening generally in these situations?
> - Who was responsible for the patients' or families' experiences in these cases?
> - How what was happening reflects your principles and values.
> - What decisions would you make about your standards of care if you were on placement in these situations.

As individual nurses we are all accountable for the decisions we make in the course of delivering nursing care. Even as a student under the supervision of a named mentor, you are accountable for what you do. Thus, you need to be clear what your limitations are, about when you should seek guidance and when you should not get involved in care which is not of the required standard and what you should do about it. This can be one of the most challenging areas for students and you will develop your skills as you grow as a professional in order to achieve progression as required by the NMC in relation to: 'Demonstrates potential to work autonomously, making the most of opportunities to extend knowledge, skills and practice'.

The NMC has the protection of the public as its prime objective and it is the NMC that investigates allegations made about registrants' fitness to practise. With around 660,000 registrants, this is a huge area of the NMC's work and the number of allegations is increasing annually. The 2008–9 annual NMC report along with all previous and future reports can be accessed at: www.nmc-uk.org/Documents/Annualreportsandaccounts/FTPannual Reports/NMC.

The key points are that:

- 2,178 allegations were made against registered nurses;
- 1,759 of these were investigated;
- 740 cases resulted in sanctions;
- 210 nurses were struck off the professional register;
- many allegations involved more than one incident and more than one type of allegation.

The most common allegations were to do with:

- physical and verbal abuse;
- failure to communicate;
- failure to respect the dignity of patients;
- incorrect administration of medicines (this accounted for 11.7 per cent of cases);
- dishonesty in 14 per cent of cases, involving, among other things; theft, fraud, falsification of records, claiming sick pay dishonestly and sleeping on duty.

You should take time to review these annual reports as you progress as they make sober reading and can help you consider and reflect on your own standards of care. When you have reviewed the reports, take some time to undertake **Activity 3.3**.

> **Activity 3.3**
>
> How do the statistics highlighted above make you feel about the nursing profession? Who do you believe owns standards of care?
>
> - The individual?
> - The managers?
> - The organization?
> - The profession?

Now let us take the issues you have considered back to your own practice. Begin with **Activities 3.4** and **3.5**.

Activity 3.4

Using Gibbs' reflective cycle (see p. 00), think of an experience in practice in which you felt that the standard of care was very good and work your way through the questions below.

- Description: what happened?
- Feelings: what were you thinking and feeling?
- Evaluation: what was good and bad about the experience?
- Analysis: what sense can you make of the situation?
- Conclusion: what else could you have done?
- Action plan: if it arose again, what would you do?

You will find it useful to go through the reflective cycle again, this time focusing on an issue from practice where the care was poor or not to the required standard.

Activity 3.5

Now compare the outcomes of these reflective activities and list the differences in each case. Go back and review your learning from earlier in this chapter and make notes about the factors that impact on the standards of care that the public are subjected to from a macro level (e.g. policy level) through to a micro level (e.g. at the level of interaction with the patient).

The impact of poor practice on patient care

The outcome of poor practice is distressing for all parties involved, whether it is recognized or not. Where poor practice is not disclosed but is experienced by patients, their carers and families who are already vulnerable, we are failing in our duty of care as we have allowed them to go on with their lives with their confidence in the services we provide compromised. In particular, nurses need to be mindful that people with learning disabilities or enduring mental illness can find it difficult to assert their views and rights. Nurses need to create opportunities for disclosure to occur in a safe environment. Therefore, nurses cannot be defensive, must be open to feedback and be non-judgemental. The ability to accept and be non-judgemental is key to reflective practice.

Student nurse behaviour

It is important to note that there are sometimes instances where student nurses' behaviour during their course does not reach the standard required. For example, students may:

- lack the knowledge base to ensure their practice is competent because they are not engaging with the theoretical learning;
- fail to acknowledge their limitations and carry out an intervention they are not competent to do;
- fail to seek appropriate guidance;
- convey unacceptable attitudes to patients, staff in clinical placements and academic staff;
- falsify records such as time sheets and clinical assessment documents;
- fraudulently claim expenses associated with practice placements.

We raise these issues not because we think that many students engage in behaviours that sit outside the required standards, but because in such instances the student may not be aware of or recognize the impact of their behaviour. The challenge for the student in this position is how they respond to the feedback provided. Students are viewed as learners who require support and guidance to take on board the standards of behaviour and practice required. However, ultimately, the student must take ownership of their behaviour, demonstrate the standards required or accept the consequences where this does not happen.

As you have worked your way through this section, you will have identified the learning that you think is most relevant to you. We will refer back to the relevant learning in the final section when we identify some of the key learning points for the chapter.

Learning to achieve high standards of care

How you approach care delivery concerns the way you interact with patients, and any others involved, as care is being delivered. Decisions about your approach reflect your personal and professional values and influence your standards of care. They are manifested through the nature of your presence at the point of delivery. **Activity 3.6** is designed to enable you to articulate the values that are important to you, and their impact on how you work with patients and own your own standards.

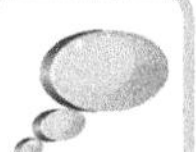

Activity 3.6

- Note down the five things you value most in your life at this time.
- Note down the five things you value most about being a student nurse.
- Note down five things you value most about being able to contribute to the care and support of service users and their families during your course.
- Note down five principles that you can use to guide your behaviour as you progress through your studies.

Key learning

- As a nurse it is important that you can identify the key principles and values that direct your standards of care.
- Be aware of any factors that might interfere with or compromise you maintaining your own standards of care according to your values and principles and the formal standards that are made explicit to you.

The importance of your role as a nurse

The key thing here is for you to become aware of the external things that affect you so you can begin to identify your learning needs in order to allow you to deal with them, but it is also about helping you begin to explore the factors within yourself that impact on your ability to maintain your standards of care. The challenge is for you to begin to notice and understand all of the things that affect you during 'real time' in practice. Mason (2002: 1) states:

> At the heart of all practice lies noticing: noticing as opportunity to act appropriately . . . [this] . . . requires three things: being present and sensitive to the moment, having a reason to act and having a different act come to mind. Consequently, one important aspect of being professional is noticing possible acts to try out in future, whether gleaned from reading, from discussion, from watching others or from personal reflection. A second important aspect is working on becoming more articulate and more precise about reasons for acting. The mark of an expert is that they are sensitised to notice things that novices overlook.

Mason is highlighting the importance of the role of your underpinning knowledge which arises from your theoretical and experiential learning. This learning gives you options for making decisions in practice and in being able to explain the reasons for your decisions. He is also suggesting that the first step in this process is being mindful within practice situations. Thich Nhat Hanh (2012) describes mindfulness as the 'energy of attention'. Being mindful in a situation is about not thinking about the past or future, what you did yesterday or what you still have to do today, or how you are going to manage to complete everything you have to do, or whether you are going to fail or succeed: it is about putting all of that aside and giving your full attention to what is happening *in the present moment as it is happening*. You actually need to make the conscious decision to engage with patients in this way – a key decision that affects the quality of the patient experience.

We become more 'mindless' when we are stressed and our minds get caught up in thinking about our worries with the result that we do not pay attention to what is going on around us. Practice environments are stressful for a whole array of reasons (Brown 2009) so it is easy to become distracted. There is evidence that effective decision-making can be compromised in dynamic environments where lots of decisions have to be made within short periods of time and the decision-makers are not taking in what is evolving as a situation unfolds (Gonzalez 2004).

To be mindful is to consciously train yourself to focus on the present moment and give it all your attention. In relation to delivering nursing care, this is about giving every patient your full attention as you work with them and consciously preventing your mind from becoming distracted by unrelated thoughts. Being a student nurse with 50 per cent of your programme in a clinical setting allows you to take a bit more time when you are delivering care to begin to practise doing so in a mindful manner.

Conclusion

In concluding this chapter, we draw your attention to the areas we have identified as being crucial to your developing an understanding of standards of care. In turn, you will now be in a position to clearly articulate how you, as a developing person and professional, *own your own standards*.

In summary:

- Standards, codes of practice, guidelines and similar statements of principles set out the values that underpin our care and the principles we use to guide it, and are used to measure our performance.
- There are ways of doing things within clinical settings that are customary and 'standard habits' need to be examined in the light of what is considered good and desirable. Students can contribute to this examination of practice with fresh eyes.
- Implementation of evidence-based practice involves ensuring that practice is informed by contemporary evidence that is discussed and debated within the practice area so that practice develops consistently and appropriately.
- Understanding and being aware of your own values and principles, and those of others, and how they impact on your behaviour, is important for ensuring you maintain high standards of care.
- Being present in the moment with the patient – being aware of how focused your attention is on the patient at the time is essential. You need to be able to judge whether you are giving the patient your full attention.
- Critical reflection on practice – at individual, team and organizational levels – is crucial in order to enable deep learning and the development of practice.
- Being open to and accepting of feedback as part of the learning and development process will enhance your ability to deliver high standards of care.

Further reading and resources

www.institute.nhs.uk. The website for the NHS Institute for Innovation and Improvement.

www.mwcscot.org.uk/publications/investigation-reports. The website for the Mental Health Commission (MWC) for Scotland.

www.scotland.gov.uk/Publications/2010/05/10102307/2. The website for the NHS Scotland Healthcare Quality Strategy.

http://bit.ly/c7Dfen takes you to the Department of Health's (DH) 2010 White Paper *Equity and Excellence: Liberating the NHS*.

www.midstaffspublicinquiry.com. The website relating to the Mid Staffordshire NHS Foundation Trust Public Inquiry conducted by Robert Frances, QC.

www.patientopinion.org.uk is a helpful site examining the experiences of service users.

References

Basford, L. and Kershaw, B. (2008) *A Key Issues Paper: Underpinning the Future of Health Professional Education in the UK*. London: University and College Union.

Brown, C. (2009) Self-renewal in nurse leadership: the lived experience of caring for self, *The Journal of Holistic Nursing*, 27(2): 75–84.

CQC (Care Quality Commission) (2011) *Review of Compliance: Castlebeck Care (Teesdale) Ltd.* London: CQC.

Frances, R. (2013) *Report of the Mid Staffordshire NHS Foundation Trust Public Inquiry*. London: The Stationery Office.

Gibbs, G. (1988) Learning by Doing: *A guide to teaching and learning methods.* Further Education Unit, Oxford Brookes University, Oxford.

Gonzalez, C. (2004) Learning to make decisions in dynamic environments: effects of time constraints and cognitive abilities, *Human Factors: The Journal of Human Factors and Ergonomic Society*, 46(3): 449–60.

House of Commons Health Committee (2003) *The Victoria Climbié Inquiry Report.* London: The Stationery Office.

Johns, C. (2010) *Guided Reflection: A Narrative Approach to Advancing Professional Practice*, 2nd edn. Chichester: Wiley-Blackwell.

Johns, C. and Freshwater, D. (eds) (2005) *Transforming Nursing Through Reflective Practice*, 2nd edn. Oxford: Blackwell.

Kabat-Zinn, J. (2004) *Wherever You Go, There You Are: Mindfulness Meditation for Everyday Life.* London: Piatkus.

Kleinman, C.S. (2006) Ethical drift: when good people do bad things, *Journal of Nursing Administration, Healthcare Law, Ethics and Regulation,* 8(3): 72–6.

Mason, J. (2002) *Researching Your Own Practice: The Discipline of Noticing.* London: Routledge Falmer.

McSherry, R., Pearce, P., Grimwood, K. and McSherry, W. (2012) The pivotal role of nurse managers, leaders and educators in enabling excellence in nursing care, *Journal of Nursing Management*, 20: 7–19.

MWC (Mental Welfare Commission for Scotland) *Starved of Care: Summary Investigation Report into the Care and Treatment of Mrs V.* Edinburgh: MWC.

NMC (Nursing and Midwifery Council) (2008) *The Code: Standards of Conduct, Performance and Ethics for Nurses and Midwives.* London: NMC.

NMC (Nursing and Midwifery Council) (2010) *Standards for Pre-registration Nursing Education.* London: NMC.

Parliamentary and Health Service Ombudsman (2011) *Care and Compassion? Report of the Health Service Ombudsman on Ten Investigations into NHS Care of Older People.* London: The Stationery Office.

Scottish Government (2010) *The Healthcare Quality Strategy for NHS Scotland.* Edinburgh: Scottish Government.

Siegel, R.D. (2010) *The Mindfulness Solution: Everyday Practices for Everyday Problems.* New York: Guildford Press.

Taylor, R. and Brannan, J. (forthcoming) Interprofessional practice, in J. Lishman and C. Yuill (eds) *Social Work: An Introduction.* London: Sage.

Thich Nhat Hanh (2012) *The Art of Mindfulness.* London: HarperCollins eBooks.

SECTION

2

Communication and interpersonal skills

4 Developing effective communication and interpersonal skills

Mary Addo and Alison Brown

Chapter contents

Introduction

This chapter is primarily concerned with helping you to develop effective communication and interpersonal skills in the context of the Nursing and Midwifery Council (NMC) (2010) *Standards for Pre-registration Nursing Education* skills clusters, required of the graduate nurse for nursing practice. The skills discussed here are inherent in all domains and competencies regardless of your field of practice. Research, evidence and health and social care policy are used to illuminate the value of why you need to be confident, compassionate and clear in your communication to patients and their families, friends and carers. The experiential exercises and case study examples will enable you to practise, reflect on and evaluate your interpersonal communication skills and their relevance in the context of your education for future professional nursing practice, as well as emphasizing the need to commit to continuing future lifelong learning for your employability. The specific domain and the relevant outcomes are summarized below.

All nurses must use excellent communication and interpersonal skills. Their communications must always be safe, effective, compassionate and respectful. They must communicate effectively using a wide range of strategies and interventions including the effective use of communication technologies. Where people have a disability, nurses must be able to work with service users and others.

Activity 4.1

- Try to remember why you wanted to become a nurse in the particular field of nursing you are studying.
- Reflect on what you thought would guide and inform about how to communicate and relate to service users, carers, families and professional colleagues as a nurse.
- Take the time to write your reflections down as a way of clearly identifying them.

The importance of communication

As social beings we are always communicating with others, be it our friends, families, peers, workmates or even strangers. Nursing is fundamentally an interpersonal profession because it concerns itself with the health and nursing care needs of society through communication and relationship-building within a professional context. Peplau (1952) redefined nursing as an interpersonal, interpretive process which laid the foundations for studying nursing as a communicative process. As far back as the 1940s Peplau was advocating that to achieve a therapeutic experience for patients, nurses need to actively work in partnership with them. She saw the crux of nursing as building on nurse–patient relationships in practice. This view is as relevant today as it was more than 70 years ago, and even more so now that the involvement of service users in the decision-making process regarding their care and treatment has become core to a raft of health care policies that guide practice (e.g. Scottish Executive 2003, 2006a, 2006b; DH 2004, 2009, 2010; Scottish Government 2005, 2010; Welsh Assembly Government 2010). Nurses cannot provide meaningful care to service users if they are poor communicators and incompetent at relating to people. Griffiths *et al.* (2012) report that what service users and their carers look for in graduate nurses is a caring professional attitude, yet sadly poor communication by clinical staff remains a major area of complaint within the NHS (Abraham 2004; Giles *et al.* 2009). It is with this knowledge that we would suggest that communication by the nurse is the most pivotal, fundamental and important skill that frames all you do as a nurse. Good, clear and professional communication is important for the delivery of high quality care.

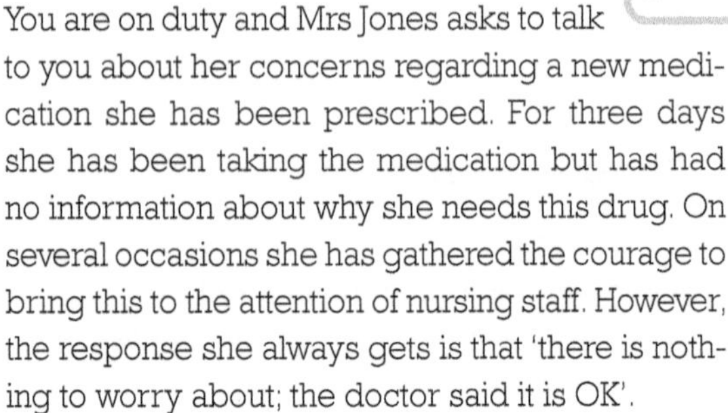

Activity 4.2

You are on duty and Mrs Jones asks to talk to you about her concerns regarding a new medication she has been prescribed. For three days she has been taking the medication but has had no information about why she needs this drug. On several occasions she has gathered the courage to bring this to the attention of nursing staff. However, the response she always gets is that 'there is nothing to worry about; the doctor said it is OK'.

- What communication issues stand out for you in this scenario?
- How will you deal with this situation and support Mrs Jones?
- Why do you think the nurses were behaving in such a manner?

Faulkner (1998: 1) states that 'to be able to communicate effectively with others is at the heart of all patient care'. When effective communication occurs, it enables the establishment of therapeutic relationships with service users, their carers and families, and increases their understanding of the treatment and care processes in which they find themselves (Silverman *et al.* 2005).

How you respond to service users in the therapeutic relationship and dialogue with them indicates the value that you place on them. The nurses' response to Mrs Jones illustrates poor interpersonal communication skills and a lack of the expected graduate attributes (NMC 2008; Griffiths *et al.* 2012). They appear dismissive of Mrs Jones' concerns, appearing unprofessional, uncaring and lacking the required, evidence-based responding qualities (Rogers 1951; Peplau 1952). An appropriate responding skill would have been to acknowledge Mrs Jones' concerns by saying, for example, 'I can understand why you are worried; I will make time today so we can talk about

 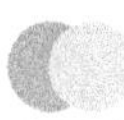

this.' A key communication issue in this scenario is the nurses' failure to listen *actively* to Mrs Jones' concerns and demonstrate that she has not just been 'heard' but *listened to* and validated.

Key learning

- It is vital to understand the importance of responding to patients and the significance of the attitude and behaviour of the nurse in this.
- Effective communication is fundamental to the delivery of quality patient care.
- Nurses' interpersonal communication skills are essential for the implementation of health care policy.

McCabe (2004) found that patients felt nurses spend more time on clinical tasks than talking to them and that nurses' communication skills needed to be improved for delivering quality patient care. This is a key point for you as a student to consider and reflect on, irrespective of what part of your programme you are on. While clinical tasks are clearly important in the delivery of patient care, they are required to be undertaken with effective communication that is both informative to the patient and reassuring.

Developing your communication skills

While your learning in the university setting will provide you with theories about and strategies for developing interpersonal and communication skills, it is within clinical practice that you will learn to apply these theories and strategies, and develop your confidence in your own skills of communication. As you begin to develop your interpersonal communication skills for professional practice, a phase of new nursing experiences will challenge those skills, which are the key determinant of patient satisfaction, compliance and recovery (Chant *et al.* 2002; Barker 2009; Kozier *et al.* 2012). For example, as a nurse you will be required to undertake an assessment of the service user's needs and the first phase of the nursing process framework. Not only will you have to demonstrate your theoretical knowledge and understanding of health, disease and illness, but also of the care and treatment interventions available that relate to the particular service user's condition. This will require effective interpersonal communication skills, without which the information needed to plan care will not materialize (Doenges and Moorhouse 2003; Arnold and Boggs 2007; Fawcett and Rhynas 2012).

Case study 4.1: Sandy Reid and his family

Sandy Reid is a 61-year-old man with Down's syndrome. Until recently he has been living in a housing complex for those with learning disabilities but this care normally comes to an end at age 60. He has now moved into a care home. His sister Jess, a widow, is 58 and comes regularly to visit him. However, she has been increasingly confused lately and has now been diagnosed with early onset dementia. She has one child, Anne, 32, who has two young children, Sophie, 4 and 18-month-old Ryan. Anne is married to John who works long hours as an on-call gas engineer and in emergencies he has been asked to travel across the country. John's parents have recently retired and are living in Dubai. They visit every few months, splitting their time between Dubai, visiting John and his family in the UK and their other son Peter and his family who live in Australia. Anne has been discussing with her mother and John the possibility that they might all live together so she can look after Jess, and maintain contact with her uncle Sandy. Nonetheless, Anne has recently been diagnosed with bowel cancer, and is having surgery later in the month for this, and has been told she will require chemotherapy. She is understandably worried not only about her own health but about her mother and children, and who will look after them if John is away. Sandy is struggling to settle himself in the care home and wants to see Jess quite often.

Activity 4.3

You are the allocated nurse meeting Sandy's family for the first time. Identify the main communication issues in this scenario, thinking about it in relation to your field-specific area.

- How would you communicate with the family?
- How would you communicate with the wider members of the multidisciplinary team?
- What communication skills do you need in this sort of situation?
- Can you address the needs of all the family members? Explain your answer.
- What do you think your responses to this scenario and these questions say about you and your values?
- What advice and support would you put in place for this family?
- How do you communicate these values and beliefs to others?

Now reflect on your responses to these questions. What have you learned about how you communicate and relate to different people, in different situations?

Defining communication

Communication is important in nursing practice and is the method by which nurses do what they do. The process for establishing, maintaining and improving human contact is interpersonal communication. Communication is an exchange between two or more people that involves the exchange of information. It also requires a sender, the message, a mode of transmission, the receiver, feedback to the sender, and can be linear, circular or both (Kozier *et al.* 2012). Communication is a complex concept with many dimensions, and therefore is not something that you can simply memorize and perform. In communicating with others meaning cannot just be transferred, but should be mutually negotiated, because it is influenced by many factors (Forchuk and Boyd 1998). Our perceptions, values, cultural backgrounds and interpretations can all affect the message we give to and receive from others (Addo 2006; Addo and Smith 2008). However, there are principles and strategies that you can learn and use in order to be therapeutically effective in your practice (Heron 2001; Arnold and Boggs 2007; Crawford and Brown 2009; Egan 2010), as outlined in the following sections of this chapter.

Types of communication

Verbal communication involves all aspects of language: words, style, grammar, content, pitch, volume, tone, pronunciation, pace, timing and the clarity and use of voice. Most of your verbal interactions when you engage with others constitute a small part of the message you are sending: a significant part of your message is conveyed through your body language, and this is known as *non-verbal communication. Personal styles* of communication are the ways in which we prefer or like to communicate, and are important in enabling facilitation of effective partnership working and mutual understanding in the helping process. Awareness of your preferred communication style will help you to prevent misunderstandings and conflicts, which can impact on teamwork, and eventually the quality of the helping process.

Activity 4.4

- How would you assess your interpersonal skills at this point in your nurse training?
- Are there aspects of your communication and interpersonal skills that you need to further develop?

It is important that as part of your ongoing learning as a professional you are able to reflect on your practice, learn from it and make changes to develop your skills, professionalism and approach to your role as a nurse.

Non-verbal communication

Non-verbal communication is more powerful than the spoken word as it communicates the meaning behind the message being sent, the real meaning intended by the sender. It is also worth noting that non-verbal communication can often carry more social meaning than verbal communication, due to individuals making inferences from your non-verbal communication when you are interacting with them (Beebe *et al.* 2011). For example, when listening to the concerns of a patient, your body language, eye contact and general way in which you conduct yourself while listening will communicate important signals. When we perceive information as giving 'mixed messages', we tend to use the sender's non-verbal cues such as their appearance, posture, gaze, touch and mannerisms to help validate what is being said, and what we think we have heard (Kozier *et al.* 2012). This is because non-verbal messages are the way we communicate our attitudes and feelings, and it therefore requires high self-awareness on the part of the nurse in relation to any non-verbal messages they may be sending when dealing with service users, patients, colleagues and members of the public.

Case study 4.2

Imagine you are on a clinical placement and as part of your learning your mentor asks you to arrange a meeting with Anne from the first case study in this chapter. She has had her surgery and made a good recovery, and preparations are being made for her discharge. You will need to elicit important information from Anne regarding her views about her impending discharge and feed this back at the weekly multidisciplinary team meeting. Your feedback will help inform the decision-making process about the care management support Anne will need when discharged.

Activity 4.5

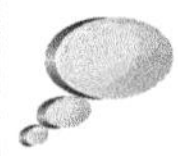

In relation to your meeting with Anne:

- What initial preparation should you make? Think about your approach, style and any non-verbal cues that may be important at this stage of Anne's care.

Good and bad communication techniques

Here are some examples of communication techniques, most good, some poor.

- **Active listening.** This is the sort of listening which demonstrates your participation and that you are attending to what is being said. It involves using verbal and non-verbal cues such as 'mmmh' and 'uh' and 'OK', while also nodding, smiling or shaking your head appropriately. This sort of listening allows you to build a relationship with the service user by demonstrating your interest in them. This leads to a trusting and respectful relationship.
- **Reflecting.** This helps to focus on the service user's perspective and promotes person-centred communication by identifying the core message and offering it back to them in your own words. Used effectively, reflecting facilitates service user/patient interaction, and builds trust, understanding and acceptance.
- **Paraphrasing.** Expressing the information received from the service user in your own words. Here the meaning remains the same but the words are different. Paraphrasing can be used to check clarity and mutual understanding of what is being communicated.
- **Silence.** This helps you communicate respect to the service user, confirms your validation of their worth, and gives you an opportunity to gather your thoughts and reflect on how best to proceed in responding to the immediacy of the issues at hand.
- **Summarizing.** An accurate summary of what has been said to you will demonstrate to the service user that you have understood them

correctly. It also allows them to address any misconceptions you may be under.

- **Open questions.** These are where you allow the person you are communicating with the opportunity to explain things to you. They normally begin with phrases such as 'What do you think . . .', Why did this . . .' or Tell me about . . .'. Such questions encourage the sharing of the individual's own story.
- **Closed questions.** This type of questioning only provides a 'yes' or 'no' response. It is used when seeking factual responses. For example, 'Are you in any pain?'
- **Probing.** This involves the use of a combination of questions in order to gain in-depth information and properly understand the service user's needs. For example, 'Could you just describe that for me?' or ' It will help me plan how to care for you if you tell me a bit more about that.'
- **Open-ended questions.** Such as those beginning with 'when', 'how', 'who', 'what' and 'where'. This approach promotes a more detailed, descriptive response: 'How long have you been feeling like this?' or 'When did this start?'
- **Clarifying.** You ask the individual to enlarge on their answer. For example, in the case study Anne may say that she feels guilty about not being able to look after everyone. Asking her *why* she feels like this should provide deeper insight into the values of the family and what is important to them. Such questions also help you to clarify things if you have been puzzled by an answer.
- **Use of touch.** Touch may be used to reassure and comfort a service user where verbal communication is insufficient. For example, holding their hand, or a gentle touch on the shoulder. However, you must be mindful of factors such as age, ethnicity, gender, cultural differences, children, elderly and vulnerable persons.
- **Leading questions.** These are questions you use to gain the answer you want, rather than the one the person wishes to give. For example you might say to Anne, 'So you would agree that until you are better your mum should go into the care home with Sandy?' Or, 'John, you are probably thinking about cutting down on your hours and asking your parents to come home aren't you?' This sort of question should be avoided if possible as it may compromise the other person's values and beliefs.

Key learning

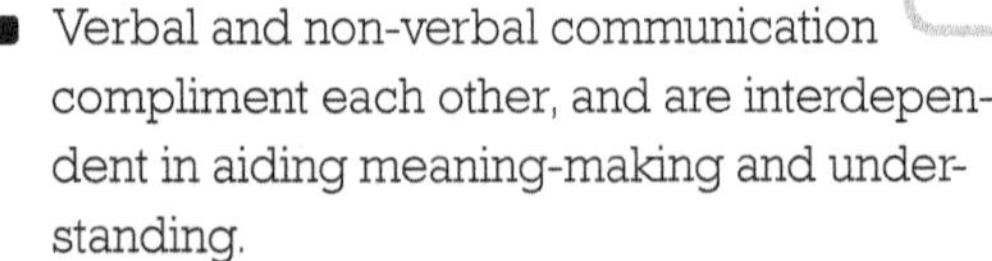

- Verbal and non-verbal communication compliment each other, and are interdependent in aiding meaning-making and understanding.
- In order to communicate with service users and others we need to prepare ourselves for our interactions and work on all aspects of our communication skills.

Activity 4.6

The aim of this activity is to help you review your use of any of the communication skills described in this chapter in your own clinical practice to date. Begin by identifying a recent interaction you had with a service user/patient, a carer or a member of staff. Now reflect on the interaction, and answer the following questions. It will help your learning if you add your answers to your reflective journal and share them with your mentor.

- What was the key intention of my interaction?
- What communication skills did I adopt during the interaction?
- Which communication skills was I comfortable with and which did I find challenging?
- Which communication skills did I not use, and for what reasons?
- What factors do I think influenced my interaction? How? Why?
- What have I learned from this interaction?
- What further communication skills do I need to develop?
- What strategies will I adopt to help develop these skills?

Interpersonal skills

Interpersonal skills are all the activities, verbal and non-verbal, that people use when interacting directly with others (Rungapadiachy 1999; Mallik *et al.* 2009). Despite variations in the literature over the actual skills that fit under this heading (Chant *et al.* 2002), various authors (e.g. Dickson *et al.* 1989; Rungapadiachy 1999; Hayes 2002; Burnard 2003) agree on the core attributes that are essential for effective interpersonal interaction: self-awareness, effective listening, questioning, helping or facilitating, reflecting, assertiveness and non-verbal cues. For example, a nursing ward report handover involves a range of different communication skills, many of which fall within the interpersonal domain, requiring the nurse to engage in active listening, discussions, monitoring the reactions of colleagues and responding appropriately to their contributions.

Barriers to effective interpersonal communication

Nurses work with people from different social and cultural backgrounds and therefore it is important to be aware of barriers to effective interpersonal communication (Luckmann 1999; Narayanasamy 2003; Addo 2006). For example:

- Language: technical and professional jargon, use of slang and metaphors.
- Cultural and gender issues: customs and beliefs of a particular people or group, gender, preconceived beliefs.
- Personal values: emotions, ignorance, ethnocentric views.
- Unsuitable environmental context: lack of privacy, noise, organizational climate.
- Inconsistencies, mistrust, power, feeling oppressed, not feeling valued.
- Attitudes, past experiences, perceptions, fear, stereotyping, stigma, defensiveness.
- Health condition of individual, disability, trauma.

Therapeutic communication strategies

Egan (2010: 135) provides a communication strategy called SOLER, comprising five key non-verbal 'micro skills', summarized below.

- **S** – sitting facing the client squarely promotes involvement and interest.
- **O** – adopting an open posture, with arms and legs uncrossed. Crossed arms and legs can be a sign of defensiveness and unwillingness to engage.
- **L** – leaning towards the person conveys to them your interest and willingness to get to know them and help.
- **E** – maintaining good eye contact, without staring. Avoidance of eye contact can signify a lack of confidence in your self or your abilities. Balance the frequency and intensity of eye contact so that the service user does not feel threatened.
- **R** – a relaxed posture enables you to appear natural in your interaction, yielding a communication.

By using this strategy you are more likely to hear what patients and service users are saying, clearly and accurately (Hamilton and Martin 2007).

Key learning 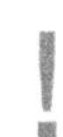

- When interacting with others you should draw on a range of communication skills.
- When communicating we need to not only consider our verbal messages but utilize SOLER when developing a therapeutic relationship.
- In any relationship you need to be aware of the barriers to communication exhibited and inherent both within yourself as a nurse and the individual you are communicating with, and the impact of the environment on you both.

Interpersonal skills and qualities of an effective nurse helper

- **Responding with empathy** is the nurse's ability to connect with service users and validate their worth, which is fundamental to the helping process (Rogers 1951).
- **Responding with respect** is about showing how much you value the integrity, autonomy and informed choices of the service user, and accepting that with appropriate person-centred

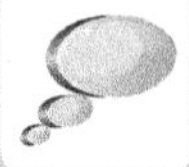

Activity 4.7

Look at the following scenario and decide which is the most empathic response, and which response lacks empathy.

A substance misuser talks to a nurse.

Service user: I feel like everything is piling on top of me. The only way I can handle it is by getting my usual fix. I know it doesn't solve anything, but it takes away the pain for a while and makes me feel in control.

Nurse:

a) Having a fix seems to be your way of dealing with life's ups and downs.
b) I know what you mean about life getting on top of you. I used to get like that a lot of years ago. It's awful, isn't it? How do you get your fix?
c) When you feel as though everything is piling on top of you, like carrying the world on your shoulders, misusing substances like drugs seems like your only answer to the problem.
d) You're lucky not to be in serious trouble with the law. Have you been checked and had an HIV test yet?

help based on involvement in the decision-making process about their care and treatment, they will be able take control of their circumstances (Watkins 2001).

- **Responding with genuineness** is your ability to be authentic, who you really are, transparent, open and honest in your interactions with people. A genuine nurse is one who works with difference of all kinds in a positive manner in order to enhance the service user's care experience (Scottish Executive 2006b).
- **Responding to immediacy** relates to attending to the here and now issues occurring for the service user within the therapeutic working relationship. This can be challenging at times, especially when negative feedback is provided by the service user on their experience of the quality of care received. How you respond will either strengthen or weaken the working relationship (Watkins 2001).
- **Responding with warmth** is closely related to empathy and respect, as you cannot show warmth in any human interaction in the absence of empathy and respect being present. The warmth that is articulated here is not 'friendly chit-chat', but rather warmth conveyed in the manner in which you communicate respect and empathy (Rogers 1951).

These qualities fit with many of the values underpinning current health care policies in the UK.

Models for developing communication strategies

There are various theoretical models to guide how you initiate, sustain and end a therapeutic dialogue with service users. For example:

- interpersonal relations model (Peplau 1952);
- client-centred therapy (Rogers 1951);
- six category intervention analysis (Heron 2001);
- the skilled helper (Egan 2010);
- the brief, ordinary and effective (BOE) model (Crawford *et al.* 2006).

Early seminal work on client-centred therapy (Rogers 1951) articulated the core conditions of acceptance, unconditional positive regard, empathy, genuineness and congruence as underpinning any helping relationship. Despite the passage of time the values described by Rogers are still relevant and pertinent to you as a professional nurse, and clearly at the heart of the thinking of today's NHS. Here we provide you with three of the models you can adopt as strategies to help facilitate effective therapeutic dialogue within your role as a nurse. There are, of course, others.

Six category intervention analysis

Heron's (2001) six category intervention model identifies six styles of helping interventions that you can adopt with service users and others. There are two basic approaches in Heron's model: 'authoritative' and 'facilitative'. These are further broken down into six core responding categories to show how you can intervene when helping a service user, their family or carer. We would suggest that to help you develop your communication skills you review Heron's work, read around the subject further and start to practise your skills. Practising communication skills in our view is as essential as practising and refining a clinical 'tasks' – so take the time to practise with a peer and then try out the approach with different clients. You may want to talk this through with your mentor so that you can gain feedback and support in your development.

Brief, ordinary and effective (BOE) health communication

The BOE model for communication in health care (Crawford *et al.* 2006) helps nurses adapt their communication within the busy dynamics of the setting. The BOE model helps to address the time constraints that often prevent nurses from spending quality time with patients when undertaking interventions and tasks. At the heart of this model is the understanding that short periods of communication can be valuable and have a big impact. It identifies for us as nurses the importance of avoiding meaningless communication and demonstrating value in our patients and the communications we have with them. While this model is not ideal for all situations, it does provides one of a range of flexible approaches and tools that can be used. A link to a useful paper by Professor Paul Crawford is provided in the resources section (p. 63).

The skilled helper

Egan's (2010) skilled helper is a useful framework for support the patient on issues that may have had an impact in their recent past or currently. It is a person-centred model and has an emphasis on empowering the individual to become more able to help themselves in their everyday lives. This requires the nurse to demonstrate the responding and communication skills described earlier in this chapter. Egan's model has three stages which are briefly described below.

Stage 1: the present – where you are at now

1. Help the client tell their story (prompts, active listening, open questions, SOLER).
2. Help the client break through any blind spots.
3. Help the client find the right problem/opportunity to work on.

Stage 2: preferred – where you want to be

1. Help the client use their imagination to spell out possibilities.
2. Help the client chose realistic and challenging goals.
3. Help the client to find incentives that will help with commitment.

Stage 3: strategies – how are you going to get where you want to be?

1. Help the client find possible actions.
2. Help the client to find 'best-fit' strategies.
3. Help the client to draft an action plan.

These helping models are relevant to all areas of nursing practice. The NMC generic standard for competence for nursing practice and communication (2010: 24) states that:

> All nurses must use excellent communication and interpersonal skills. Their communications must always be safe, effective, compassionate and respectful. They must communicate effectively using a wide range of strategies and interventions including the effective use of communication technologies. Where people have a disability, nurses must be able to work with service users and others to obtain the information needed to make reasonable adjustments that promote optimum health and enable equal access to services.

Relationship of communication to personal values and professionalism

The values we hold are based on the fundamental beliefs we have and we use them to guide our actions. Beliefs can be thought of as those things which we hold to be true. Values are those beliefs we consider to be important (refer to Chapter 2). The values we adopt give us guidance in determining right from wrong, good from bad. They become our standards as to how we behave, and how we expect others to behave. However, we all have different kinds of values, and here we will focus on those which are personal or professional in their nature. Our personal values come from a variety of sources: our parents, our upbringing, our schooling, our religion, our political beliefs, our peers and the media. Horton *et al.* (2007) have identified the core values of a nurse as being:

- respect;
- caring;
- responsibility;
- honesty;
- patient participation;
- preservation of wholeness and humanity;
- patient autonomy;
- dignity;
- making a difference;
- versatility;
- altruism;
- nurturing;
- integrity;
- supporting and empowering individuals;
- reciprocal trust;
- sound knowledge;
- clinical competence;
- relationships;
- continuity;
- homogeneity;
- self-sacrifice;
- hard work;
- control;
- diversity;
- patient choice.

As nurses we are expected to abide by the NMC *Code* but are also guided in our actions by various policies which detail the values we should demonstrate. Yet, if we do not subscribe to the values and beliefs shown by others, including those we look after, then conflict can arise.

In the first case study of this chapter we saw the conflict that can often arise within a service user's family. However, such conflict resolution can be achieved with effective interpersonal and communication strategies between the health professionals and the family, requiring that you develop awareness and clarification of your personal and professional values and those of others. Reflecting on your practice gives you the opportunity to disassemble and examine a situation to make sense of it, in light of your own values and those of others.

The importance of interpersonal communication as a lifelong approach to delivering quality patient care

The importance of teaching and learning about communication with patients is well established within nursing (Chant *et al.* 2002). According to Sheldon *et al.* (2006: 141) 'communication is a cornerstone of the nurse-patient relationship'. The value of effective interpersonal communication skills in health care practice has been extensively researched and evidenced (Hack *et al.* 2005; Thorne *et al.* 2006). However, most complaints consistently made against the NHS in the UK relate to poor interpersonal, inter- and intraprofessional communication skills, as reflected in the investigation of The Bristol Royal Infirmary Inquiry (2001) regarding the high mortality rates in a paediatric surgical unit, where 'strained' communication was a key factor.

Compassionate engagement with service users and maintaining their dignity cannot be achieved where nurses remain incompetent in their interpersonal and communication skills (RCN 2008; NMC 2010; Scottish Government 2010; Sharples 2011). Therefore your commitment to lifelong continuing professional development to maintain your credibility and integrity for practice as a nurse remains paramount.

Conclusion

This chapter has emphasized the importance and relevance of the graduate attributes of an effective communicator and interpersonally skilled nurse in the context of health care delivery, and in upholding nursing's professionalism. It is important that developing your communication and interpersonal skills is perceived as a lifelong commitment to quality enhancement in your professional nursing practice. Remember that it is only by practising these skills and obtaining feedback that you will perfect their use. You will know how effective you are from feedback given by service users.

In summary:

- Be self-aware in your approach and keep the patient as the central point for all you do.
- Effective communication and interpersonal skills are essential for quality patient care.
- Be active in your listening to service users to explore how you can work with their views.
- Adopt effective communication skills in your work with peers, colleagues and external agencies.
- Be aware of the barriers to effective communication in the work environment and seek appropriate support.

Further reading and resources

We suggest that you look at the following material to enhance and develop your knowledge and awareness of communication and interpersonal skills.

Bach, S. and Grant, A. (2009) *Communication and Interpersonal Skills for Nurses*. Exeter: Learning Matters Ltd.

Hamilton, S.J. and Martin, D.J. (2007) Clinical development: a framework for effective communication skills, *Nursing Times*, 103(48): 30–1.

Harrison, A. and Hart, C. (2006) *Mental Health Care for Nurses: Applying Mental Health Skills in the General Hospital*. London: Blackwell.

A useful paper by Professor Paul Crawford can be found at www.wales.nhs.uk/sites3/docopen.cfm?orgid=415&id=162430.

You can learn more about Herons' six category intervention analysis at: www.mindtools.com/CommSkll/HeronsCategories.htm.

References

Abraham, A. (2004) Lack of communication affects the care of patients and families, *Professional Nurse*, 19(6): 351–3.

Addo, M. (2006) Culture, spirituality and ethical issues in caring for clients with a personality disorder, in *Forensic Mental Health Nursing: Interventions with People with 'Personality Disorder'*. London: Quay Books.

Addo, M. and Smith, I. (2008) Equality and diversity: respecting the person with a learning disability, in *Forensic Mental Health Nursing: Capabilities, Roles and Responsibilities*. London: Quay Books:

Arnold, E. and Boggs, K.U. (2007) *Interpersonal Relationships: Professional Communication Skills for Nurses*. Philadelphia, PA: W.B. Saunders.

Barker, P. (2009) *Psychiatric and Mental Health Nursing: The Craft of Caring*. London: Arnold.

Beebe, S.A., Beebe, S.J. and Redmond, M.V. (2011) Interpersonal Communication: Relating to Others, 6th edn. San Marcos, TX: Pearson.

Bristol Royal Infirmary Inquiry (2001) *The Report of the Public Inquiry into Children's Heart Surgery at the Bristol Royal Infirmary 1984–1995: Learning from Bristol*. London: DH, available at: www.bristolinquiry.org.uk/final_report/report/, accessed 14 April 2012.

Burnard, P. (2003) Ordinary chat and therapeutic conversation: phatic communication in mental health nursing, *Journal of Psychiatric and Mental Health Nursing*, 10: 678–82.

Chant, S., Jenkinson, T., Randle, J. and Russell, G. (2002) Communication skills: some problems in nursing education and practice, *Journal of Clinical Nursing*, 11: 12–21.

Crawford, P. and Brown, B. (2009) Communication, in M. Mallik, C. Hall and D. Howard (eds) *Nursing Knowledge and Practice: Foundations for Decision Making*, 3rd edn. London: Elsevier: London.

Crawford, P., Brown, B. and Bonham, P. (2006) *Communication in Clinical Settings*. Cheltenham: Nelson Thornes.

DH (Department of Health) (2004) *The NHS Improvement Plan: Putting People at the Heart of Public Services*. London: The Stationery Office.

DH (Department of Health) (2009) Report on the National Patient Choice Survey. London. The Stationery Office.

DH (Department of Health) (2010) *Equity and Excellence: Liberating the NHS*. London: The Stationery Office.

Dickson, D.A., Hargie, O. and Morrow, N.C. (1989) *Communication Skills Training for Health Professionals: An Instructor's Handbook*. London: Chapman & Hall.

Doenges, M.E. and Moorhouse, M.F. (2003) *Application of the Nursing Process and Nursing Diagnosis*, 4th edn. Philadelphia, PA: F.A. Davis.

Egan, G. (2010) *The Skilled Helper: A Model for Systematic Helping and Interpersonal Relating*. Pacific Grove, CA: Brooks Cole.

Faulkner, A. (1998) *Effective Interaction with Patients*, 2nd edn. London: Churchill Livingstone.

Fawcett, T. and Rhynas, S. (2012) Taking a patient history: the role of the nurse, *Nursing Standard*, 26(24): 41–6.

Forchuk, C. and Boyd, M.A. (1998) Communication and therapeutic relationship, in M.A. Boyd *Psychiatric Nursing: Contemporary Practice*, 4th edn. Philadelphia, PA: Lippincott.

Giles, S.J., Morris, M. and Cook, G.A. (2009) An in-depth analysis of complaints in an orthopaedic department in the NHS, *Clinical Risk*, 15(4): 146–50.

Griffiths, J., Speed, S., Horne, M. and Keeley, P. (2012) 'A caring professional attitude': what service users and carers seek in graduate nurses and the challenge for educators, *Nurse Education Today*, 32: 121–7.

Hack, T.F., Degner, L.F. and Parker, P.A. (2005) The communication goals and needs of cancer patients: a review, *Psychooncology*, 14(10): 831–45.

Hamilton, S.J. and Martin, D.J. (2007) Clinical development: a framework for effective communication skills, *Nursing Times*, 103(48): 30–1.

Hayes, J. (2002) *Interpersonal Skills at Work*, 2nd edn. Hove: Routledge.

Heron, J. (2001) *Helping the Client – A Creative Practical Guide*, 5th edn. London: Sage.

Horton, K., Tschudin, V. and Forget, A. (2007) The value of nursing: a literature review, *Nursing Ethics*, 14(6): 716–40.

Kozier, B., Erb, G., Berman, A., Snyder, S., Harvey, S. and Morgan-Samuel, H. (2012) *Fundamentals of Nursing – Concepts, Process and Practice*. London: Pearson.

Luckmann, J. (1999) *Transcultural Communication in Nursing*. New York: Delmar Publishers.

Mallik, M., Hall, C. and Howard, D. (2009) *Nursing Knowledge and Practice: Foundations for Decision Making*. London: Elsevier.

McCabe, C. (2004) Nurse–patient communication: an exploration of patients' experiences, *Journal of Clinical Nursing*, 13: 41–9.

Narayanasamy, A. (2003) Transcultural nursing: how nurses respond to cultural needs, *British Journal of Nursing*, 12(3): 185–95.

NMC (Nursing and Midwifery Council) (2008) *The Code: Standards of Conduct, Performance and Ethics for Nurses and Midwives*. London: NMC.

NMC (Nursing and Midwifery Council) (2010) *Standards for Pre-registration Nursing Education*. London: NMC.

Peplau, H. (1952) *Interpersonal Relations in Nursing*. New York: Putnam.

RCN (Royal College of Nursing) (2008) *Dignity at the Heart of Everything We Do*. London: RCN.

Rogers, C.R. (1951) Client-centred Therapy: Its Current Practice, Implications, and Theory. Boston, MA: Houghton Mifflin.

Rungapadiachy, D.M. (1999) *Interpersonal Communication and Psychology for Health Care Professionals: Theory and Practice*. Edinburgh: Butterworth-Heinemann.

Scottish Executive (2003) *Partnership for Care*. Edinburgh: Scottish Executive.

Scottish Executive (2006a) *Rights, Relationship and Recovery: The Report of the National Review of Mental Health Nursing in Scotland*. Edinburgh: Scottish Executive.

Scottish Executive (2006b) *The 10 Essential Shared Capabilities for Mental Health Practice*. Edinburgh: Scottish Executive.

Scottish Government (2005) *Delivering for Health*. Edinburgh: Scottish Government.

Scottish Government (2010) *The Health Care Quality Strategy for NHS Scotland*. Edinburgh: Scottish Government.

Sharples, K. (2011) *Successful Practice: Learning for Nursing Students*. Exeter: Learning Matters Ltd.

 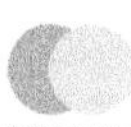

Sheldon, L.K., Barrett, R. and Ellington, L. (2006) Difficult communication in nursing, *Journal of Scholarship in Nursing*, 38(2): 141–7.

Silverman, J., Kurtz, S. and Draper, J. (2005) *Skills for Communicating with Patients*. Oxford: Radcliffe Publishing.

Thorne, S.T. Gregory, H., Kuo, M. and Armstrong, E.A. (2006) Hope and probability: patient perspectives of the meaning of numerical information in cancer communication, *Qualitative Health Research*, 16: 318.

Watkins, P. (2001) *Mental Health Nursing: The Art of Compassionate Care*. Oxford: Butterworth Heinemann.

Welsh Assembly Government (2010) *Doing Well, Doing Better: Standards for Health Services in Wales*. Cardiff: Quality Standards and Safety Improvement Division.

5

Developing skills in solution-focused interactions

Steve Smith

Chapter contents

Introduction

This chapter discusses solution-focused interactions, a specific approach to communication which is based on 'solution-building' (as opposed to 'problem-solving'), which you can utilize across all fields of nursing and implement within your clinical practice. It will explore the theory and skills of solution-focused interactions and provide an understanding of how they can be used. The chapter will draw on examples from various fields of nursing, including from a public health context, to demonstrate the strength of this approach across a range of settings. In addition it builds on the core skills from the previous chapter.

This chapter is relevant to the following Nursing and Midwifery Council (NMC) competencies.

Domain 2: Generic standard for competence

1 All nurses must build partnerships and therapeutic relationships through safe, effective and non-discriminatory communication. They must take account of individual differences, capabilities and needs.

4 All nurses must recognise when people are anxious or in distress and respond effectively, using therapeutic principles, to promote their wellbeing, manage personal safety and resolve conflict. They must use effective communication strategies and negotiation techniques to achieve best outcomes, respecting the dignity and human rights of all concerned.

5 All nurses must use therapeutic principles to engage, maintain and, where appropriate, disengage from professional caring relationships, and must always respect professional boundaries.

6 All nurses must take every opportunity to encourage health-promoting behaviour through education, role modelling and effective communication.

We begin with a case study which will help to illustrate the communication skills and approaches required to understand and adopt a solution-focused approach to nursing care.

Case study 5.1: Mark and Janeczka

Mark is 24 and suffered a traumatic amputation of his lower left leg in a motorcycle accident. He also sustained a complicated fracture of his left wrist. His girlfriend, Debbie, was killed in the accident. He is currently being cared for in a surgical ward, as his stump wound is infected and failing to heal. Mark is frequently verbally aggressive and abusive towards nursing staff; at other times he complains of extreme pain in his wrist and phantom pains in his leg. He does not get on with other patients and is being nursed in an individual room.

Janeczka is a nurse working on the surgical ward where Mark is being cared for. On this particular morning she is re-dressing Mark's stump wound. She is aware that he is 'difficult' to work with; today he has sworn at her several times, complained she is causing him pain, and insulted her East European heritage. Janeczka is on the verge of walking away from Mark, casting the experience off as 'just another failed attempt to help him'; however, in desperation and frustration she suddenly asks him, 'What is wrong with you?' The following conversation ensues while Janeczka gathers together the equipment used for Mark's dressing.

M: What do you think's wrong with me?
J: I don't know; there are so many things that could be wrong with you, I can't begin to imagine. But if I don't know what it is, I can't do anything to help.
M: Yeah, and what are you gonna do?
J: I don't know what I can do.
M: Exactly; just more goody-goody claptrap. Just leave me alone, I don't need your help.
J: If there was something I could do, just one thing, what would it be?
M: I don't know!
J: Suppose you did know . . . what would you say?
M: [pause] Bring Debbie back . . . that would be it.
J: How would that help?
M: It would just be . . . I feel so guilty. I've never seen her mother . . . I wouldn't know what to say to her . . . just her face . . . would kill me. She always said Debbie shouldn't ride on the back; she never liked the bike at all. 'If Mark had an accident, he could be injured and you could be killed' she used to say, and we laughed, 'How come Debbie was always the one that got killed and I only got injured'; that seemed funny at the time . . . Now who's got the last laugh? Nobody, nobody's laughing now . . .
J: What difference would it make if Debbie was here now?
M: I'd have something to get better for, I'd have a reason to get out of here.
J: Hmmn . . . what else?
M: I'd be looking forward to seeing her, and getting out, and doing things.
J: What sort of things?
M: I dunno, just getting out, getting back on a bike, getting . . . I don't know . . . just getting back to normal; maybe yeah, getting back on a bike someday, or going to rallies, or just doing stuff . . . going to the pub, y'know, normal stuff.
J: Yeah. What else would be different?
M: I wouldn't feel so guilty all the time.
J: What would you feel?

M: Determined . . . Strong. Like I was gonna get out of here.
J: What would be different about you? What would I see different?
M: Oh, I don't know. How do I know what would be different?
J: Okay, yeah. Let me ask you this though. How close are you to feeling like that? Say '10' stands for you're feeling strong and determined, and ready to fight your way back out of here, and '0' is sort of the exact opposite; you're just gonna surrender and give in to everything. Where are you just now, between '0' and '10'?
M: [sigh] . . . I dunno . . . about '2' I'd say.
J: Okay . . . how have you managed that?
M: I dunno, I just block the whole thing out my mind sometimes.
J: And that helps?
M: Well, for a little while . . .
J: What else have you done?
M: Nothing, I don't think . . .
J: So you've just got to '2' by blocking things out for a while and letting things happen?
M: Yeah, I guess.
J: How will you know when you've got to '3'?
M: I dunno . . . I'll be able to think about it without blocking it out.
J: What will you do instead . . . instead of blocking it out?
M: I dunno, just accept it, accept that it's happened.
J: And would that help?
M: Yeah, I suppose it must. [pause]
J: Is that what you're doing now?
M: Yeah, I suppose it is . . .
J: How have you managed to do that?
M: I dunno, just you asking these questions . . . I don't want to do this . . .
J: What do you want to do?
M: I dunno, I suppose I have to . . .
J: So . . . if you're thinking about this just now, and accepting how it is . . . is this you at '3' at the moment?
M: Yeah, I suppose it is. [looks vaguely surprised at this]
J: Well done. '3'.
M: Hmmn!
J: Look; if you want to talk again, give me a shout. In the meantime . . . what would '4' look like?

Activity 5.1

Consider how you might have responded to Mark's initial outburst in the conversation above. If you were in Mark's position, what do you think '4' would look like?

Analysing the conversation

In the above conversation there are several points where Janeczka may have regretted getting into the conversation, and felt like running away from Mark's pain. Having taken the plunge and asked Mark, in realistic terms, what was wrong with him, Janeczka could easily have been swamped by the enormity of his answer. Given his situation, where would she begin to list his potential problems? However, Janeczka did something that nurses (and most other health professionals) rarely do: she admitted that she 'didn't know'. We are, as a profession and as professionals, 'trained to know'. Our knowledge base is the root of our professional identity, and as professional practitioners it is the application of our knowledge to a given situation that defines our practice. So it often goes against all we have been taught, and all we have learned from practice, to say 'I don't know'. Which is unfortunate, because in most situations (or at least in most situations involving subjective experiences) we don't know what our patients are experiencing. So, in this situation, Janeczka admitted that she 'didn't know', which was not only an honest response, but invited Mark to continue in the conversation.

Key learning !

- By adopting a 'not knowing' position in our conversation we can often encourage patients to give us more information, and in greater detail, about how they are feeling and what they are thinking, than if we assume that we know what they mean.
- 'Not knowing' is a technique used by skilled practitioners to enable patients to explore their own thoughts and feelings; it doesn't necessarily reflect what the nurse actually knows or understands about a particular situation.

Again, Janeczka may have felt overwhelmed when Mark asked her directly what she was going to do to help him. Given his list of potential problems, where could she begin to help him? In light of this (so far) brief interaction, Janeczka might well have felt that Mark's derisive comments were justified, and again felt some regret at rushing into this conversation. However, she knows that she is not offering to 'solve' Mark's problems, she's only asking 'what she would have to do' to solve his problems; in other words, her question is a hypothetical one aimed at discovering what it is Mark wants. Mark, naturally enough, finds it very difficult to answer this question, and so Janeczka, bearing in mind the hypothetical nature of the conversation, encourages him to use his imagination, to 'think outside of the box'.

Sometimes, gently asking someone, 'Suppose you did know?' allows them to think things they have not been allowing themselves to think about previously; sometimes it's just such a strange question that prompts the person to look afresh at the situation being discussed; either way, it can gently encourage someone to look beyond 'I don't know'.

When Mark does look again at what would help, his answer could well have left Janeczka stuck in her tracks. Bringing Mark's girlfriend back to life is an understandable response, but one that is clearly beyond Janeczka's power to deliver, and one that conveys some of the enormity of his loss and grief. Janeczka is able to 'hold' Mark's grief for a moment, because she knows that she doesn't have to 'sort it out'; instead, she continues to ask Mark what difference that would make. In all of this, Janeczka is asking rather than telling, and in the asking she is enabling Mark to begin to describe the world as he would like it to be. Clearly, Debbie is not going to come back, but there may well be a time at some point in the future where Mark begins to feel more able to confront the world and begin to move forward. This is in essence what Mark is describing – a future in which things are more positive. Note that in all of this conversation, Janeczka only makes three statements; everything else she says is a question. By asking 'not knowing' questions, Janeczka encourages Mark to explore his own solutions, rather than those which she might try to offer up to him in response to her understanding of his problem. Because the focus of this type of communication is on the patient's description of their solution (rather than their problem) it is often described as a 'solution-focused' conversation.

Activity 5.2

Watch Insoo Kim Berg, one of the founders of the solution-focused approach, working with a teenage girl and her parents via the video link given below. Notice how she listens to the mother using only minimal 'not knowing' questions, and changes the focus of the conversation from Sarah's deficits to her assets by asking what she has 'going for her' at the end of the first session. You can access the video on YouTube at: http://bit.ly/YDyR8L.

The background to solution-focused interactions

Solution-focused interactions developed out of the work in solution-focused brief therapy (SFBT) of a husband and wife team, Steve De Shazer and Insoo Kim Berg, and their colleagues at the Brief Family Therapy Centre in Milwaukee, Wisconsin (De Shazer and Dolan 2007). De Shazer and Berg's background was in problem-solving; however, they came to realize that the people they were working with made quicker progress the less they spoke about their problems. In other words, less time spent talking about problems, and more time spent on talking about what people wanted out of life, made for more effective communication. Where the typical number of sessions required for other forms of therapy was between 12 and 20 (and sometimes many, many more) the average number of sessions required by the team at the Brief Family Therapy Centre was less than 5 (De Shazer *et al.* 1986). Although SFBT originated in family therapy, it was quickly adopted by other practitioners in a variety of fields. It has been utilized in settings as diverse as couples therapy, substance misuse, sex therapy, individual counselling work, group work and self-help books, as well as settings such as social care, education, prison populations and business systems (Iveson 2002; Trepper *et al.* 2006; Walsh 2006).

In particular, nurses quickly recognized the potential benefits from this approach and began to incorporate solution-focused interactions in nursing practice (Webster 1990; Wilgosh *et al.* 1993; Montgomery and Webster 1994; Iveson 1995; Hillyer 1996). Webster (1990) argued that SFBT provided a framework that was congruent with both traditional nursing values and feminist ethics. Montgomery and Webster (1994) developed this further when they argued that solution-focused approaches provide a framework to promote a shift from a cure-orientation to a care-orientation in health care, and particularly in nursing. They argued that brief therapeutic approaches enabled nurses to re-engage with their patients, concluding that working within a solution paradigm, nurses could respond to their patients' vulnerability, as opposed to their pathology, and could reduce 'the mystique of our own power and knowledge', in order to 'give them a sense of their own power and help them rediscover their resources' (p. 296). McAllister (2007) takes this further, and argues that solution-focused nursing represents a 'practical philosophy' emphasizing the importance of exploring solutions as well as problems, a focus on strategies for working with patients and not on them, and the need to be cautious of dominant ways of thinking. Bowles *et al.* (2001) found that nurses working in a solution-focused way experienced less stress and anxiety, and reported being more confident in their work. Similar outcomes were reported by Boscart (2009) for nurses working in a continuing care setting, and by Neilson-Clayton and Brownlee (2002) and Smith *et al.* (2011) for nurses working in cancer care and surgical care respectively. In all these papers, nurses utilizing a solution-focused style of communication were able to care for their patients in a less authoritative manner, giving patients more opportunity to take responsibility and make decisions about their health care.

Values and principles of solution-focused interactions

Some of the values and principles which underpin solution-focused interactions are:

- sensitivity to individual and cultural differences;
- maintaining human dignity;
- promoting self-care;
- recognizing and enhancing patients' strengths;
- a health, rather than illness, focus;
- endeavouring to reduce pain and discomfort;
- reintegrating patients into helpful social systems;
- emphasizing the pragmatics;
- promoting a safe environment;
- mobilizing patient hope and agency.

Webster (1990) argues that these same principles underpin traditional nursing values. Given the very close links between the ethics and practice of nursing and the principles underpinning solution-focused interactions, it is not surprising that working in a solution-focused way can be seen to operationalize some of the NMC competencies relating to communication and interpersonal skills. In particular, nursing from a solution-focused perspective enhances the nurse's ability to ensure that communication is 'safe, effective, compassionate and respectful'. We have seen how Janeczka used solution-focused skills to listen to Mark in an empathic way. This is central to the NMC expectations, and indeed Domain 2, Competency 1 states that all nurses 'must build partnerships and therapeutic relationships through safe, effective and non-discriminatory communication'. In the example above, it can be seen that Janeczka's practice met these standards, in that she didn't tell Mark what to do, rather she facilitated a conversation that helped him identify his 'problem' and begin to build a solution to it. This principle crosses all domains of nursing; in the next conversation note how Anne, a children's nurse, enables David, an 8-year-old boy who has Type 1 diabetes, to maintain his sense of independence and engage in the decision-making process.

Case study 5.2: David and Anne

David's previously well managed diabetes has become unstable in the last year. It is thought this is due to his increasing reluctance to follow a regular dietary regime, which he is unable to do as he is spending more time with friends from school than he did previously. While his family are keen to promote normal social interactions, they are worried that David's desire to be 'the same as everyone else' is at odds with his diabetes management.

Anne works in a unit specializing in the care of children and young people with diabetes. David has been referred by his GP to a nurse-led clinic within the unit. Anne begins by talking to David about his life: what he enjoys, his favourite sports and his favourite television programmes. In carrying out this 'problem-free talk' Anne is both learning something about David's wider life, and letting him know that she sees him as more than just a problem or just another case. She then goes on to ask David how he sees the problem. In this period of 'problem talk' Anne listens to David describe how he sees the problem from his perspective. David talks at some length about how his mum gets onto him for not eating the 'right food' at the 'right time' and how it's not fair, because all he wants to do is play with his school friends and it's not his fault about the diabetes. Throughout this period, Anne simply listens and acknowledges that she understands what David is telling her; specifically, she offers no opinions or advice on what David is telling her. In this respect, solution-focused communication differs from other forms of professional communication Anne might employ as a nurse, in which she might provide health education information, or take the opportunity

 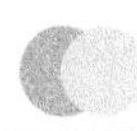

to explore David's feelings more deeply. Here, she simply listens (T.K., one of my students on a solution-focused training course, described the approach as 'more of a listening therapy than a talking therapy', which I thought very apt). Anne then asks David how she can help him deal with his problem – i.e. how can she help him stop his mum 'getting on to him'. In doing this she is both addressing David's problem (as opposed to his doctor's problem or his family's problem) and using the words that David used to describe the problem to her. Not surprisingly, David doesn't have many ideas how she could do this. Here's an extract from their conversation.

D: You could tell her she doesn't need to worry about me.
A: Would that help, do you think?
D: Probably not.
A: Let me ask you a question then, David. [Anne pauses] Suppose . . . just suppose that later . . . after you leave here and go home and do the things you're going to do for the rest of the day . . .
D: I'm going out to play with Gavin at the park.
A: Right; so you go out to play with Gavin at the park . . . and then you come home . . . and when it get's to bed-time, you go to bed. Now . . . while you're sleeping . . . something amazing happens . . . and the problems you've been telling me all about . . . are gone. Just like that! You don't understand how it's happened, but they're gone. But . . . you're asleep, right?
D: Yeah . . .
A: So . . . because you're asleep, you don't know that this thing has even happened. So . . . what will be the first thing that tells you in the morning that something is different? Can you draw me a picture of what it will be like when things are different, and this problem's gone? [Anne then provides David with paper and a large selection of coloured pencils and pens]

It can be seen here that Anne and David are essentially 'telling a story'; Anne is providing most of the story but readily incorporates the parts David provides. She makes good use of pauses; allowing David time to imagine what that part of the story is like. In asking David to draw a picture of his ideal day rather than describing it in words, Anne is recognizing that it is often easier for young children to use visual communication, as opposed to verbal communication, to express their ideas. This approach can also be used when asking scaling questions (**Figure 5.1**).

Note also that Anne doesn't say, 'Can you draw me a picture of what it would be like when things are different', or 'what it will be like if things are different', instead she uses pre-suppositional language to suggest that things not only can be different, but will be different. David then goes on to draw a picture of his family in the kitchen on the morning after his problem is gone.

Different media for scaling questions

0 ———————— 10
Typical adult scale / numeric scale

☹ ———————— ☺
Emotive / child friendly scale

Bad ———————— Good
Simple construct scale

□ ———————— ■
Simple visual scale

Note that in all cases the nurse must define what each end of the scale represents.

Figure 5.1 Different media for scaling questions

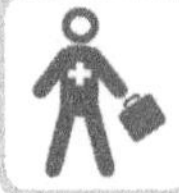

Case study 5.2: continued

A: So, what's here?

D: This is me, sitting in the kitchen, and I've got my football top on.

A: Right, so, what day is it?

D: It's Saturday, 'cause I'm going out to play. I'm going to play football with Gavin and Tom, and we're going to the park.

A: Right. What else?

D: We'll buy sweets.

A: Okay; what else is happening in the picture?

D: The dog's wagging his tail, 'cause he's happy . . . and I'm smiling 'cause I'm happy too. And Mum's smiling, 'cause she's happy.

A: Right! So everyone's happy. What else is happening?

D: I'm having my breakfast, I'm having sausage and eggs, that's the egg there, and I'm having juice to drink.

A: Wow, okay. What else is there?

Anne goes on to get David to describe how this particular story ends and David, knowing the rules about stories, provides a suitable happy ending as he sees it. In doing this, Anne is helping David describe his 'positive future scenario'. The capacity to tell a story with a happy ending is something that is not lost to us as we grow older; we can all describe a positive future scenario given the right encouragement. However, no matter how happy the ending, this is still just a story. Anne continues to encourage David to add detail to his story by asking him what his mum would notice different about him on this day ('I'd be all happy and talking to her') and eliciting detail about this, and what his Dad would notice different about him ('I'd finish my breakfast quick, and clear away the plates'); even what the dog would notice different about him ('Ha ha; he'd get a really big walk and we'd go to the park, and he'd get a bone. He'd know I was happy 'cause I'd give him a big hug'). In every case, Anne elicits as much detail from David as he can provide about what would be happening and what each person (or pet) would notice. In doing this, David creates more and more detail, and his story becomes more and more 'real' as a result. It is though, still a story; which is why Anne then brings the story back to reality.

A: Wow . . . what a great picture. But, I'm wondering . . . have there been any times you can remember when any of that's actually happened? Any time you've all been happy, or you've gone out with the dog, or even given him a big hug?

D: Well . . . we're happy sometimes . . . and the dog's always wagging his tail, and we take him out for walks and stuff.

A: Wow . . . how do you manage to do that? I mean with all these problems you were telling me about; with all that going on, how do you manage to be happy sometimes and take the dog out?

D: Well . . . it's not always like that . . . Mum's not always getting on at me . . . mostly she's okay.

A: How do you manage that . . . how do you get your mum not to be getting on at you?

D: I don't know . . . it's only when I'm messing about with my diet that she gets mad . . .

A: So what do you do to stop her getting mad?

D: Well . . . I just keep to my diet really.

A: Oh right . . . Okay . . . How do you do that?

D: Well, it's quite easy really. I've got a thing here, look . . .

David then goes on to explain his diet regime to Anne. Note that throughout Anne is asking 'not-knowing' questions, using David's words wherever possible, and looking at the situation from his point of view. In doing this she helps David create a meaningful positive future scenario, and then helps him to recognize that *parts* of it are happening already; not only does he not need a miracle to bring about his positive future scenario, but parts are already happening and he wasn't even aware of it! This highlights a basic principle of solution-focused interactions; *it's not our job to change the patient's life*. Our job is to help the patient recognize where change is already happening in their life, and they haven't noticed it yet, and to do more of what has helped bring about that change. Most of the key principles of solution-focused practice can be grouped under four interconnected headings, which we examine in the next section after **Activity 5.3**.

Activity 5.3

- Consider for a moment how solution-focused interactions might enable you to practise in accordance with the NMC competencies within your own area of practice.
- Make a note of a recent clinical situation you were involved in, and think of how you could have applied solution-focused interactions in that situation.
- Make links from this to the specific NMC competencies you would be demonstrating were you to have responded in that way.

Some key principles of solution-focused interactions

If it's not broken, don't fix it

Patients come to us with problems; they are not the problem themselves. We often hear other practitioners (and, truth be told, we sometimes do it ourselves) speak about 'problem patients' or refer to patients using a diagnostic label; in other words, defining patients by what is wrong with them. While there is, obviously, an element of logic to this process, it is very likely to encourage us to see our patients in terms of their deficits, and to focus our attention on what they *can't* do. In solution-focused interactions we make a deliberate attempt to build on what is healthy and functioning about the patient. We see patients as being inherently competent, and having the necessary resources to change and adapt to whatever problems are occurring in their lives. Therefore we focus on what is going well in the patient's life (while not ignoring their presenting problem) and what they have at the moment that they would like to keep in the future. These are the patient's assets and strengths, and these are the things that they are going to have to rely upon in order to overcome whatever difficulty they are experiencing at the moment.

Activity 5.4

Take a piece of A4 paper and fold it in half. On the left-hand side write down any problems you have been experiencing recently (equally you can note any problems a patient you have been working with has been experiencing); make a list of between three and five aspects of the problem. On the right-hand side of the paper, write down opposite each part of the problem the skills, strengths or attributes which you (or your patient) have brought to bear in dealing with that problem. Now tear the paper in half along the fold you made earlier. Throw away the left-hand panel, and look at the right-hand panel; where did you get these strengths and abilities from? Consider how they have helped you in the past, and think of how they might be useful in helping you in the immediate future. What other strengths, skills and positive attributes do you possess?

If it's working, do more of it

This might seem like a really obvious statement, but very often people respond more to what they think they 'should be doing', rather than what they know to work. In order to know if something is working, we have to know where we are going or what it is that we want to happen. Often, particularly in times of distress, we focus on feelings of 'I don't want this to happen' without necessarily thinking what it is 'I do want' to happen. In Mark and Janeczka's story, Janeczka helps Mark move from what he doesn't want to be happening to what he does want, by asking him 'What would you feel?'. Mark then begins to describe what it is he would like to be happening instead. Janeczka then helps him measure how well his efforts at getting to where he wants to be are working by asking him to scale his progress, and even to identify a 'next step'. Similarly, Anne enables David to describe what he wants to be happening and then helps him to describe what it is he is doing already 'that works'. Again, it is not Anne's or Janeczka's job to tell their patient what they should be doing, it's their job to help their patient identify what they are already doing that works, and then to encourage them to do more of it.

If it's not working, stop doing it

If the previous point seemed pretty elementary, this key principle should be even clearer. However, there are many times when we all continue to do things that aren't helping us, even when we are clear what we want from a situation. Sometimes we are unaware of the connection between what we are doing and a lack of positive change, sometimes we tend to think that we're just not doing what we think will be helpful 'hard enough', and sometimes we just like doing something even though we know it isn't helpful. In all three cases it isn't our role to lecture our patients on what they should, or shouldn't be doing, but rather we can take a 'not knowing' posture and ask them to explain to us how what they are doing is helpful to them. By asking questions like, 'Does that help?', or 'How is that good for you?' we can encourage our patients to explore the impact of what they are doing, and to recognize that if something isn't helping the first time you do it (or certainly by the third or fourth time), it's unlikely to help at all. We can then ask, 'What else can you do that will be helpful?' It's important to recognize that, sometimes, a patient might benefit from permission from a nurse, or other perceived authority figure, to stop doing something that isn't working (e.g. to stop responding to a violent partner, or to stop 'grieving' for a loss); however, the recognition that it isn't working must come from the patient before we can respond to it in a helpful way.

Big problems don't need big solutions

Most people are pretty good at solving the problems of daily life; we regularly overcome any number of problems on a daily basis. 'Where are my shoes?', 'How do I address this assignment?', 'How can I tell my friend that I can't meet her tomorrow night?': these are all the types of problems that most of us deal with every day. However, the problems that our patients often bring to us are of a different order: 'How can I live my life with the impact of injury, disease, disability and loss?' These are the kinds of problems that can feel overwhelming to us as nurses, and we often resort to 'on the surface' responses that fail to respond to the patient's underlying need for help. However, from a solution-focused perspective we take the view that problems and solutions are not as closely connected as we might think. We don't have to 'solve' the patient's problem; we only have to help them see it in a different way, in order that they can find their own way of dealing with (or solving) their problem. In helping people see things in a different way, encouraging them to make a small change in their lives is often more effective that asking them to make a major change. A small change in the way a person behaves is frequently enough to bring about further changes in their life and in the way people around them behave towards them.

 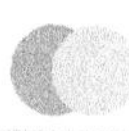

Activity 5.5

The diagram below describes the solution-building process. See if you can link the parts of the process to what you have learned about solution-focused interactions so far.

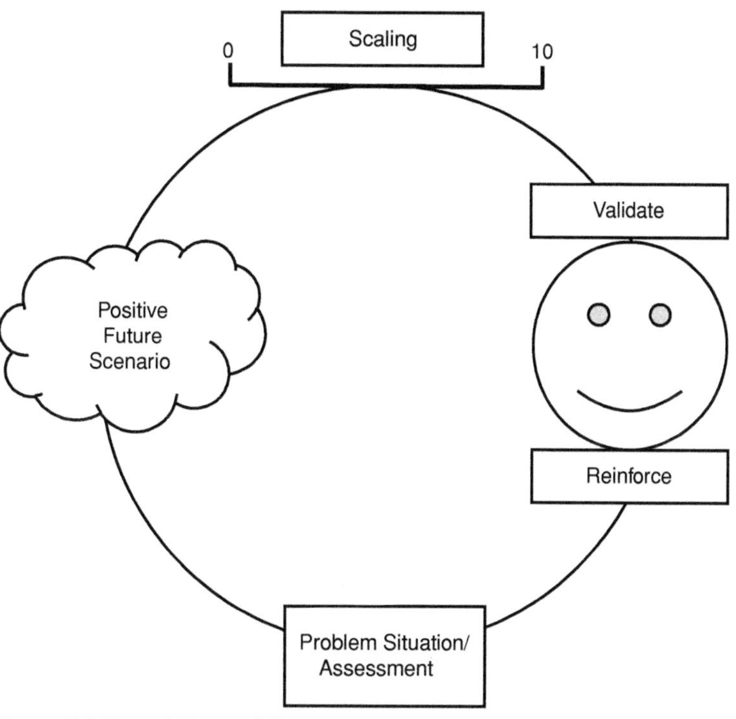

Figure 5.2 The solution-building process

Key learning

The process of solution building begins with hearing the patient's account of 'the problem'. We then help the patient describe their positive future scenario, and scale how close they are to achieving that goal. We then validate the steps the patient has taken towards achieving their goal and reinforce the things that are 'working'. In doing this we are guided by the principles of:

- if it's not broken, don't fix it;
- if it's working, do more of it;
- if it's not working, stop doing it;
- big problems don't need big solutions.

Solution-focused interactions in the 'non-clinical' setting

Some of these key principles have been seen in the clinical scenarios presented above. However, solution-focused interactions can also be used in non-clinical situations such as team meetings, staff appraisals and planning meetings. The same techniques of 'not knowing', 'asking rather than telling', 'focusing on assets rather than deficits', and the use of scaling and a 'positive future scenario' can all be utilized in moving professional conversations away from a problem focus to a solution focus. The NMC generic standard for competence in communication and interpersonal skills states that, 'all nurses must use excellent communication and interpersonal skills. Their communications must always be safe, effective, compassionate and respectful'. This standard does not only apply to communication with patients but equally to professional communications – for example, with members of the multiprofessional team. Solution-focused interactions can provide a framework for engaging in effective communication in a range of difficult situations. Where, increasingly, the registered nurse's role encompasses that of mentor and coach to junior staff, the skills of solution-focused interactions can be utilized to facilitate respectful, yet effective, coaching across the domains of professional practice.

Conclusion

No single approach can be seen as a panacea for all nursing practice; however, solution-focused interactions are an important addition to the 'tool-box' of knowledge and skills possessed by the contemporary nurse practitioner. Whether practising in adult, children's, learning disabilities or mental health nursing, all practitioners are required to demonstrate competency in communication and interpersonal skills. This requirement not only crosses all domains of practice, but also crosses communication with patients and clients, relatives, colleagues, and anyone the nurse comes into contact with. Solution-focused interactions provide a framework for nurses to communicate in a safe, respectful, compassionate and effective manner, recognizing the traditional values of nursing and promoting patient independence and well-being. Several examples of the techniques being used in clinical practice have been discussed, and further reading is suggested below.

In summary:

- It can be seen that solution-focused interactions are structured around a process of:
  - hearing the client's definition of their particular problem;
  - helping the client construct a positive future scenario;
  - scaling how close the client is to achieving their goal and their next small step;
  - delivering a solution-focused intervention.
- These questions provide a structure within which we can then address the NMC competencies in relation to communication and interpersonal skills.

Further reading and resources

Connie, E. and Metcalf, L. (eds) (2009) *The Art of Solution Focused Therapy.* New York: Springer.

De Shazer, S. and Dolan, Y. (eds) (2007) *More than Miracles: The State of the Art of Solution-focused Brief Therapy*. London: Routledge.

Hanton, P. (2011) *Skills in Solution Focused Brief Counselling and Psychotherapy*. London: Sage.

MacDonald, A. (2011) *Solution-focused Therapy: Theory, Research and Practice*. London: Sage.

McAllister, M. (ed.) (2007) *Solution-focused Nursing: Rethinking Practice.* Basingstoke: Palgrave Macmillan.

References

Boscart, V. (2009) A communication intervention for nursing staff in chronic care, *Journal of Advanced Nursing,* 65(9): 1823–32.

Bowles, N., Mackintosh, C. and Torn, A. (2001) Nurses' communication skills: an evaluation of the impact of solution-focused communication training, *Journal of Advanced Nursing*, 36(3): 347–54.

De Shazer, S. and Dolan, Y. (eds) (2007) *More than Miracles: The State of the Art of Solution-focused Brief Therapy*. London: Routledge.

De Shazer, S., Berg, I.K., Lipchik, E., Nunnally, E., Molnar, A., Gingerich, W. and Weiner-Davis, M. (1986) Brief therapy: focused solution development, *Family Process*, 25(2): 207–22.

Hillyer, D. (1996) Solution oriented questions: an analysis of a key intervention, *Journal of the American Psychiatric Nurses Association*, 2(1): 3–10.

Iveson, C. (1995) Solution focused brief therapy: a tool for health visitors, *Health Visitor*, 68(6): 236–8.

Iveson, C. (2002) Solution-focused brief therapy, *Advances In Psychiatric Treatment*, 8: 149–57.

McAllister, M. (ed.) (2007) *Solution-focused Nursing: Rethinking Practice.* Basingstoke: Palgrave Macmillan.

Montgomery, C. and Webster, D. (1994) Caring, curing and brief therapy: a model for nurse psychotherapy, *Archives of Psychiatric Nursing*, 8(5): 291–7.

Neilson-Clayton, H. and Brownlee, K. (2002) Solution-focused brief therapy with cancer patients and their families, *Journal of Psychosocial Oncology*, 20(1): 1–13.

Smith, S., Adam, D., Kirkpatrick, P. and McRobie, G. (2011) Using solution-focused communication to support patients, *Nursing Standard*, 25(52): 42–7.

Trepper, T.S., Dolan, Y., Mccollum, E.E. and Nelson, T. (2006) Steve De Shazer and the future of solution-focused therapy, *Journal of Marital and Family Therapy*, 32(2): 133–9.

Walsh, T. (2006) Two sides of the same coin: ambiguity and complexity in child protection work, *Journal of Systemic Therapies*, 25(2): 38–49.

Webster, D.C. (1990) Solution focused approaches in psychiatric/mental health nursing, *Perspectives In Psychiatric Care*, 26(4): 17–21.

Wilgosh, R., Hawkes, D. and Marsh, I. (1993) Session two and beyond – or, 'what do you say after you say "hello" again?' *Context*, 9: 31–3.

Communication in difficult situations

6

Kay Townsend, Beth Sepion and Delia Pogson

Chapter contents

Introduction

It is possible to argue that communication underpins the majority of the Nursing and Midwifery Council (NMC) competencies. However, we have identified the key issues in each domain and competency that we think are significant when discussing communication in difficult situations. While other chapters in this book focus on highlighting specific aspects of communicating in practice situations, this chapter focuses on the difficult conversations that patients and carers face throughout their care experience with us. Of course these conversations are difficult for us too.

No matter which field of nursing you are studying, you will on occasions find yourself in situations where you feel that you just don't know what to say. The situation we think most likely to prompt this reaction, and one which is common to all fields of nursing, is when someone is dying or has been bereaved. To enable you to consider how you can develop your competence in communication we will use end-of-life care as the theme for this chapter. There is no one, single, way to communicate with people who are coming to the end of their lives. Just as all end-of-life situations are unique, so is the way that you will feel.

However, the following three things can help you deal with difficult situations:

- thinking about these situations before you find yourself in them;
- having good practice knowledge to fall back on;
- being able to reflect on them afterwards.

This chapter is not a recipe for success, it's a resource to allow you to improve your practice. It is also not an in-depth analysis of communication at the end-of-life – for this we recommend Duke and Bailey's chapter in Payne's book, *Palliative Care Nursing: Principles and Evidence for Practice* (Payne *et al.* 2008).

Communicating in difficult situations: NMC competencies (NMC 2010)

Domain 1: Professional values

2 All nurses must practise in a holistic, non-judgemental, caring and sensitive manner that avoids assumptions, supports social inclusion, recognises and respects individual choice; and acknowledges diversity. Where necessary, they must challenge inequality, discrimination and exclusion from access to care.

The key issues for communication in difficult situations raised by this competency include avoiding assumptions, respecting choice and individuality, and challenging others.

Domain 2: Communication and interpersonal skills

1 All nurses must build partnerships and therapeutic relationships through safe, effective and non-discriminatory communication. They must take account of individual differences, capabilities and needs.

The key issues raised here are the virtues of care and compassion, the moral wisdom you use to make judgements and the account you take of another person's values (which may be different to your own).

2 All nurses must use a range of communication skills and technologies to support person-centred care and enhance quality and safety. They must ensure people receive all the information they need in a language and manner that allows them to make informed choices and share decision making. They must recognise when language interpretation or other communication support is needed and know how to obtain it.

The key issues here is the *variety* of ways information can be provided and the wisdom to choose an appropriate method of communication with each individual.

3 All nurses must use the full range of communication methods, including verbal, non-verbal and written, to acquire, interpret and record their knowledge and understanding of people's needs. They must be aware of their own values and beliefs and the impact this may have on their communication with others. They must take account of the many different ways in which people communicate and how these may be influenced by ill health, disability and other factors, and be able to recognise and respond effectively when a person finds it hard to communicate.

The key issues raised here are understanding the impact of illness on the whole person and their family, the impact of your own values and beliefs on your attitudes and behaviours, and the wisdom to make a decision based upon another individual's values rather than your own.

4 All nurses must recognise when people are anxious or in distress and respond effectively, using therapeutic principles, to promote their wellbeing, manage personal safety and resolve conflict. They must use effective communication strategies and negotiation techniques to achieve best outcomes, respecting the dignity and human rights of all concerned. They must know when to consult a third party and how to make referrals for advocacy, mediation or arbitration.

The key issues here are acknowledging and responding to distress, and understanding and acknowledging your own limitations.

5 All nurses must use therapeutic principles to engage, maintain and, where appropriate, disengage from professional caring relationships, and must always respect professional boundaries.

The key issues here are sensitivity, understanding the limits of the relationship, and the need for 'closing' in conversations and relationships.

Communication and end-of-life care

Why use end-of-life care as the theme for this chapter? 'How we care for the dying is an indicator of how we care for all sick and vulnerable people. It is a measure of society as a whole and it is a litmus test for health and social care services' (DH 2008: 2). In the next 20 years, with an increasingly elderly population, the health care workforce will be more involved in end-of-life care (National End-of-Life Care Programme 2011a), and as nurses spend more time with patients than any other health care professionals, you are likely to be present when someone is facing death. While caring for dying patients, and their families, can be a stressful experience for student nurses (Cooper and Barnett 2005) it can also be a profoundly influential experience (DH 2008). Thinking about end-of-life care, how you support others and what makes you anxious can help reduce the stress of these situations, and improve your own well-being as well as the care you give (Melo and Oliver 2011).

There are other chapters in this book that will help you to think about some important concepts with respect to communication in different practice settings and we suggest that you refer to these as well. Chapter 2 looks at professional values and this strongly links to how we communicate and interact with others. Chapters 4 and 5 explore other specific practice opportunities related to you developing effective communication, interpersonal skills and competencies.

Caring and communication

Activity 6.1

Think about what makes you feel cared for and cared about. How does the way someone behaves, what they say and what they do, convey this to you?

Theories about caring in nursing emphasize the importance of the relationship between the nurse and the person being cared for, as well as harmony, wholeness, comfort and the broad spectrum of human living beyond health. When considering communication in end-of-life care it is worth revisiting the five interrelated concepts of caring (Morse *et al.* 1990):

- a human trait;
- an ideal;
- an interpersonal relationship;
- a therapeutic intervention;
- an affect.

The way that we value others and the way that we are with others have an impact on the way people feel cared for. Research and literature about what are important characteristics for nurses help us understand the things that we should reflect upon as we engage in care: moral behaviour, ethical reasoning and decision-making (Skisland *et al.* 2012); being (not acting) virtuous (Putman 2012); comforting and encouraging (Hwang *et al.* 2012); integrity (Ekeberg 2011); respect for equality (Kangasniemi 2010); moral courage (LaSala and Bjarnason 2010); being 'amenable' (Jonasson *et al.* 2010); and compassion (McLean 2012). How many of these things featured in your reflection about what makes you feel cared for?

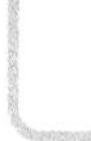

Key learning

- Nurses are likely to care for people who are dying or are bereaved.
- Being caring is fundamental to the experience other people have in any situation, including end-of-life care.

Caring, but difficult, conversations

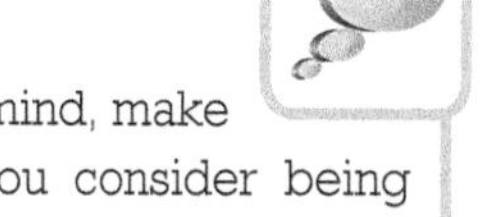

Activity 6.2

With your field of nursing in mind, make a list of conversations that you consider being difficult, or have seen as being significant.

The situations you have listed in **Activity 6.2** will in all likelihood have a common feature of very significant change: difficult conversations are often about telling someone that the future they pictured is not how they have been picturing it or hoping it will be. This is often called 'breaking significant news', and a model that may help you with this is discussed later in the chapter. Models are very useful, but they do depend on the person using them having some key skills, and these will be explored first.

Earlier chapters, in particular Chapter 4, have explained that communication difficulties are *not only* about what is *said*, either by you or by the person being cared for or their family members, but are also about the *non-verbal* messages. Although body language has been discussed, we think it is important, and want to remind you about some key facts. According to Donnelly and Neville (2008), approximately:

- 7 per cent of what we communicate relies on the words being used;
- 38 per cent is communicated by the tonality of the voice;
- 55 per cent is communicated by body language.

We rely very heavily on our body language, particularly in situations such as the end-of-life. We rely on active listening skills and empathy, so it is helpful to more consciously consider what these mean to us. Body language is an aspect of our behaviour that we often forget about until, or after, we are in a difficult situation. Many communication models describe the components of body language or non-verbal communication (e.g. Donnelly and Neville 2008; Atherton and Crickmore 2011; Hannon and Clift 2011), but consider **Activity 6.3**. We think that theory is useful and necessary to appreciate why things happen the way they do. The only way you can appreciate the reality for people you speak to is to listen to them and think about the impact that good and bad communication skills have on the way they feel.

Activity 6.3

With your field of nursing in mind, talk to a family member, friend or neighbour about their experience of a health care conversation. What helped them and what did not?

Try writing about this experience in the form of a short story and share it with your tutor group. Are there common themes that you notice that you could explore in the literature?

The person you speak to in **Activity 6.3** may have mentioned:

- facial expressions (movement of eyebrows, frowning, smiling, crying);
- eye contact (contact or not, staring);
- voice (volume, rate of speech, silence, tone);
- posture (sitting or standing);
- body movements (fidgeting, nodding, gestures);
- proximity (physical closeness or distance).

Being aware of your own body language and the often unintentional signals it sends is part of the emotional labour of nursing that creates a clear message that ensures people feel safe and cared for (Horschild 1983, cited in Gray 2008).

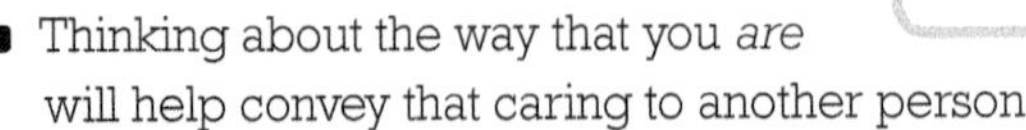

Key learning

- Thinking about the way that you *are* will help convey that caring to another person.
- Thinking about the things that make you anxious about end-of-life care can help improve the way you feel as well as the care you give.
- It takes energy (emotional labour) to create an outward expression of caring in your facial expressions, tone of voice, posture and positioning.

What contributes to difficulty in conversations?

Communication difficulties for the person you are speaking to

A difficulty when communicating with individuals, in particular on first meeting them and when forming new relationships, is finding out how much the person understands and if they have any existing communication difficulties (Hannon and Clift 2011). Their level of understanding or any existing communication difficulties may make the communication interaction more complex, for you or for the other person. On first meeting with someone it may be obvious that they have an existing communication difficulty, such as lack of or altered speech, or expressing difficulty in understanding you ('Say it again?' or 'Oh yes' in response to an open question). There will be many other situations where it may *not* be so obvious and you will be in a position of trying to identify whether the person has a specific difficulty. Hannon and Clift (2011: 104) suggest some possible indicators when communicating with people with learning disabilities, but these could apply equally when communicating with other individuals, such as children, people with cognitive impairments, people with sensory impairments, people experiencing mental health difficulties and people whose first language is not English.

Activity 6.4

With your field of nursing in mind, consider the following and reflect on those occasions when you have experienced similar situations in your practice. Consider whether those situations were well managed, and if not, why not?

The person you are speaking to:

- has difficulty in finding the right words to express their thoughts and emotions;
- uses words but does not appear to fully understand them;
- demonstrates confusion, especially when more than one person is talking – for example when staff and family members are present;
- is acquiescent – giving you the answer they think you want;
- repeatedly asks the same question;
- talks about everyday things but not about emotions;
- has family members that talk instead of them.

Conversations about dying: fears, misconceptions and beliefs

As well as specific difficulties in their communication, people also have to overcome other barriers to communication. These barriers are faced by all people in the conversation and are put there by both the person and the professional. For the *person in the end-of-life situation* there are all sorts of reasons that make it difficult for them to approach you and share their worries and needs. The challenges for a person needing care in end-of-life situations are compounded by the challenges the *professional* feels (see **Table 6.1** next page).

Finding the words

A difficulty for many nurses when communicating to patients that they are dying is deciding what to tell everyone involved. There is a natural initial response to 'not tell' as a means of protecting them. Much can be learned from the literature about communicating about dying in children's nursing. This knowledge can be transferred into many adult, mental health and learning disability nursing situations.

What to tell children who are dying

The evidence indicates that children are never too young to be told what is happening to them (Silverman 2000). Children of all ages are astute observers who pick up on parents' emotions and anxieties. They read non-verbal communication, compare it with the verbal and try to make sense

Table 6.1 Common fears, beliefs and challenges that hamper effective communication (adapted from National End of Life Care Programme 2011b)

Fears of people being cared for	**Fears of professionals**
■ Of being stigmatized ■ Of being judged ungrateful or inadequate ■ Breaking down and crying ■ Burdening health and social care staff ■ Causing distress to others ■ Not being able to find the words	■ Unleashing strong emotions ■ Making things worse ■ Saying the wrong thing ■ Facing difficult questions ■ Taking up too much time ■ Facing our own failure
Beliefs of the person being cared for	**Beliefs of professionals**
■ Problems are an inevitable part of illness so health and social care staff should anticipate them ■ Problems cannot be alleviated ■ Professional people are only interested in certain types of problems ■ This is not the 'right' professional person to talk with ■ Professional staff are too busy	■ Emotional problems are inevitable and nothing can be done about them ■ It's not my role to discuss such things ■ There's no point talking about problems that cannot be solved ■ They don't understand what's happening ■ They don't need to know
Challenges perceived by the person being cared for	**Challenges perceived by professionals**
■ It's hard to find the right words ■ The right questions weren't asked by the professional ■ Problems hinted at are not picked up by the professional ■ Not communicating in first language ■ Cognitive impairment	Lack of skills or confidence ■ Starting end-of-life discussions ■ Exploring concerns ■ Handling difficult questions – saying the 'right' thing ■ Closing the conversation sensitively Workplace ■ Lack of support from colleagues or managers ■ Lack of privacy ■ Time constraints ■ Noise and distractions ■ Nowhere to refer to for psychological support ■ No training or supervision in communication skills

of it. Piaget (1929) describes this as 'accommodation and assimilation': comparing what is known and matching the unknown within this to make sense. However, some things will not make sense and will be interpreted as being 'at odds', causing children to feel concerned and not involved (e.g. when the parent is crying and distressed but says everything is fine). This can lead to a concept of 'mutual pretence': the parent's reluctance or distress holds them back from talking to the child about the potential of death or the seriousness of the situation. Recognizing the distress, the child attempts to protect the parents by not asking questions that they think may cause further distress. The parents interpret this as 'they do not need to know' and thus a situation of *mutual pretence*, that both are 'OK', develops (Bluebond-Langner 1978).

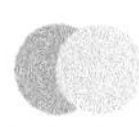

However, we know that children have to make sense of everything (see **Case study 6.1**). Asking questions is how they learn and fantasy and make-believe are tools that children use to help make sense of unfamiliar, unknown or frightening situations. When did I last see my mummy cry? What makes daddy so angry? At a time when they would ask mummy or daddy they feel unable to do so. Understanding why parents try to avoid these conversations, and what benefit the conversation may have for a child, can help you support the parents in their decision-making (see **Table 6.2**).

The nurse is in a challenging situation when supporting and communicating with a family where a child is dying. It is necessary to be able to act as the patient's advocate while at the same time meeting the needs of the family. Kübler-Ross (1969) states that everyone has a right to know that they are dying but not everyone *needs* to know, and the thing to bear in mind is that parents know their child best and therefore their views must be taken seriously. The parents' decision to not tell their child needs to be explored sensitively, utilizing the skills explored in this chapter. Whatever decision is made, it is important that parents are encouraged to respond to a child's questions in a composed and relaxed manner. This can help the child to feel secure and supported (Faulkner 1998). Honesty is a key element when communicating with family members (Heyland *et al.* 2006).

Case study 6.1: Ben

Ben was 8 years old and had been diagnosed with an osteosarcoma when he was aged 7. A routine follow-up scan three months after the completion of treatment confirmed that the tumour had regrown. The results of this test were shared with his parents and a decision regarding no further active treatment was agreed upon. However, Ben's parents requested that he should not be told the results as they felt he would not be able to cope with this news.

While the team were with his parents Ben asked a nurse who was recording his observations, 'Am I dying?' She sat next to him and asked why he had asked this question. He described how, when he was diagnosed, it was explained to him that he had a tumour, that it would not get better on its own but there was treatment to help. He continued, 'I have had the treatment but it has not gone away so I must be going to die.' The nurse explored this with him and he told her that he had things that he wanted to do, and asked how long he had to live. He didn't want to ask his parents because he knew that they would be upset. He was relieved that the nurse suggested sharing this with his parents, and together they were able to plan his end-of-life care.

Table 6.2 Understanding parents and children in end-of-life care

Why parents may be reluctant to tell their child that they are dying	Why children need to know
Impression of giving up on their child	They may have questions
Need to maintain hope	They may be frightened
Don't know what to say	They may already have an idea (expert patient)
Child doesn't need to know	They may have unfinished business – things they want to do or say
They won't understand	They may want to make a will if they are over the age of 12, or give instructions about their belongings in a less formal way
They wouldn't be able to cope	They may want to plan their funeral
They might ask difficult questions	They may want to say goodbye

> **Key learning**
>
> - The fears and beliefs of people both being cared for and acting as the carer will create barriers and challenges in end-of-life care conversations.
> - Situations of 'mutual pretence' and collusion create tensions in care for all concerned and need to be managed with honesty and sensitivity.

The power of language

Reluctance to communicate due to fear, having false beliefs and misconceptions, or assuming that you know what the question is about are some of the reasons that communication can break down. If such problems are not identified and resolved it can lead to a chain reaction of communication breakdown between yourself and the person or family members (Bunning 2011). This is described as a breakdown process – from the initial communication struggle through to the outcome and possible social implications, such as withdrawal and social isolation. This chain reaction and the potential outcomes highlight the crucial nature of consciously reflecting upon *all* aspects of any communication interaction, and this includes the words that you choose to use. Thinking about these before the situation arises can help you to be a little more prepared and to feel a bit more confident.

Euphemisms can make communication more complex or distressing, either at the time or subsequently when the true meaning becomes clear. Euphemisms can represent a struggle to express ideas; they can create a complex starting point when we consider all the terms and euphemisms that are associated with dying and death. Some euphemisms that have led to distressing conversations include 'he went to sleep' which resulted in a fear of falling asleep; 'he's gone to heaven' which raises questions about heaven and hell; 'he's with the angels' – so why them and not me?; 'the tumour/lump/mass' – but that's not *cancer*! There are many more examples like this, and you should try to avoid them. Most people can identify their own difficulty when trying to talk about dying and death, in particular with specific individuals such as children and people with cognitive impairments, but there are some other situations we want you to prepare for, and these are addressed in **Activity 6.5**.

> **Activity 6.5**
>
> With your field of nursing in mind, think about some of the ways that 'dying' and 'dead' are explained and the possible difficulties these terms may pose. Write down (and try saying out loud) the exact phrase you would use to explain someone is dying if talking to:
>
> - an elderly relative with a hearing impairment;
> - a school-age child, grandchild or sibling (5–10-year-old);
> - a pre-school age child, grandchild or sibling (2–4-year-old);
> - a teenager with a cognitive impairment;
> - someone with dementia;
> - someone with a learning disability;
> - a son or daughter with a mental health difficulty.

The key thing you are trying to achieve is mutual understanding – do you and the other person understand what is being communicated? Remember that in practice settings, communication is not only about the person understanding you and other staff, but also about you understanding the other person and their family members.

> **Key learning**
>
> - A person's current level of understanding or difficulties in communicating must be assessed.
> - Indicators may help you identify those who have a communication difficulty.

 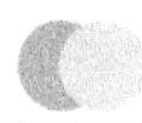

Impact of difficult communication situations on emotions

If communication breaks down, you must consider how this makes the person *and yourself* feel and behave. Behaviours demonstrated in difficult situations are often a way of expressing one's underlying emotions (e.g. frustration, anger, anxiety, fear, sadness, disappointment, grief). At times like this, we are once again in a position of considering the expression of communication by means of our body language and trying to understand the underlying communication message (Donnelly and Neville 2008).

Emotions are a normal physiological and psychological reaction to many complex health care situations, and that means our own emotions as well as those of others. The following points may help you in complex situations such as end-of-life care.

- Consider your own emotional state and your response to the other person's emotions – are you feeling upset, anxious, frightened, angry, sad, worried? How are you displaying these feelings to the other person?
- Acknowledge the emotion – recognize it and try to support, manage or diffuse it – emotions should not be ignored. For example, strong negative emotions such as anger may need to be diffused.
- Try to find out the cause of the emotion – it may not be what you think it is.
- Empathize with the other person – imagining what it must be like to be in their situation.
- Use your body language and speech – remember that earlier we mentioned that the largest part of what is communicated is by body language and then by voice, with only a small percentage by our actual words.
- Draw upon the humanistic models, such as Rogers (1951), Egan (1986) and Heron (1999). The three qualities advocated by Rogers are evident in humanistic models and highlight the complexity of interpersonal interactions, particularly in difficult situations. They are:
  - unconditional positive regard;
  - warmth and genuineness;
  - empathy.

Activity 6.6

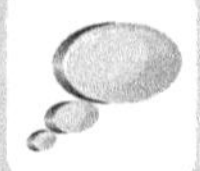

What is meant by the three qualities below suggested by Carl Rogers?

- Unconditional positive regard means . . .
- Warmth and genuineness means . . .
- Empathy means . . .

With your field of nursing in mind, identify a practice experience that you have been involved in or observed where these qualities were evident.

- What was it about this experience that highlighted unconditional positive regard for the other person?
- How did you or another person demonstrate empathy, warmth and genuineness?

Communicating and giving emotional support

Thinking about and adopting a humanistic model can help develop skills of *emotional support,* which along with *information* is one of the two essential elements of a health care conversation (Duke and Bailey 2008). These will depend on the context of the situation and the nature of the problem, but both must be there in the conversation to some degree or another for it to be a successful one. And another consistent feature of end-of-life conversations is the courage to be with people in distress, to offer empathy and try to 'hold' the distress with the person. It may seem obvious to say that you need to be kind, yet this is one of the things that patients and relatives complain about – that empathy is apparently lacking in their relationships with nurses (Kunyk and Olson 2001). Stories about lack of compassion or care make devastating reading (Triggle 2011).

The shape of the conversation

The structure of the conversation is as important as the tone. The shape of a *good* conversation contains a greeting, a farewell, an ending. Have you ever felt upset about someone walking away before the conversation seemed to have ended, or when someone has hung up the phone without saying goodbye? Again, it seems obvious, yet stories of poor practice – such as the visitor who asks a patient 'Who was that?' after a doctor's round only to be told 'I don't know' – are common. And nurses are no less guilty – we start conversations with 'I'm just here to take your blood pressure' without saying 'Hello' or 'How are you', or 'May I?'

As well as the greeting and the farewell, there are other interconnected stages in a health care conversation that will help to make it successful. A good conversation will normally have five stages (Duke and Bailey 2008):

- greetings and introductions;
- listening to and understanding the other person's story;
- exploring how this story might change and what this possibility feels like;
- agreeing a plan to manage the things that might cause the story to change;
- summarizing, providing follow-up and contact details, saying goodbye.

A good starting point when you are communicating with a patient about end-of-life care is to use some open-ended questions, but not too many. This enables you to develop an understanding about the person's perceptions and views. These are the sort of questions you can ask:

- What do *you* think might help the situation?
- What would *you* like to do?

The answers to such questions can help you as the professional to avoid assuming that you know what the person is feeling or needs, or jumping in with an unwelcome or untimely suggestion. These key supportive strategies are incorporated into models such as the Sage and Thyme model for supporting people in distress (Connolly *et al.* 2010), and using a model like this in one of the licensed training sessions can help staff develop confidence in emotional situations (**Box 6.1**).

Box 6.1 Sage and Thyme model

Setting – If you notice concern – create some privacy – sit down
Ask – 'Can I ask what you are concerned about?'
Gather – Gather all of the concerns – not just the first few
Empathy – Respond sensitively – 'You have a lot on your mind'
AND
Talk – 'Who do you have to TALK to or to help you?'
Help – 'How do they HELP?'
You – 'What do YOU think would help?'
Me – 'Is there something you would like ME to do?'
End – Summarize and close – 'Can we leave it there?'

Key learning !

- Conversations should contain the five essential elements: greeting, listening to the story, thinking about how things may change, agreeing a plan and summarizing the conversation before saying goodbye.
- Conversations need to contain both emotional support and information.
- Emotions are a normal reaction, but thinking about and recognizing the emotion before, during and after a conversation can help in the delivery of good care.

Breaking bad news

The Sage and Thyme model is useful when acknowledging, managing or containing distress, but is not a model for the breaking of significant bad news. For this, the SPIKES model (Baile *et al.* 2000) is the appropriate one. While the intent of these two models is different and they should not be confused with one another, they both contain the essential components of a good health care conversation identified by Duke and Bailey (2008).

Box 6.2 The six steps of SPIKES

- STEP 1: S – SETTING UP the interview
- STEP 2: P – Assessing the patient's PERCEPTION
- STEP 3: I – Obtaining the patient's INVITATION
- STEP 4: K – Giving KNOWLEDGE and information to the patient
- STEP 5: E – Addressing the patient's EMOTIONS with empathic responses
- STEP 6: S – STRATEGY and SUMMARY

Using models such as Sage and Thyme and SPIKES assumes that you have some key skills such as being able to reflect questions back to the person so that you can be certain the answer to their question really is what they're after. This is particularly important when being asked a question such as 'Am I dying?' You may want to respond to this question by asking, 'Can you tell me why you ask that?' This can help to clarify what is actually being asked. When the reply is 'I'm scared to go to sleep' or 'I need to make things better with my brother who I haven't spoken to for 20 years' you might find the response you were rehearsing ('Yes, I'm sorry but I think you have less time now than when we spoke at the end of your treatment'), is not where this conversation was going at all! While standard answers are not suitable for these situations there are certain skills that will help. **Figure 6.1** offers examples of how these might be phrased.

Key learning

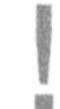

- Thinking about the words you choose to use before a situation arises can be helpful.
- Avoid euphemisms, which can cause misunderstandings and anxiety in others.
- Finding out what the person wants or thinks is key to supporting them.
- Using a model for a particular situation may be helpful in guiding the conversation and ensuring all the key things are thought about and addressed.

How can I manage to do all of this?

> Nurses' emotional commitment to their patients goes beyond what they may feel personally, and this contributes to the quality and excellence of nursing care . . . Experiencing emotions is considered essential for nurses to cope with morally difficult clinical situations (e.g. patients who refuse medical treatment) and to interact ethically and meaningfully with people in distress.
>
> (Huynh *et al.* 2008: 196)

What you will find is that this all takes effort, and the concept of emotional labour is wisely named, for labour it is. It can certainly be very demanding or draining to maintain an outward expression of calm safety while feeling uncertain and out of your depth (Gray 2008). Spontaneous emotional reactions to a situation need to be transformed into expressions of emotion that are acceptable both to society and the organization you are working in. This should lead you to think about the way you present yourself as a professional person, your 'work personna', and the way you express not just reactions to circumstances but also the deliberate

People respond to people who respond

STOP, LOOK, THINK
Resist the temptation to run!
Make eye contact and pay attention - *you are important*
Negotiate: 'Are you able to say what's worrying you?' = *I am willing to listen, but I can see it's hard and I don't want to distress you*

LISTEN, RESPOND
Silence: don't be afraid to be quiet and let the person gather their thoughts
Open questions: 'How are you feeling/what do you think about that?' = *I am interested/concerned*
Educated guesses: 'I imagine that came as quite a shock' = *I have an idea about how you might be feeling, do you want to talk to me about it?*
Prompt: 'Yes, go on' = *I'm still listening*
Acknowledge and reflect: 'You've had a rotten time by the sound of it' or 'You look/sound upset' = *how you feel matters, I can see you're upset, it's OK to tell me about it, I want to help*
Clarifying: 'What are the things about it that upset you?' = *I'd like to understand exactly what the problem is*

MAKE A PLAN, END THE CONVERSATION
Paraphrasing to sum up: 'Being ill has been really distressing/you really want to get some answers about this' = *I want you to know I've heard and I'm checking I've got it right*
Open directive questions: 'What's most important to you right now?' = *I think you might have concerns/needs and I want to help*
Summarizing: 'So what's most important is ... [list of things said]' = *I've heard you, have I got it right, have I missed anything out?*
Permission: 'Can I talk to someone about this?' = *I think you need more help than me, but I'd like your permission first*
Remember to close: 'I'm glad you talked to me, would you like me to come back/let you know when I've done...' = *it was all right to talk to me, you've given me things to do on your behalf and I know that you need to know when I do them*

©Kay Townsend, University of Southampton, 2011. Adapted from National End of Life Programme *Finding the Words*

Figure 6.1 Managing difficult conversations

expression of more deeply felt emotions (Huynh *et al.* 2008). This concept is relatively underdeveloped in nursing, but having a sense of what it is about may help you manage the labour it entails.

Activity 6.7

- Who helps you think about your work persona?
- Make a list of the people that you talk to about difficult situations, and how they help (e.g. listen, challenge, guide).
- Who do you help and support with their developing work persona?
- How often do you reflect on difficult situations from practice? What guides your reflections?

A work 'persona' helps nurses engage in emotional labour (Truc *et al.* 2009). Knowing what your work persona is like, that is, how it appears to others, what helped to form this 'nurse version' of you, and what influences the way your persona manages situations, will all help you develop your ability to labour emotionally. Social norms in work and the support you receive will help your persona develop, as will your work experience, your skills, how you view the nursing profession and of course the situation you work in, what sort of demands are made of you, how much you work alone or in a team and how complex your work is.

Conclusion

The guidance in this chapter has aimed to help guide your practice in difficult times. Remember that it takes courage to just 'be with someone', not talking or carrying out tasks. One of the most complex and difficult areas of practice is end-of-life conversations. Such communication can provoke a range of emotions both for you and the other person/people involved. The difficulties may be around fears, beliefs and misconceptions; both yours and the other person's. Having good conversations with those facing death and dying requires both preparation beforehand and reflection during and after the conversation. Communication is not only about you being understood by others, but about you understanding other people.

Communication involves the synchronization of what you are thinking, how you are feeling, and the expression of these thoughts and feelings in the words you use and your body language. It's not just what you say but the way that you say it. Body language is a major element in communication and your tone of voice and facial expressions will be remembered. Prevent confusion and misunderstanding by avoiding euphemisms.

Make sure you greet people, listen to their story and consider how their life is changing and how that makes them feel. Leave people with a sense that there is a plan, then summarize the conversation and make sure you say goodbye.

Importantly, look after yourself. Consciously think about your 'work persona', how it is perceived, how it is developing and how it helps you in your emotional labour.

Further reading and resources

Beale, E.A., Baile, W.F. and Aaron, J. (2005) Silence is not golden: communicating with children dying from cancer, *Journal of Clinical Oncology*, 23: 3629–31.

Duke, S. and Bailey, C. (2008) Communication: patient and family, in S. Payne, J. Seymour and C. Ingleton (eds) *Palliative Care Nursing: Principles and Evidence for Nursing*. Maidenhead: Open University Press.

Lambert V., Long T. and Kelleher, D. (2012) *Communication Skills for Children's Nurses*. Maidenhead: Open University Press.

McPherson, A. (2010) Involving children: why it matters, in S. Redsell and A. Hastings (eds) *Listening to Children and Young People in Healthcare Consultations*. Oxford: Radcliffe Publishing.

Petrie, P. (2011) *Communication Skills for Working with Children and Young People*. London: Jessica Kinglsey.

References

Atherton, H.L. and Crickmore, D.J. (eds) (2011) *Learning Disabilities Toward Inclusion*. Philadelphia, PA: Elsevier.

Baile, W., Buckman, R., Lenzi, R., Glober, G., Beale, E. and Kudelka, A. (2000) SPIKES – a six step protocol for delivering bad news: application to the patient with cancer, *Oncologist*, 5: 302–11.

Bluebond-Langner, M. (1978) *The Private Worlds of Dying Children*. Princeton, NJ: Princeton University Press.

Bunning, K. (2011) Let me speak – facilitating communication, in H.L. Atherton and D.J. Crickmore (eds) (2011) *Learning Disabilities: Toward Inclusion*. Philadelphia, PA: Elsevier.

Connolly, M., Perryman, J., McKenna, Y., Orford, J., Thomson, L., Shuttleworth, J. and Cocksedge, S. (2010) SAGE & THYME: a model for training health and social care professionals in patient-focussed support, *Patient Education and Counseling*, 79(1): 87–93.

Cooper, J. and Barnett, M. (2005) Aspects of caring for dying patients which cause anxiety to first year student nurses, *International Journal of Palliative Nursing*, 11(8): 423–30.

DH (Department of Health) (2008) *End of Life Care Strategy: Promoting High Quality Care for all Adults at the End of Life, Executive Summary*. London: The Stationery Office.

Donnelly, E. and Neville, L. (2008) *Communication and Interpersonal Skills*. Newton Abbot: Reflect Press.

Duke, S. and Bailey, C.D. (2008) Communication: patient and family, in S. Payne, J. Seymour and C. Ingleton (eds) *Palliative Care Nursing: Principles and Evidence for Practice*. Maidenhead: Open University Press.

Egan, G. (1986) *The Skilled Helper*. Pacific Grove, CA: Brooks/Cole.

Ekeberg, V. (2011) Mature care and the virtue of integrity, *Nursing Philosophy*, 12: 128–38.

Faulkner, A. (1998) Communication with patients, families and other professionals, in M. Fallon and B. O'Neill (eds) *ABC of Palliative Care*. London: BMJ Books.

Gray, B. (2008) The emotional labour of nursing – defining and managing emotions in nursing work, *Nurse Education Today*, 29(2): 168–75.

Hannon, L. and Clift, J. (2011) *General Hospital Care for People with Learning Disabilities*. Chichester: Wiley-Blackwell.

Heron, J. (1999) *The Complete Facilitators Handbook*. London: Kogan Page.

Heyland, D.K., Dodek, P., Rocker, G. *et al.* (2006) What matters most in end-of-life care: perceptions of seriously ill patients and their family members, *Canadian Medical Association Journal*, 174(5): 627–41.

Huynh, T., Alderson, M. and Thompson, M. (2008) Emotional labour underlying caring: an evolutionary concept analysis, *Journal of Advanced Nursing*, 64(2): 195–208.

Hwang, H.-L., Tu, C.-T., Chen, S. and Wang, H.-H. (2012) Caring behaviours perceived by elderly residents of long-term care facilities: scale development and psychometric assessment, *International Journal of Nursing Studies*, 49: 183–90.

Jonasson, L., Liss, P., Westerlind, B. and Berterö, C. (2010) Ethical values in caring encounters on a geriatric ward from the next of kin's perspective: an interview study, *International Journal of Nursing Practice*, 16: 20–6.

Kangasniemi, M. (2010) Equality as a central concept of nursing ethics: a systematic literature review, *Scandinavian Journal of Caring Sciences*, 24: 824–32.

Kübler-Ross, E. (1969) *On Death and Dying*. London: Macmillan.

Kunyk, D. and Olson, J.K. (2001) Clarification of conceptualizations of empathy, *Journal of Advanced Nursing*, 35(3): 317–25.

LaSala, C. and Bjarnason, D. (2010) Creating workplace environments that support moral courage, *Online Journal of Issues in Nursing*, 15.

McLean, C. (2012) The yellow brick road: a values based curriculum model, *Nurse Education in Practice*, 12: 159–63.

Melo, C.G. and Oliver, D. (2011) Can addressing death anxiety reduce health care workers' burnout and improve patient care? *Journal of Palliative Care*, 27(4): 287–95.

Morse, J.M., Solberg, S.M., Neander, W.L., Bottorff, J.L. and Johnson, J.L. (1990) Concepts of caring and caring as a concept, *Advances in Nursing Science*, 13(1): 1–14.

National End of Life Care Programme (2011a) *Finding the Words. Communication Skills Workbook*. London: The Stationery Office.

National End of Life Care Programme (2011b) *Talking About End of Life Care: Right Conversations, Right People, Right Time*. London: The Stationery Office.

NMC (Nursing and Midwifery Council) (2010) *Standards for Pre-registration Nursing Education*. London: NMC.

Payne, S., Seymour, J. and Ingleton, C. (eds) (2008) *Palliative Care Nursing: Principles and Evidence for Practice*. Maidenhead: Open University Press.

Piaget, J. (1929) *The Child's Conception of the World*. London: Routledge & Kegan Paul.

Putman, D.A. (2012) A reply to 'Skepticism about the virtue ethics approach to nursing ethics' by Stephen Holland: the relevance of virtue in nursing ethics, *Nursing Philosophy*, 13: 142–5.

Rogers, C.R. (1951) *Client Centered Therapy*. Boston, MA: Houghton Mifflin.

Silverman, P.R. (2000) *Never too Young to Know: Death in Children's Lives*. Oxford: Oxford University Press.

Skisland, A., Bjørnestad, J.O. and Söderhamn, O. (2012) Construction and testing of the Moral Development Scale for professionals, *Nurse Education Today*, 32: 255–60.

Triggle, N. (2011) NHS: elderly care dossier shows 'shameful attitudes'. BBC, London, available at: www.bbc.co.uk/news/health-15639046, accessed 7 May 2013.

Truc, H., Alderson, M. and Thompson, M. (2009) Emotional labour of nursing care: an evolutionary concept analysis, *Rech Soins Infirm*, 97: 34–49.

SECTION

3

Nursing practice and decision-making

An introduction to clinical decision-making in practice

7

Mary-Jane Baker

Chapter contents

Introduction

People make decisions all the time. What to eat, when to go to bed, what to wear . . . the list is endless. Some decisions we make without really thinking about them, but others prove more difficult, prompting us to consider options and make judgements about what might be the best decision in the circumstances presented.

Professional health care practice requires much decision-making and when you first start a programme of study leading to registration as a nurse, it can seem complex and confusing. It may be reassuring to understand that even experienced practitioners have difficulty in deciding what the right course of action might be at times, because caring for people can be complicated. However, complicated does not mean impossible, or even difficult – it just means that you have to observe carefully and think hard about what is going on and what you and others need to do. Making the right decision is very important as decisions have consequences – not only for you but also for colleagues and most importantly for those you care for.

In this chapter the NMC generic standard for competence in decision-making will be explored.

Domain 3: Nursing practice and decision-making Generic competence

All nurses must practise autonomously, compassionately, skilfully and safely, and must maintain dignity and promote health and wellbeing. They must assess and meet the full range of essential physical and mental health needs of people of all ages who come into their care. Where necessary they must be able to provide safe and effective immediate care to all people prior to accessing or referring to specialist services irrespective of their field of practice. All nurses must also meet more complex and coexisting needs for people in their own nursing field of practice, in any setting including hospital, community and at home. All practice should be informed by the best available evidence and comply with local and national guidelines. Decision-making must be shared with service users, carers and families and informed by critical analysis of a full range of possible interventions, including the use of up-to-date technology. All nurses must also understand how behaviour, culture, socioeconomic and other factors, in the care environment and its location, can affect health, illness, health outcomes and public health priorities and take this into account in planning and delivering care.

Regardless of your field of practice, this chapter will facilitate your understanding of the value of making appropriate decisions in clinical settings and what resources need to be accessed to help you make the best decision in the many and varied situations you will come across. It is not the intention to give you a series of answers to all clinical problems, but rather a toolkit for you to use as a professional resource for action. It may be useful to have a pencil and paper handy as you work through the chapter as you may wish to record your responses to the exercises offered. Indeed, if you have not already started to record your nursing activities, feelings and thoughts in a reflective log or journal of some kind, now may be a good time to begin.

Remember that this is a generic domain but it takes on field-specific qualities when applied to the needs of the particular client group you will encounter in your field of practice: child, adult, mental health and learning disability – as specified by the Nursing and Midwifery Council (NMC 2010). Additionally, further scrutiny of the other NMC domains will identify that decision-making is a core component of practice and central to the provision of excellent care.

What is clinical decision-making and what is the decision-making process?

To decide something means that you have reached a conclusion or determined an end point to your deliberations. According to Gambrill (1990), clinical decision-making is concerned with managing a range of information from diverse sources, to make professional judgements. Dowie (1993: 8) puts it more simply by explaining that judgements are 'the assessment of alternatives' whereas decisions require that one 'chooses between the alternatives presented'.

A variety of models which explain and clarify the decision-making process are available (Banning 2008). Of these, the hypothetico-deductive model described by Taylor (1997) has been a popular choice in nursing. It offers decision-making as a process in four stages, as shown in **Box 7.1** opposite.

A different model for clinical decision-making is offered by Junnola *et al.* (2002) who indicate that clinical decision-making is a process operating in two phases, starting with a diagnosis of a problem and moving on to problem management or action (see **Box 7.2** opposite).

Whatever model is used, it is clear that collecting information, assessing that information and making choices for action are all key aspects of the clinical decision-making process. See Junnola's 2 phase process.

The complexity of the context of decision-making

The number of activities involved in clinical decision-making, together with the added dimensions of critical thinking and problem-solving (Wainwright *et al.* 2011) give some insight into the breadth of skills required to do it well. Also, it must be remembered that decisions are made in a specific context and the influencing factors of any practice situation offer additional information, but with that, additional complexity. Gillespie (2010) helpfully divides the contextual influencing factors which are encountered when making nursing decisions into three levels (see **Box 7.3** p. 100). When starting out as a student nurse, it is likely that you already

Box 7.1 The four stages of the hypothetico-deductive model (Taylor 1997)

1 **Picking up available cues:** for example, this may include observing the patient for signs that tell you something about them, noting their age, facial expression, how ill they appear, any disabilities and how dependent or independent they are. In addition, patients can report symptoms to you, such as thirst or pain.

2 **Making hypotheses from those cues:** as your experience in clinical practice grows you will be able to make use of multiple cues to assess what is going on. You may begin to be able to assess what the underlying problem or issue is, or at least consider one or two possibilities which may be causing the patient's problem.

3 **Obtaining further information about each hypothesis to validate or invalidate them:** for example, while taking routine post-operative observations, you might note that a female patient has dry lips and looks flushed. She may be in pain and feeling nauseous and therefore unable to drink, making her become dehydrated. Questioning can help you better assess the situation, along with observations, noting fluid chart data and when analgesia was last given to the patient. Together this information will help you to form an idea of what is happening to the patient.

4 **Evaluating each hypothesis and then reaching a final diagnosis:** at this point you may decide the patient requires pain relief and an antiemetic that has been prescribed to solve the problems you have noted. As a student nurse you may find it helpful to check your diagnosis with your colleagues, mentor or a qualified practitioner.

have some experience of all these factors but perhaps the area where you feel most 'comfortable' and 'independent' initially is at the micro level.

By virtue of the fact that all interventions of care are derived from the decision-making process, it is easy to see why it has been described as the 'cornerstone of practice' (Flannery *et al.* 2011). To care for patients safely and effectively, it is essential that health care professionals understand the component parts of the decision-making process, their role in that process and the means to improve or attain skills to complete the process well and in different situations, time and time again. Looking at decision-making, in practical terms, the key stages of the process are summarized in **Box 7.4** opposite.

Key learning !

- An understanding of how decision-making is defined, the process involved in reaching a decision and evaluating that decision are central to providing effective and high quality care.

Box 7.2 Clinical decision-making as a two-phase process (Junnola *et al.* 2002)

Phase one	**Diagnostic**	■ Observation of the patient episode ■ Collection of data ■ Processing of data ■ Diagnosis or identification of the problem
Phase two	**Management**	■ Draw up a plan of action

Box 7.3 Influencing factors (Gillespie 2010)

Micro level	**The nurse–patient relationship** All patients are individuals and knowing about the person, their preferences and responses to care, including their own resources, will be important and impact on clinical decisions made. In addition, as a student, your own experience, confidence, along with knowing your own strengths, limitations and learning needs will be significant in how you approach making decisions.
Meso level	**The working environment and other personnel** As a student, communicating and collaborating with other appropriate staff in the working environment is important and an understanding of the clinical environment and culture will be needed. There may be challenges in terms of constraints, such as workload and other interruptions, or limitation of time and resources which will impact on what decision is possible to carry through.
Macro level	**Professional and political factors** As a student you will need to be aware of the NMC competencies and code of practice (NMC 2008) which impact on what you do in practice and on the decisions you make. It is worth remembering that there are many factors which will impact on and influence priorities in health care decision-making which relate to other professional, political and social drivers.

Box 7.4 Key stages of the decision-making process

- Interpret the context (i.e. ask 'What is happening?')
- Identify the purpose or goal (i.e. ask 'What do I want to happen?')
- Consider what resources are available (i.e. ask 'What do I already know about the person/the context/the situation?')
- Clarify what other resources you need (i.e. ask 'What else do I need to know and where can I get this information/help?')
- Gather your resources together
- Evaluate your resources (i.e. ask 'Is this evidence relevant to the situation and if it is relevant, is it useful?')
- In cases where you have more than one useful resource, decide which resource/piece of evidence is *most* useful *now* to attain your goal/purpose
- Confirm to yourself why this is the case
- Inform the patient and everyone else involved what you intend to do
- Receive feedback and adapt your actions accordingly
- Reflect on the decision-making process (i.e. ask yourself 'Did that event go well/badly/as expected?')

 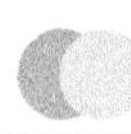

> **Activity 7.1**
>
> - Consider an activity in which you made some decisions today and involved other people (such as a conversation, a journey or a shared meal).
> - Can you frame that activity so that it becomes a scenario with a beginning and an end (e.g. I felt hungry, I ate something and I did not feel hungry any more)?
> - Now, apply the stages **Box 7.1** to your scenario and see what you come up with.

In **Activity 7.1** it is likely that the first two stages did not take you very long to do, but what about the others? The first two stages are in the diagnostic phase of decision-making and the rest are in the management phase. In a situation where something is so familiar, like having a meal, it may be strange to break down the activity in this way but hopefully you defined some actions that uncover the intricacies of the decisions we make without really thinking about them (e.g. what you ate, why you ate the amount you did at the time you did, and so on).

> **Activity 7.2**
>
> Now look at the following scenario and apply the stages again.
>
> Catherine Lessing is a 62-year-old who was admitted earlier today on your ward. You are asked to take and record Mrs Lessing's observations. You have not met Mrs Lessing before. When you go up to see her, she is sitting on her own by her bed and you notice that she is crying.

In applying the stages in **Activity 7.2** you may have come up with a number of alternative plans of action and also have some questions that need to be answered with more detailed information. Perhaps your process includes the factors and considerations suggested in **Table 7.1** on the next page.

Reflecting on your decision-making processes

In your response to **Activity 7.2**, you may have given some rationale for your thoughts (as in the example) but it is interesting and important to note what factors influence *your* decision-making. What you have just done in the activity is a process called 'thinking aloud' (Ness *et al.* 2010) which is a particularly useful way to clarify your purpose, the situation and your resources and consider how they fit together. Interestingly, the process of decision-making in this scenario necessitated a change of purpose from the original one planned. This, in turn, meant that pre-planned resources needed to be altered and new ones added to ensure the best outcome at this time. This 'shifting situation' can often happen in clinical practice and the speed with which you decide to act in such circumstances is dependent on your skills and experience in considering the factors influencing the situation and in doing a number of activities, seemingly simultaneously (see **Box 7.5** p. 103).

> **Activity 7.3**
>
> In considering your ability in each aspect, try to offer an example from your practice that supports your assertion. How skilled are you at changing practice situations? Look at **Box 7.5**, p. 103 and take a few moments to give yourself a score out of 10 for each of the activities listed, where '10' means that you have considerable skill and '1' denotes an area that you feel you do not do well at the moment. If you give yourself a score of 70 (i.e. 10/10 for each activity) you have done very well. However, there is always something new and useful to learn and everyone can extend their competence in decision-making, so please complete the activity honestly and then read on.

Table 7.1 Possible stages of decision-making

Stage	**Thoughts**	**Level of influencing factors (Gillespie 2010)**
Interpret the context: what do you observe and what does it mean? (i.e. ask 'What is happening'?)	The patient is crying. I do not know the reason for this.	Micro
Identify the purpose or goal (i.e. ask 'What do I want to happen'?)	I want to introduce myself and find out why the patient is crying. I want to take and record her observations.	Micro
Consider what resources are available (i.e. ask 'What do I already know about the person/context/situation?')	I know the name and age of the patient and what she has been admitted for (as I heard this at handover). I know that she has been admitted today. She is sitting on her own but her bed is in a six-bedded area and other patients occupy the other beds.	Micro and meso
Clarify what other resources you need (i.e. ask 'What else do I need to know and where can I get this information/ help?')	I need to know why she is crying to see if I can help her. I need to give the patient some privacy. I may be able to ask the patient. I may be able to find information out from her charts and care plan at the end of the bed. I still need to do her observations so should I get the equipment for this ready? I may need to get the help of another member of staff.	Micro and meso
Gather your resources together	I am a resource as I have a legitimate reason to talk to and have some limited knowledge of the patient. The patient is distressed but appears able to speak. There is a box of tissues on the patient's locker. There are curtains that could be pulled around the bed space. The patient's care plan and charts are available at the end of the bed. The necessary equipment to take and record the observations is with me. There is a call bell by the bed. My mentor knows that I am with this patient.	Micro, meso and some macro (with professional accountability issues acknowledged)
Evaluate your resources (i.e. ask 'Is this evidence relevant to the situation and if it is relevant, is it useful?')	All the resources I have identified are relevant to the situation but I am not sure how useful the equipment for taking and recording the observations is at this time. I do not think that this is an emergency at the moment so I may not need to use the call bell.	Micro and meso
In cases where you have more than one useful resource, decide which resource/piece of evidence is *most* useful *now* to attain your goal/purpose	I think that there are a few very useful resources at this time: the patient, myself and the curtains around the bed.	Micro and meso

Table 7.1 Possible stages of decision-making (*Continued*)

Stage	**Thoughts**	**Level of influencing factors (Gillespie 2010)**
Confirm to yourself why this is the case	The resources are helpful because my overriding purpose now is to find out why the patient is crying and to try to help her	Micro
Inform the patient and everyone else involved what you intend to do	I will approach the patient gently, asking if I can sit with her. I will introduce myself and state that I have noticed that she appears to be upset. I will offer to close the curtains around her bed. I may hold the patient's hand.	Micro and meso
Receive feedback and adapt your actions accordingly	Hopefully the patient will acknowledge and accept my presence but if not, I would have to act on her cues and take action accordingly (go back to the beginning of the decision-making process)	Micro
Reflect on the decision-making process (i.e. ask yourself 'Did that event go well/as expected?')	If the patient is able to tell me what is upsetting her I may be able to help her and I would say that the process had gone well, particularly if I knew I had given her the required privacy, listened to her, acted professionally and with kindness and taken further action as a result of what she told me.	Micro, meso and macro

Box 7.5 Skilled activities in changing practice situations

	Your score
• Picking up cues by making detailed observations of the situation (the scenario started with these). • Having a sense of purpose (your intervention intention/tentative hypothesis). • Clarifying what resources are available to you – what you know, what you may know and what you need to know (about the situation, the possible outcomes and the subsequent possible course(s) of action). • Focusing on the specifics of the situation and organizing your resources into some order. • Setting priorities and making choices with confidence. • Practising skilled two-way communication. • Reflecting on (in or before) practice. **Total score =**	

Key learning

- Understanding what you are already good at and what you might do better at is the first step to understanding how to make good decisions in clinical practice.

The chapter now explores some of the specific concepts already outlined, offering practical tips which will support you in clinical practice and help you consider what can be improved when you have clinical decisions to make.

Picking up cues

The clinical decision-making process is initiated when the nurse recognizes or picks up cues from a patient or clinical situation. These can take the form of something expected or unexpected and provide data for the nurse to process. Cues enable a situation to be understood more fully and it may sound easy, but consider **Activity 7.4** and identify the important cues or information for you to be able to decide the best course of action.

Activity 7.4

A patient complains of feeling nauseated and seems distressed and agitated. From what you already know about the patient, this is unusual. They have no dietary or fluid restrictions and appear to have eaten a normal lunch. They have taken their prescribed medication. It is visiting time on the unit.

- List the pieces of data you can gather from this scenario.
- What do you consider the possible reasons for the patient's condition?
- From the information you have, what would you do next?

The problem with the scenario in **Activity 7.4** is that, of course, you do not have enough information and your first action would probably be to find out more by assessing the situation with the patient (Standing 2007). That includes talking and listening to them, looking at patient notes and records and conferring with other members of staff. This highlights the value and importance of communication as a skill to access and share the information you require.

However, it is also possible to have too much information. Certainly when you start your nursing career, you may feel bombarded with information and until you get to a point where you can discriminate between useful and non-useful information, the number of cues or data you collect can be vast and confusing. Being discerning with cue collection is an important skill but one that must be balanced with care, so that you collect enough information and avoid jumping to conclusions. For instance, as a nurse, I may have omitted to note that the medication taken by the patient had been newly prescribed (and nausea may be a common side-effect) or that I was unaware that the patient was anxious about an expected visit of a relative.

In practical terms then, to maximize your ability for cue collection, you need to use skills of communication to collect as many cues as you can, but try to place these into some semblance of order of importance based upon:

- where you got the information from (the source);
- whether the cue has the breadth to encompass the activity in the scenario (the scope);
- whether the cue is relevant; and
- whether the cue reminds you of a previous experience (pattern recognition) to help you assign meaning to the current situation.

Having a sense of purpose/being clear in your plan

Florence Nightingale identified the essential nature of knowing the outcome of each intervention to be able to plan effective care (1946). The hypothetico-deductive model described

earlier identifies this stage of the decision-making process as hypotheses formation. An hypothesis is a proposal or something you believe may be a possible outcome to a situation. Previous experience of a similar situation may help you here but you cannot experience everything, therefore you require skills to be able to build a picture of possibilities (Huckabay 2009).

At a basic level you may only be able to offer a 'best guess' in a situation but even in these circumstances you must ensure that a safe outcome results. To do this you must, wherever possible, involve the patient and/or others in the plan to get guidance and support that the chosen action is acceptable and patient focused. Involvement of others offers the opportunity for more options (which you may or may not think you want), but as a collaborative process is one that enables the acknowledgement of the ethical requirements of decision-making (Trede and Higgs 2003) and keeps the process 'real' (Elwyn and Miron-Shatz 2009). It also gives the opportunity for 'rehearsal' (Ness *et al.* 2010) which diminishes aspects of risk through trial and error and promotes the choice of safe options.

Key learning !

- When making any decision it is helpful to clarify your purpose, the situation and the available resources and to consider how they fit together.

Identifying available sources of knowledge

Botti and Reeve (2003) support the work of Tanner *et al.* (1987) who suggest that knowledge is the best resource that one can access when making clinical decisions and the more knowledge one has the better should be the skills in both cue collection and hypothesis formation. However, there are different types of knowledge; so you need to have an understanding of how knowledge is classified. A seminal paper by Carper (1978) described that nurses knew more than they could communicate to others. Carper was doubtful that scientific or factual knowledge alone could explain all aspects of nursing practice. Recognizing that the complexities of nursing practice had not been well explained in the past, Carper offered a new way to illuminate the patterns of knowing that nurses operated within. Although Carper's paper is dated, the patterns of knowing in **Table 7.2** (on the next page) have been added to by authors such as Munhall (1993), White (1995) and Chinn and Kramer (2008), and still reflect contemporary practice.

In summary these ideas are intended to highlight the fact that when decisions are made in clinical practice, you will have a broad range of knowledge bases on which to draw. Sometimes this can make it feel difficult to know what is the 'best action' in any particular situation. There may also be times when as a student you may be challenged to appreciate the decisions made by patients, relatives, professional colleagues and even government policies. For example, the decision of a patient to refuse treatment such as a blood transfusion, or the difficulty of deciding how best to provide care for a group of elderly clients when there is a limited financial budget.

Key learning !

- Knowledge acquisition, utilization and recognition is complex.
- Nurses must personally declare what knowledge they use, identify if the use of any sources of knowledge has been neglected and consider how they can enhance the utilization of new/different forms of knowledge to nurture clinical curiosity and engender confidence in using resources effectively within clinical decision-making processes.

Table 7.2 Patterns of knowing

Pattern of knowing	Description	Author(s)
Empirical	Based on the assumption that what is known can be measured and tested scientifically. Reality exists and can be demonstrated through observation. When making decisions in clinical practice nurses can draw on factual information such as that derived from research studies and theory.	Carper 1978
Ethical	Based upon experiential knowledge of social values and ethical reasoning that guides and directs the conduct of practice. Ethical knowing requires nurses to have an understanding of ethical matters (e.g. obligation and consequentially) and the philosophical positions of deontology (duty), autonomy and social justice.	Carper 1978
Personal	Nurses have personal knowledge based on self-awareness and use of self in practice. It is dynamic and continues to be developed and extended through reflection on their practice, and remains open to learning more about ourselves through new experiences. Personal knowledge is demonstrated in nurses' personal attitudes and attributes.	Carper 1978
Aesthetic	Nurses have a deep understanding of the whole situation, and can develop the ability to bring together both the science and the art of care and interaction to implement confident, competent and skilled performance.	Carper 1978
Unknowing	Unknowing specifically concerns the understanding of the patient's perspective and a setting aside of personal beliefs and values until the patient's view is known.	Munhall 1993
Sociopolitical	This pattern of knowing was added by White to acknowledge the political and social context of care influenced by economic constraints and government policy. Issues of power are involved, not only in whose voice is heard but whose voice is silent. When a decision is made, do you acknowledge the patient voice or the governmental voice?	White 1995
Emancipatory	Based on the assumption that, through critical reflection, nurses can understand and use all the patterns of knowing to deliver and achieve holistic patient care.	Chinn and Kramer 2008

 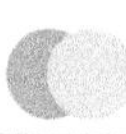

Activity 7.5

Consider a scenario from your recent practice where you were caring for a patient or client. Write it down as a story about what happened (taking care not to mention the names of patients or clinical settings). It does not need to be very long, in fact limit your writing to just one intervention/episode of care that you were involved in. Now look at what you have recorded.

- What was the intervention?
- How did you 'decide' what to do?
- Identify how you 'knew' what was the correct course of action
- Was it because you had been taught what to look out for?
- Did you use a specific type of knowledge or way of knowing?
- What were the ethical dimensions in the decision-making process?
- How did you collaborate with the patient?
- How did you use yourself (your personal knowledge) in the interaction?

Now decide which form of knowledge you used most and which form you used least, or not at all. If there are aspects of knowledge that you do not regularly use when making clinical decisions, write these down to act as an *aide-mémoire* and think how you might incorporate different 'ways of knowing' to build your knowledge repertoire.

It is hard to analyse one's own practice but in doing so one can discover areas that require further attention in order to offer a balanced approach to making decisions confidently and competently.

Using evidence in decision-making for care

In making person-centred judgements, nurses must use up-to-date knowledge and evidence to assess, plan, deliver and evaluate care, communicate findings, influence change and promote health and best practice (NMC 2010: 26). The move towards evidence-based practice (EBP) in health care is demonstrated in the evidence used to underpin protocols and procedures and this is seen as a positive means to offer equitable and safe care for all patients. With regard to decision-making, the use of protocols has been found to be most helpful for novice/new nurses in making decisions, as it enables standard hypotheses or diagnoses to be described for specific cases, together with accompanying guidance for the access, choice and use of resources in the form of knowledge and evidence (Manias *et al.* 2005). As such, these standard cases and responses limit the range of possible options for action (cue acquisition, hypothesis formation and resource/evidence selection) and provide novice nurses with 'certainty' and confidence to proceed. This is understandable given that errors in decision-making usually occur in previously unknown situations and without specialist knowledge and experience (Flannery *et al.* 2011).

Nevertheless, nurses must be aware of the dangers of following protocols and procedures unthinkingly, for in so doing may lie the road to complacency and a lack of awareness of confounding factors that make a usual situation unexpected or unusual. Unthinking decision-making denies the nurse the opportunity for taking the wider view (Manias *et al.* 2005; Kinchin *et al.* 2008) and complacency is the enemy of skilled nursing in that it can stifle clinical curiosity and diminish the ability to problem-solve. Nurses have access to many different forms of knowledge which they should utilize to care for patients holistically. You must access and use these to keep an open mind and to provide the breadth of care options that best benefit the patients in your care (Kinchin *et al.* 2008; Thompson and Kagan 2011).

Key learning

- Using best evidence to inform decision-making in practice can be supported by the use of protocols and procedures when used appropriately.

Decision-making: being organized in your thoughts and actions

In clinical decision-making, being organized is largely dependent on clear thinking about the specifics of:

- why you are doing something;
- what needs to be done to complete the task; and
- what constraints (such as time or concurrent activities) may impose upon the situation.

This clarity of thought is what makes the difference between those who are organized and those who are disorganized – being single-minded about a specific goal and the actions to achieve it. However, the unpredictable and fast-paced environment of clinical practice offers a different arena where 'clear thinking' may be hard work for everyone, particularly when, as a student, you are trying to learn the ropes. Translating actions to be taken into problems to be solved has been suggested as a useful mechanism to throw specific situations into relief and provide some shape and boundary to them (Standing 2007), thus providing a more manageable structure within which to arrange one's thoughts.

Experienced practitioners or 'experts' who have been working in practice for some time may seem to be 'more organized' than less experienced colleagues or student nurses. Sometimes student nurses are referred to as 'novices' or 'advanced beginners' and certainly there is a wealth of literature and much debate on this subject (Benner 1984; Rashotte and Carnevale 2004; Bakalis and Watson 2005; Flannery *et al.* 2011). For the purposes of relating it to decision-making here, it is understood that experienced practitioners are usually more able to see problems clearly and quickly because they recognize them as similar to, or reminiscent of, something they have encountered before. This 'pattern recognition' or intuitive practice is something that you may have witnessed or indeed experienced yourself, and its benefits include the ability to clarify specific problems and quickly identify the resources needed.

If you find it hard to 'see the wood for the trees', ask for help (Ladyshewsky 2002). Peer and mentor support can help you to organize your thoughts and actions, for example to clarify the scope of a problem and identify the specific resources required to resolve it. This can be invaluable while you develop your own portfolio of experience and confidence in this area. Meanwhile, consider the organizational attributes you already hold and those you need to hone.

Setting priorities and making choices

Deciding on what to do first indicates that there is an order of activity in all situations. When you are caring for a number of patients or clients your caseload or list of activities needs to be organized and prioritized in some way. Even when you are caring for one client at a time, the care they require will need to be managed in a way that makes best use of the resources available and provides efficient, effective and safe care.

The parameters for applying priorities to care are usually influenced by two main factors: the *critical nature* of the situation and *time* (Hendry and Walker 2004). In an emergency situation, these two factors are synonymous as the overriding priority is patient safety and the order and timeliness of nurses' interventions take on particular significance. However, considerations of time can have individual significance for care, even when the situation is not critical – i.e. when getting a patient bathed and dressed. Deciding upon priorities of care in a clinical situation requires skill in assessing risk and the ability to take appropriate steps to minimize the predicted risk by timely intervention. When setting priorities it is important to recognize that practice will always have elements of certainty and uncertainty. Where there is certainty and risk may be accurately predicted, protocols and procedures may objectify the logical reasoning process and assist in setting priorities of care, however, where the clinical situation is less certain, individual and locally tailored clinical judgement may need to operate.

To enhance your skills for accurate risk assessment and sound clinical decision-making

 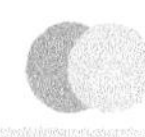

it is important to be aware of your personal attributes – strengths and shortcomings that you bring to the decision-making process – and learn to identify opportunities that help you make good decisions in clinical practice (e.g. people, clients, research, evidence or experiences). This self-knowledge of what might influence your decision-making is important, but remember that seeking and using help and support to build your confidence is invaluable, not only as a student but during your professional career (Thompson *et al.* 2007).

Key learning

- While developing your skills in making clinical decisions you can always invite others to support you by asking them for comments on your diagnosis of the situation and your plan for action.

Communication, reflection and decision-making

It is assumed that you come to this section of the chapter with knowledge of both the theory and practice of skilled communication as detailed in earlier chapters. The emphasis of communication in relation to clinical decision-making is one of collaborative working and inclusivity where all parties involved in the situation should also be involved in the decision-making process. The involvement of patients and your ability to work with them in the decision-making process is vital for the following key reasons:

- it allows you to gain necessary consent for procedures;
- it enables cooperation when giving care;
- the patient can contribute to goal-setting and achievement;
- the patient can offer their own knowledge and expertise.

For collaboration to be achieved successfully, clear two way communication is key.

The systematic processes offered by models of reflection offer practitioners the opportunity to articulate, scrutinize and document their decision-making practice in detail. The relevance of this activity is illuminated by Boud *et al.*'s (1985) definition of reflection as an opportunity to turn experience into learning, a sentiment that is echoed by the work of Johns (1995). According to Rashotte and Carnevale (2004) this notion of transformational learning for individuals who have had clinical experience is fundamental for good decision-making in practice. The practical benefits of reflection are outlined by Huckabay (2009), who highlights that nurses cannot experience every situation, yet working in the changing context of practice they must develop a repertoire for transferring learning from one situation to another. Reflection offers you an opportunity to build a portfolio of experience as a means of surfacing and articulating experiential knowledge that may be recorded and reviewed. It is always valuable to reflect on cases where your decision-making has resulted in positive outcomes for the patient and/or others, in order to critically analyse and learn from them and apply that learning to future situations.

There are a number of models of reflection which take you step-by-step through the deconstruction, scrutiny and reconstruction phases at varying levels of complexity. The model by Driscoll (2000) operates within a simple framework using three headings, as illustrated in **Table 7.3**.

By engaging with reflective processes, your practice will enter a new domain, for by constantly scrutinizing and questioning your own practice you will develop the clinical curiosity and observational skills that are so vital to decision-making. Also, deeper engagement with practice may provide you with the realization that, as a health care professional, at whatever stage in your pre-registration programme, you are playing an integral and vital role in increasingly complex health care situations.

Table 7.3 Stages of reflection model (Driscoll 2000)

Stage	**Explanation**	
What	Description of the details of what happened in the scenario	Deconstruction
So what?	Critical exploration of the details described (feelings/actions/ consequences)	Investigation
Now what?	Identification of the implications for future practice (learning) with rationale	Reconstruction

Moving forward

Looking back at your progress through the chapter, I hope you can see how gaining competence in clinical decision-making involves understanding yourself, understanding how you learn and a rehearsal of the component parts of the decision-making process. To take this work forward you may find the following suggestions helpful.

- Consider how you learn; your personal learning style.
- Hone your skills of patient observation and clinical assessment in practice.
- Don't jump to conclusions. Take time to consider the possibilities and options open to you and the care of your patients.
- Get help if necessary but don't necessarily go for the quickest option.
- Use your peers. Problem-solving, particularly priority-setting, is often better done in a group.
- Choose to work with people who challenge and test you. Mentors are very important to help you hone your decision-making skills – try to get a good one who you may observe in action making sound decisions and then ask them to uncover why they chose the decision they did.
- Keep up to date with new developments and nurture a critical stance. Botti and Reeve (2003) linked academic achievement with better ability to reach a reasonable and swift decision – certainly in simple cases but particularly in complex ones where confounding factors were present to 'test' the decision-making process.
- Consolidate what you know. Getting to know a clinical setting and the associated care options of patients within that setting enables nurses to focus and add depth to their knowledge of particular specific clinical situations (Bakalis and Watson 2005). Consolidation of knowledge in a setting can offer personal and professional confidence in decision-making in that setting.
- Look after yourself. Bakalis and Watson (2005) propose that psychological stress is potentiated in high stress areas such as critical care where decisions are high risk due to the complexity of illness, new technology (keeping up to date) and increased morbidity and mortality.
- Keep a reflective journal or log. Use a mind map within your reflective log to identify the influencing factors involved in the scenarios (Kinchin *et al.* 2008). Journal entries will help to build a record of experience. Reflection on these entries will assist you to uncover the knowledge sources you access and the subsequent outcomes from action.

In summary:

- This chapter has offered you the opportunity to review the component parts of clinical decision-making as a process.
- It has enabled you to consider your own decision-making abilities in relation to each component part.
- Your use of the activities within the chapter will start, or maintain and continue, your reflective journey through understanding what you know and what you need to know to develop and nurture your increasing competence and confidence in decision-making in practice.

Further reading and resources

Standing, M. (2011) *Clinical Judgment and Decision Making for Nursing Students.* London: Sage.

http://shareddecisionmaking.health.org.uk. This resource centre is designed to support individuals and teams to put shared decision-making into practice through systems and processes, skills and behaviours of staff, social marketing and patient support. It offers a 'one stop' portal for shared decision-making, and advice on navigating these resources, based on learning from the UK and linked to international research.

References

Bakalis, N.A. and Watson, R. (2005) Nurses' decision-making in clinical practice, *Nursing Standard,* 19(23): 33–9.

Banning, M. (2008) A review of clinical decision making: models and current research, *Journal of Clinical Nursing*, 17(2): 187–95.

Benner, P. (1984) *From Novice to Expert: Excellence and Power in Clinical Nursing Practice.* Menlo Park, CA: Addison-Wesley.

Botti, M. and Reeve, R. (2003) Role of knowledge and ability in student nurses' clinical decision-making, *Nursing and Health Sciences*, 5: 39–49.

Boud, D., Keogh, R. and Walker, D. (eds) (1985) *Reflection: Turning Experience into Learning.* Abingdon: Routledge.

Carper, B. (1978) Fundamental patterns of knowing in nursing, *Advances in Nursing Science*, 1(1): 13–23.

Chinn, P. and Kramer, M. (2008) *Integrated Theory and Knowledge Development in Nursing*, 7th edn. St Louis, MO: Mosby Elsevier.

Dowie, J. (1993) Would decision analysis eliminate medical accidents? in C. Vincent, M. Ennis and R. Audley (eds) *Medical Accidents.* Oxford: Oxford University Press.

Driscoll, J. (2000) *Practising Clinical Supervision.* Edinburgh: Bailliere Tindall.

Elwyn, G. and Miron-Shatz, T. (2009) Deliberation before determination: the definition and evaluation of good decision making, *Health Expectations*, 13: 139–47.

Flannery Wainwright, S., Shepard, K., Harman, L. and Stephens, J. (2011) Factors that influence the clinical decision making of novice and experienced physical therapists, *Physical Therapy*, 91(1): 87–101.

Gambrill, E. (1990) *Critical Thinking in Clinical Practice.* Oxford: Jossey-Bass.

Gillespie, M. (2010) Using the situated clinical decision-making framework to guide analysis of nurses' clinical decision-making, *Nurse Education in Practice*, 10: 333–40.

Hendry, C. and Walker, A. (2004) Priority setting in clinical nursing practice: a literature review, *Journal of Advanced Nursing*, 47(4): 427–36.

Huckabay, L. (2009) Clinical reasoned judgement and the nursing process, *Nursing Forum*, 44(2): 72–8.

Johns, C. (1995) Framing learning through reflection within Carper's fundamental ways of knowing in nursing, *Journal of Advanced Nursing*, 22(2): 226–34.

Junnola, T., Eriksson, E., Salantera, S. and Lauri, S. (2002) Nurses' decision-making in collecting information for the assessment of patients' nursing problems, *Journal of Clinical Nursing*, 11: 186–96.

Kinchin, I., Cabot, L. and Hay, D. (2008) Using concept mapping to locate the tacit dimension of clinical expertise: towards a theoretical framework to support critical reflection on teaching, *Learning in Health and Social Care*, 7(2): 93–104.

Ladyshewsky, R. (2002) A quasi-experimental study of the differences in performance and clinical reasoning using individual learning versus reciprocal peer coaching, *Physiotherapy Theory and Practice*, 18: 17–31.

Manias, E., Aitken, R. and Dunning, T. (2005) How graduate nurses use protocols to manage patients' medications, *Journal of Clinical Nursing*, 14: 935–44.

Munhall, P. (1993) 'Unknowing': towards another pattern of knowing in nursing, *Nursing Outlook*, 41(3): 125–8.

Ness, V., Duffy, K., McCallum, J. and Price, L. (2010) Supporting and mentoring nursing students in practice, *Nursing Standard*, 25(1): 41–6.

Nightingale, F. (1946) *Notes on Nursing. What it is and What it is Not.* Philadelphia, PA: Lippincott.

NMC (Nursing and Midwifery Council) (2008) *The Code: Standards of Conduct, Performance and Ethics for Nurses and Midwives.* London: NMC.

NMC (Nursing and Midwifery Council) (2010) *Standards for Pre-registration Nursing Education*. London: NMC.

Rashotte, J. and Carnevale, F. (2004) Medical and nursing clinical decision making: a comparative epistemological analysis, *Nursing Philosophy*, 5: 160–74.

Standing, M. (2007) Clinical decision-making skills on the developmental journey from student to registered nurse: a longitudinal inquiry, *Journal of Advanced Nursing*, 60(3): 257–69.

Tanner, C., Padrick, K., Westfall, U. and Putzier, D. (1987) Diagnostic reasoning strategies of nurses and nursing students, *Nursing Research*, 36: 358–63.

Taylor, C. (1997) Problem solving in clinical nursing practice, *Journal of Advanced Nursing*, 26(2): 329–31.

Thompson, C., Bucknall, T., Estabrookes, C., Hutchinson, A., Fraser, K., de Vos, R., Binnecade, J., Barrat, G. and Saunders, J. (2007) Nurses' critical event risk assessments: a judgement analysis, *Journal of Clinical Nursing*, 18: 601–12.

Thompson, H. and Kagan, S. (2011) Clinical management of fever by nurses: doing what works, *Journal of Advanced Nursing*, 67(2): 359–70.

Trede, F. and Higgs, J. (2003) Re-framing the clinician's role in collaborative clinical decision making: re-thinking practice knowledge and the notion of clinician-patient relationships, *Learning in Health and Social Care*, 2(2): 66–73.

White, J. (1995) Patterns of knowing: review, critique and update, *Advances in Nursing Science*, 17(4): 73–86.

8

Advanced decision-making: involving patients and relatives in decisions on care

Jackie Bridges

Chapter contents

Introduction

> When confronted with complex or unfamiliar clinical situations, novice nurses frequently respond by drawing on theoretical knowledge and psychomotor skills, rather than enacting decision-making that addresses the complex and multidimensional nature of the situation. Further, when novices lack confidence in the clinical setting, they may rely excessively on more experienced nurses and avoid situations that require them to make decisions.
>
> (Gillespie and Paterson 2009: 164)

If this passage rings any bells with you and reflects in any way your own experiences in decision-making, be assured that with time and effort clinical decision-making will get easier. As your experience grows, and as you effectively draw out learning from reflecting on your experiences, your own skills will improve, enabling you to make the best decisions for, and with, your patients and their families. However, the way we make decisions can remain prone to errors, regardless of how experienced we become. In addition, we need to consider how to effectively involve patients and their families in decisions about their care and treatment, and not just assume that we know what is best for them.

Throughout this chapter, you will be able to build on what you have read and learned in Chapter 7 and specifically can:

- find out how experts make decisions;
- explore the concept of bias and how it can influence your clinical decision-making;
- identify how you can effectively involve patients and families in decisions about treatment and care.

This chapter addresses Nursing and Midwifery Council (NMC) competencies 1, 2, 3, 4, 8 and 10.

Domain 3 Nursing practice and decision-making (NMC 2010: 17–19)

1 All nurses must use up-to-date knowledge and evidence to assess, plan, deliver and

evaluate care, communicate findings, influence change and promote health and best practice. They must make person-centred, evidence-based judgements and decisions, in partnership with others involved in the care process, to ensure high quality care. They must be able to recognise when the complexity of clinical decisions requires specialist knowledge and expertise, and consult or refer accordingly.

2 All nurses must possess a broad knowledge of the structure and functions of the human body, and other relevant knowledge from the life, behavioural and social sciences as applied to health, ill health, disability, ageing and death. They must have an in-depth knowledge of common physical and mental health problems and treatments in their own field of practice, including co-morbidity and physiological and psychological vulnerability.

3 All nurses must carry out comprehensive, systematic nursing assessments that take account of relevant physical, social, cultural, psychological, spiritual, genetic and environmental factors, in partnership with service users and others through interaction, observation and measurement.

4 All nurses must ascertain and respond to the physical, social and psychological needs of people, groups and communities. They must then plan, deliver and evaluate safe, competent, person-centred care in partnership with them, paying special attention to changing health needs during different life stages, including progressive illness and death, loss and bereavement.

8 All nurses must provide educational support, facilitation skills and therapeutic nursing interventions to optimise health and wellbeing. They must promote self-care and management whenever possible, helping people to make choices about their healthcare needs, involving families and carers where appropriate, to maximise their ability to care for themselves.

10 All nurses must evaluate their care to improve clinical decision-making, quality and outcomes, using a range of methods, amending the plan of care, where necessary, and communicating changes to others.

How experts make decisions

Much has been made in the professional nursing literature of the 'intuition' that expert nurses use in making decisions. However, studies that have looked closer at this intuition have identified that there is in fact a logic underpinning such apparently seamless decisions. Experts do not instinctively know what to do but through their experiences have learned how to rapidly and unconsciously process the available cues to select the option that is likely to create the best outcome (Elstein and Bordage 1988; Harbison 2001; Bond and Cooper 2006). There is no consensus in the nursing literature on the model that best describes how expert nurses make decisions, but in this section the concept of recognition-primed decision-making (Klein 1993) is used to explain expert decision-making.

Recognition-primed decision-making

The recognition-primed decision-making model does not reflect that experts consider the full range of available options before acting (Klein 1993). Instead it reflects that they use prior experience to recognize and classify a situation and they then know from the classification they make what the most workable option for action is. Any available time is then used to evaluate how feasible that selected option is before they implement it. If they foresee problems, then they modify the option or implement the next most workable option. This model strongly focuses on assessment of the situation and Klein (1993: 142) notes four important aspects of this assessment:

1. Understanding the *types of goals* that can be reasonably accomplished in the situation.
2. Increasing the salience of *cues that are important* within the context of the situation.

3. *Forming expectations* which can serve as a check on the accuracy of the situation assessment.
4. Identifying the typical *actions to take*.

While the recognition-primed decision-making model is based on research from outside nursing, Bond and Cooper (2006) have identified it as a relevant model to explain decision-making in nursing. The model highlights the value of experience in informing decision-making and sets out the steps that experts take to make decisions, often in urgent or emergency situations and over a very short space of time see example in **Box 8.1**.

A final point to make here is that experience does not necessarily equal expertise (Bond and Cooper 2006). Just because someone has many years of nursing experience, it does not automatically mean that they make good decisions. The next section looks more closely at the errors that can be made by decision-makers, regardless of length of experience.

Key learning

- Expert nurses use their experience to recognize and classify a situation and to use this classification to select the most workable option.

Bias and its impact on decision-making

Judgement errors are 'a natural consequence of limitations in our cognitive capacities and of the human tendency to adopt short cuts in reasoning' (Elstein and Schwarz 2002: 732). Making decisions rapidly can be helped by cognitive shortcuts known as heuristics, but these shortcuts can make decisions prone to errors (Klein 2005). In addition, bias can also limit our ability to make the best decision. This section looks more closely at the cognitive errors that decision-makers are prone to, and offers suggestions on how to minimize their impact.

Box 8.1 Example of recognition-primed decision-making

John, who is a fragile elderly patient, is observed slipping off his chair onto the floor. The ward manager, Sue, sees this happening.
1 GOALS. Sue knows what needs to be achieved in terms of limiting damage and injury to John – the goals. The fall may not be prevented and intervention during John's slipping to the floor may cause further damage to anyone intervening. Instead John could possibly be helped to slowly descend to the floor and possibly a blanket or pillow could be used to soften the fall. The aim is to avert or deal with any adverse impact of the fall.
2 CUES. Sue will recognize the pain, anxiety and distress John will experience physically and mentally and begin to observe and monitor these.
3 EXPECTATIONS. It is likely that Sue will anticipate the worst possible outcomes resulting from the fall for John in order to prepare for action to manage and deal with all possible injuries occurring.
4 ACTIONS. Sue will ask for assistance and ensure she has resources brought to John to monitor his condition, assess the pain and manage any bleeding, bruising or other injury sustained. Intervention may be required but she will not rush to lift him off the floor until his condition is assessed and he is safely stabilized.

Activity 8.1

Take a look at the following two scenarios (Brannon and Carson 2003: 202) and follow the instructions.

- You are working in a hospital and you notice a male lying down in the waiting room. When doing your assessment you notice the following: slurred speech, uneven gait and a weakness in his right arm. What is your best diagnosis (list only one, no combinations or qualifications)? You may focus on whatever information you want. If you're not sure, please make your best guess.
- You are working in a hospital and you notice a male lying down in the waiting room. When doing your assessment you notice the following: smell of alcohol on his breath, slurred speech, uneven gait and a weakness in his right arm. What is your best diagnosis (list only one, no combinations or qualifications)? You may focus on whatever information you want. If you're not sure, please make your best guess.

You'll notice that the scenarios in **Activity 8.1** are identical except for the presence or absence of the information about the smell of alcohol on the man's breath. Nurses and student nurses (n = 182) were presented with one of the above scenarios in the study by Brannon and Carson (2003). Of the participants who read the scenario that included the smell of alcohol on the man's breath, 72.73 per cent attributed the symptoms to inebriation and 27.27 per cent to a physical illness. Just 1.96 per cent of participants who read the scenario without the mention of the smell of alcohol attributed the symptoms to inebriation, with 98.04 per cent attributing them to a physical illness. A similar pattern was seen with a different scenario, participants being more likely to give less weight to the physical symptoms when contextual information was provided. These findings are reflected in other studies and throw important light on how we make decisions and how the weighting we give to certain information can lead us away from taking the right decision. This scenario is a good example of a pitfall known as the 'representativeness heuristic' (Klein 2005) or, in other words, the assumption that if A is similar to things in category B, then it can be categorized as B. In the scenario, we see the tendency for people to attribute all of the symptoms to inebriation just because of the piece of information about the smell of alcohol. While this example seems most relevant to adult nursing, nurses in all fields of practice are susceptible to the representativeness heuristic. Nurses can counter it by being aware of how common particular events are and to avoid giving undue weight to single pieces of information. This links to the NMC requirement that nurses 'have an in-depth knowledge of common physical and mental health problems and treatments in their own field of practice, including co-morbidity and physiological and psychological vulnerability' (NMC 2010: 17).

Common pitfalls for decision-making when making assessments

Klein (2005) usefully outlines five pitfalls in decisions about diagnosis and prescribing, the first of which is the representativeness heuristic. Klein's paper is primarily directed at a medical audience, but all practitioners in health care are equally prone to the pitfalls. The second pitfall identified by Klein is the 'availability heuristic'. This is the tendency to use recently encountered or easily remembered information to make assumptions about a current situation. Klein gives the example of people choosing to travel by car after a major train crash because they incorrectly believe it is safer. The availability heuristic means that the risk of something occurring, such as being involved in a train crash if you travel by train, tends to be overestimated and wrongly used to inform the course of action. Nurses can counter the availability heuristic by being aware of what information may be influencing a decision, and questioning whether that information is representative of the current situation, or if it just reflects recent or memorable experiences.

The third pitfall identified by Klein is overconfidence. There is a human tendency to overestimate what we know and this can give us misplaced confidence in our judgements. This means we are less likely to seek alternative explanations or to ask for help when we need it. It also underlines the importance of making decisions in teams, a point covered in the previous chapter. Overconfidence can be countered by being aware of your shortcomings, and seeking the opinion of colleagues.

Confirmatory bias is the fourth pitfall. Klein (2005: 782) defines this as 'the tendency to look for, notice, and remember information that fits with our pre-existing expectations' and also points out that information that contradicts these expectations can be ignored or dismissed. This can mean that gathering information can be used to confirm the expectation that a particular problem exists and that information-gathering can cease too early before key information is identified. Klein recommends countering confirmatory bias through remaining vigilant to information that may contradict your interpretation of what is happening and giving such information careful consideration. Be aware of alternative explanations for a situation and challenge your interpretation to check that it's the best interpretation of the evidence available (Klein 2005). Thorough assessment is clearly key here, taking account of 'relevant physical, social, cultural, psychological, spiritual, genetic and environmental factors' (NMC 2010: 18).

The fifth pitfall is illusory correlation, defined by Klein (2005: 783) as 'the tendency to perceive two events as causally related, when in fact the connection between them is coincidental or even non-existent'. One example of this from nursing would be the use of brandy and egg white by nurses to treat nappy rash in infants. Nurses who used this treatment believed that the brandy would clean the skin and the egg white would provide a protective barrier. When the nappy rash healed this provided evidence to the nurses that the treatment apparently worked, thus increasing the likelihood that they would use it again. The brandy used would, in addition to being very painful against excoriated skin, also have probably dried the skin out leading to further breakdown, but if nurses were using illusory correlation to guide them, they would have discounted the harmful effects of the treatment in favour of the perceived benefits. Illusory correlation can be minimized by being aware of available evidence as to cause and effect of particular interventions. Klein also recommends keeping a written record of events that you believe to be correlated.

So there are a number of pitfalls which can make nurses prone to errors in interpreting a situation and in identifying the right course of action. People who are prone to these cognitive biases are also more likely to believe that they are good decision-makers, so self-awareness is key here! Being aware of what these pitfalls are can help to avoid them. This remains the case, however experienced you are as a practitioner. In Brannon and Carson's (2003) study, qualified nurses were as prone to representativeness bias as student nurses. If you are aware of your own particular pitfalls, whatever your level of experience, you are more likely to question your decisions, to seek alternative explanations and more information, and crucially to ask for help in making decisions when you need it.

Key learning

- Even experienced practitioners are prone to errors in judgement but there are methods that nurses can use to reduce the likelihood of errors.

Involving patients and relatives in decisions

Now let's take a look at a case study to try and apply some of the principles outlined in the above section. The true story below is told by a patient in her own words, although her name has been changed.

Case study 8.1: Anna Brown

My name is Anna Brown and I am 92. I live on my own at home and since my stroke have a home help and meals-on-wheels. Five weeks ago, I tripped at home and hurt my wrist. The doctor visited and said I'd broken it and needed to go to the hospital. He arranged for a taxi to take me there. The taxi driver helped me out of the taxi and walked me into the hospital . . . I walk so slowly without my frame and that was at home. You will have to excuse me, since my stroke it's affected my speech you see. Oh, I was lost without my frame really.

Then I think they came and took me along then to the receptionist. She asked me some questions, I cannot remember everything, there was lots of noise. I could not hear the lady very well. I don't think she understood me very well either, but she was in a rush . . . I think you can understand me because I can take my time. If I get flustered it seems worse. I waited and waited and then I was taken in my chair into another department. Eventually the nurse came and took me into the room. She looked at my wrist and asked me questions. I had taken the list of my tablets that the doctor prepared for me . . . I gave the paper to the nurse. She said she was pleased I had taken it. Oh . . . I was tired but she was kind and she wanted me to have some pain tablets but I said no, they make me feel unwell and I did not want to have nausea. She said I had to have an X-ray. The young lady . . . she pushed me in the chair and I had to wait and wait again. Then I went in for the test and then they told me I would have to wait again . . . then have another X-ray. I was taken back to the first department or was it the second? She looked at my tests and said it was broken and I had to go back to the first place, so I was pushed back there and I was waiting and waiting . . . again.

The problem was I did not know what was going to happen . . . it was the noise . . . lots of rushing about and people talking . . . lots of people everywhere . . . I can't explain it somehow . . . Just before they came to get me, I heard a voice behind me say 'What are you doing here?' and it was the man from next door. He was told I was there you see. He was going to visit his cousin in the hospital, so he came to find me. He stayed with me and brought me home in the afternoon. I was so pleased. I was feeling very anxious and so very frustrated not knowing what was happening . . . I had been there for hours. Straight away it was better. He stayed with me for a long time . . . we waited and waited. After some time I was seen again and a doctor looked at the test . . . he said I had a clean break . . . across here . . . and that I would have to have a plaster on my wrist, he said I had to go to another department for that. They told my neighbour where to go . . . he had to push me up a long corridor in the wheelchair . . . ohh it was a long, long, long way and up a hill too. Then we had to stay by some green chairs to have the plaster put on . . . we had to wait and wait again.

At the time I just wanted to go home, I was so tired and thirsty . . . I had not had anything all day. I hurt my wrist early in the morning and the doctor came after half past twelve you see. I didn't think about how much more difficult it would be to manage at home at the time, to use my frame and pick things up, and turn the tap on and things like that, I am right-handed you see . . . and you do not think how much you use this hand . . . even when I cannot do an awful lot anyway. Anyway . . . finally I had my plaster put on. The lady was nice. She smiled at me. It was nice, made me feel better. By then, I was worried about my neighbour because he had been with me for such a long time . . . and he had to go back to his family. I was tired. I needed to go to the toilet. I didn't want to be a nuisance, everyone was rushing about and I could not ask my neighbour. So I tried to hold on until I came home. It was alright. When we got home my neighbour looked after me. He made me a sandwich then and a cup of tea. After he left, I managed to get to the toilet. I didn't use my frame. I held onto whatever I could. I had a sling around my neck you see. The doctor said I had to keep it on for a few days. I had a slight accident, but I managed with this hand and the home help came in the morning and was able to do the laundry.

(Bridges 2008)

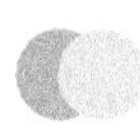

Activity 8.2

Now answer these questions:

- What information does Mrs Brown provide that is relevant to decisions about her treatment and care during and after her hospital visit?
- What information about Mrs Brown did staff appear to use when deciding on her care while she was in the department, her treatment and her discharge? What information did not appear to have been used?
- What pitfall(s) do the staff appear to have been prone to?
- Can you identify an incident from your own field of practice that you have witnessed or read about where staff took too narrow a focus with regard to a patient's care and treatment? Identify the related pitfall(s).
- Using Mrs Brown's story or your own example, identify what decisions and actions would have optimized the patient outcomes.

Let's stay with Mrs Brown for a while longer. From her account of events, it appears that she had rather a passive role during her hospital visit. She took along a list of her medications which was welcomed but she didn't feel able to ask for a cup of tea or help in going to the toilet. Being in a hospital environment or other health care setting, especially in conjunction with a worrying illness or injury, can make patients of any age feel disempowered. Even if they are confident people outside of the health care environment, many patients feel unable to express important needs, share pertinent information, ask questions or disagree with what is being proposed. Their reliance on relatives and friends is often very important and you may often find out there is a problem when approached during visiting hours by a relative concerned for their next of kin. Both patients and their relatives depend on nursing staff to sort out their illness or injury and keep them informed and involved in decision-making. Too often an appreciation of high staff workloads can compound patients' feelings of being disempowered and make it too difficult for them to ask for help.

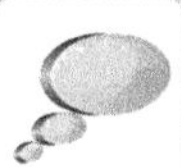

Activity 8.3

Think about a time when you or someone close to you was a patient.

- Did you know who each member of staff was who you met?
- Did you feel you understood what was happening?
- Did staff keep you informed of what would be happening next?
- Did you feel you had an opportunity to share relevant information or to ask questions?
- Did you feel able to ask for help if you needed it?
- If there were key decisions to be made, how involved did you feel?
- If there were shortcomings in your experience, list the staff actions that could have made a difference.
- If you felt involved by staff throughout your experience, list the staff actions that enabled this.

Advocating for patients who are making decisions

As patient advocates, nurses have an important role to play in helping patients feel in control of what is happening. The NMC competencies specify the need for nurses to empower children and young people to express their views and preferences, but this need applies to patients and service users across all fields. Many people will need nurses to use proactive measures to help them be in control of their care and treatment. This may for example include issuing explicit invitations such as 'It might seem that I'm busy today, but please stop me and ask if you need my help getting to the toilet or if your glass needs filling up. That's what I'm here for.' Understanding how best to involve someone can mean putting yourself in their shoes to anticipate their needs or preferences. It means establishing a relationship with them so they feel able to be open with you. And it means negotiating with them each step of the way what information they need and supporting them to make the decision that feels right to them.

These principles don't just apply to the big decisions such as a significant change in the medical management of a mental health need, but to everyday decisions such as what time an individual would like to wake up, what they like for their breakfast, how much milk they like in their tea, when they have a wash, or what clothes they'd like to wear. Being in receipt of nursing care can mean that people's ability to be in control of these everyday things can be disrupted by, for instance, having to wait in for the community nurse to visit, or being subject to ward routines. Again, as patient advocates, nurses have to proactively address this risk in order to preserve the patient's control. This involves providing and honouring choice whenever this is possible and challenging aspects of health care such as routine or traditions that unnecessarily disrupt an individual's needs being met.

In a systematic review I carried out with colleagues, we looked at qualitative research that reported older people's experiences in acute care hospitals (Bridges *et al.* 2010). The review identified the importance of the interactions between staff and patients in shaping patients' experiences. It also reported that what older people want is for staff to:

- 'See who I am': recognize and acknowledge who I am as a person and what is important to me.
- 'Connect with me': establish a warm and caring connection with me that makes me feel respected and enables me to be open with you.
- 'Involve me': establish what involvement I want, and support and advocate for my choices.

While the review focused on research with older people, these messages apply across client groups in health and social care. The review also looked at research that reported older people's relatives' experiences and found that they also need staff to see who they are, to connect with them and to involve them. Relatives or other important people in the patient's life can play a crucial role in maintaining that person's health and well-being. Some nurses are very skilled at making relatives feel a part of what is happening, and in drawing on the expertise of patients and their relatives, especially for patients with a long-term condition. When people cannot communicate their wishes themselves, then their relative or loved one can be an important consultee for what the patient would want if they were able to make a decision, and communicate it.

Activity 8.4

Think about your most recent clinical placement and the patient that you had the most involvement with.

- Who were the important people in that patient's life?
- What involvement did they have in maintaining that person's health and well-being?
- If they were a carer for the patient (or the parent of a child patient or young person), what strategies were used by you or other nurses to acknowledge and draw on their carer or parent role, to establish their support needs, to enable them to ask questions and ask for help, to help them feel involved? What other strategies would have helped?

Key learning

- It is really important to involve all patients in decision-making as it acknowledges and recognizes their personhood.

Patients who are unable to be fully involved in making decisions

Involving patients in decision-making is not always straightforward, especially if the person has impaired communication or capacity, or if they are judged too young to make a decision for themselves. Have a look at the resources in **Activity 8.5** that provide some useful guidelines, including for making decisions with children and young people.

Activity 8.5

- Review the following information on capacity and consent.

Resources on capacity and consent

NMC advice on consent, including consent for people aged under 16 years can be found at: http://bit.ly/9bnNhQ.

The British Medical Association (BMA) has also produced some detailed guidance on working with children and young people that includes guidance on consent and capacity issues. You can find this guidance at: http://bma.org.uk/practical-support-at-work/ethics/children/children-and-young-people-tool-kit.

The Department of Health (DH) has produced a useful guide on capacity and consent for people working with people with learning disability: http://bit.ly/14oeqxL.

The Social Care Institute for Excellence (SCIE) website has a range of resources on the Mental Capacity Act: http://www.scie.org.uk/publications/mca/index.asp.

- Talk to your mentor in your current/next clinical placement about how decisions are made in that clinical setting for people who lack capacity (or who are deemed by law to lack capacity such as those aged under 16 years), and ask to see any local policies and procedures related to this.
- Participate in the care of a patient who has impaired, fluctuating or absent capacity to consent, and evaluate how decisions are made as their care and treatment are planned and delivered. Note when decisions are straightforward to make and when they are more difficult. Helpful questions to ask yourself about this patient's involvement might be:

  What do I or others do to help this person understand what is happening (e.g. verbal/non-verbal communication, actions)?

  How do I or others know the person has understood what is happening?

  How do I or others know that what is happening is what the person wants or what they would want if they were able to make a decision?

  What happens if the person resists the planned care or treatment?

- Make a written note of your observations in practice and discuss them with a fellow student.

Some health care professionals take decisions on other people's behalf if they think they know what's best for them or if finding out what they want takes time and skill they feel they don't have. Some avoid getting involved in difficult situations or talking about difficult things with patients and families. Others recognize their shortcomings and work hard to establish the best course of action. Some health care professionals are enormously skilled at talking about difficult subjects (such as death and dying) with patients and families and at handling complicated family situations (e.g. when there is disagreement among family members as to the best course of action). You will come across such individuals in your clinical placements and in your practice after qualifying. Ask to shadow them, encourage them to talk about how they do what they do, watch them at work and learn from them.

Key learning

- Nurses need to take proactive steps to empower patients to express their needs and preferences and to help them to feel in control of what is happening.

Conclusion

We have seen in this chapter how experts use their experience to recognize and classify a situation and to use this classification to select the most workable option. Regardless of previous experience, the chapter has also identified strategies that nurses can use to reduce the likelihood of making errors in decisions:

- Carrying out comprehensive and systematic assessments.
- Being knowledgeable about the likelihood of different patient problems.
- Avoiding giving undue weight to single pieces of information.
- Being aware of what information is influencing a decision and questioning whether the information represents the current situation.
- Being knowledgeable about the evidence base for common nursing interventions in their field of practice.
- Being aware of shortcomings and seeking other opinions in complex situations.
- Revising plans in the light of further relevant information becoming available, including information about an individual's response to an intervention.

The chapter has also illustrated that nurses need to take proactive steps to empower patients to express their needs and preferences and to help them feel in control of what is happening. Involving relatives or other important people in the patient's life is also an important part of ensuring the best patient outcomes and of making sure that carers get the right support. The chapter has reflected on the importance of nurses understanding how to work with issues of capacity and impaired communication. Finally, the chapter has underlined that nurses can build their skills in patient and family involvement by learning from colleagues with advanced skills in handling difficult topics and difficult situations.

Further reading and resources

Bridges, J., Flatley, M. and Meyer, J. (2010) Older people's and relatives' experiences in acute care settings: systematic review and synthesis of qualitative studies, *International Journal of Nursing Studies*, 47(1): 89–107.

Elstein, A.S. and Schwarz, A. (2002) Clinical problem solving and diagnostic decision making: selective review of the cognitive literature, *British Medical Journal*, 324(7339): 729–32.

Klein, J.G. (2005) Five pitfalls in decisions about diagnosis and prescribing, *British Medical Journal*, 330(7494): 781–3.

www.city.ac.uk/bpop. Look at the CD on this site for guidelines on how to apply patient and relative involvement principles to care for older people in acute settings.

References

Bond, S. and Cooper, S. (2006) Modelling emergency decisions: recognition-primed decision making. The literature in relation to an ophthalmic critical incident, *Journal of Clinical Nursing*, 15(8): 1023–32.

Brannon, L.A. and Carson, K.L. (2003) The representativeness heuristic: influence on nurses' decision making, *Applied Nursing Research*, 16(3): 201–4.

Bridges, J. (2008) *Listening Makes Sense*. London: City University, available at: www.city.ac.uk/listeningmakessense, accessed 2 August 2012.

Bridges, J., Flatley, M. and Meyer, J. (2010) Older people's and relatives' experiences in acute care settings: systematic review and synthesis of qualitative studies, *International Journal of Nursing Studies*, 47(1): 89–107.

Elstein, A.S. and Bordage, G. (1988) Psychology of clinical reasoning, in J. Dowie and A.S. Elstein (eds) *Professional Judgment: A Reader in Clinical Decision Making*. Cambridge: Cambridge University Press.

Elstein, A.S. and Schwarz, A. (2002) Clinical problem solving and diagnostic decision making: selective review of the cognitive literature, *British Medical Journal*, 324(7339): 729–32.

Gillespie, M. and Paterson, B.L. (2009) Helping novice nurses make effective clinical decisions: the situated clinical decision-making framework, *Nursing Education Perspectives*, 30(3): 164–70.

Harbison, J. (2001) Clinical decision making in nursing: theoretical perspectives and their relevance to practice, *Journal of Advanced Nursing*, 35(1): 126–33.

Klein, G.A. (1993) A recognition-primed decision (RPD) model of rapid decision making, in G.A. Klein, J. Orasanu, R. Calderwood and C. Zsambok (eds) *Decision Making in Action: Models and Methods.* Norwood, NJ: Ablex.

Klein, J.G. (2005) Five pitfalls in decisions about diagnosis and prescribing, *British Medical Journal*, 330(7494): 781–3.

NMC (Nursing and Midwifery Council) (2010) *Standards for Pre-registration Nursing Education*. London: NMC.

SECTION

4

Leadership, management and team working

Effective leadership, management and team working skills

9

Yvonne Middlewick

Chapter contents

Introduction: NMC competencies

This chapter will help you focus on your understanding of leadership, management and teamworking within health care settings. Every day in practice nurses lead and manage care of their patients and as a student you are expected by the Nursing and Midwifery Council (NMC 2010) to show your competence in leading and managing others in the health care team. In this chapter there will be an exploration of the concepts of leadership and management, considering the similarities and differences in the qualities and skills required to be a good leader and manager. You will be prompted to explore your role as a leader and manager wherever you are on your pre-registration student journey. The chapter goes on to explore the attributes of successful and less successful teams and the potential impact these can have on patient care.

The term 'patient' has been chosen for this chapter. Service user, client, child, young person or people could equally have been used. It is suggested that you choose a term appropriate for your field of practice and use this whenever you read 'patient'.

It is important not to view the skills required to fulfil the competencies within Domain 4 in isolation. They are closely linked to the other three domains: professional values, communication and interpersonal skills, and nursing practice and decision-making, all included in this book.

This chapter is relevant to the following NMC competencies.

Domain 4: Leadership, management and team working

1 All nurses must act as change agents and provide leadership through quality improvement and service development to enhance people's well-being and experiences of health care.

3 All nurses must be able to identify priorities and manage time and resources effectively

to ensure the quality of care is maintained or enhanced.

4 All nurses must be self-aware and recognize how their own values, principles and assumptions may affect their practice. They must maintain their own personal and professional development, learning from experience, through supervision, feedback, reflection and evaluation.

5 All nurses must facilitate nursing students and others to develop their competence, using a range of professional and personal development skills.

7 All nurses must work effectively across professional boundaries, actively involving and respecting others' contributions to integrated person-centred care. They must know when and how to communicate with and refer to other professionals and agencies in order to respect the choices of service users and others. Promoting shared decision making, to deliver positive outcomes and to coordinate smooth, effective transition within and between services and agencies.

Nursing management and leadership

Leadership and management can be defined as separate entities, however, when you begin to try to explore these it becomes more challenging because the terms overlap and are frequently used interchangeably (Mullins 2007; Warriner 2009; Curtis *et al.* 2011a). Within the nursing literature there is also no agreed definition of what nursing leadership and nursing management are (Warriner 2009; Stanley and Sherratt 2010). This can make it challenging to understand exactly what is required from nurses at different levels in an organization and may suggest that leadership and management is only for those in more senior positions. It may also lead student nurses to believe that these elements are not part of their role until later in their education when in fact student nurses may be well placed to influence the development of care from the beginning of their journey to becoming a registered practitioner.

What is clear is that in the complex world of health care there is a need for nurses who have leadership and management skills. As nurse education has developed, the focus on these skills has been highlighted. This is also in alignment with the focus on high quality leadership and management in the NHS (Darzi 2008; National Leadership Council 2012). This is to ensure the delivery of high quality services continues to develop to reflects local need and the financial climate. It is therefore important that you consider how to develop or enhance these skills throughout your education and beyond. This will help you gain confidence to deliver first-class services as a registered nurse (RN).

Management

Activity 9.1

Before reading this section take a few minutes to reflect on management. Consider someone you think is a great manager:

- What qualities do they have?
- What do they do that makes them a particularly good manager?

'Management' is a broad term that can encompass a number of different perspectives, making it difficult to find an agreed definition in the literature (Mullins and Christy 2010). Before focusing on a definition related to management in nursing, a starting point to enable you to begin to compare your answers in **Activity 9.1** is the definition in *Collins English Dictionary*:

1. the members of the executive or administration of an organization or business
2. managers or employers collectively
3. the technique, practice, or science of managing, controlling or dealing with [issues]
4. the skillful or resourceful use of materials, time, etc
5. the specific treatment of a disease, disorder, etc

The lack of consensus about a definition of management means that many authors focus on the responsibilities and behaviours expected in management to explain the meaning. Fayol (1916 cited in Sullivan and Decker 2009: 55) states that management functions are 'planning, organizing, directing and controlling'. This view is supported by Curtis *et al.* (2011b). Following their review of the literature they found that the important functions of management were viewed as planning, finance, managing people and staffing. Mullins (2007: 364) describes management as 'getting things done through other people in order to achieve stated organizational objectives'. He goes on to suggest that the manager may have a tendency to be reactive in situations, focusing on solving short-term problems rather than proactively considering the longer-term implications of situations.

Compare the answers you gave to the questions in **Activity 9.1** to the views expressed above. Did you have similar things on your list? You may find that your answers are dependent on the context in which you have experienced management. Keep hold of this list for the next section where leadership will be explored. This will allow for a comparison of your views in relation to these terms. From the perspective of nursing it could be argued that all of the above are applicable in ensuring people receive appropriate and timely care. However, this chapter will focus on the management qualities and skills required within the context of the role of a student nurse.

Management qualities

Adair (2003: 62) considers managers embody the following qualities:

> reliable, responsible, trustworthy, hard-working, thrifty with scarce resources, plan ahead, keep to agreed procedures or systems, prompt in business, open minded to change, knowledgeable in their specialties, meticulous over detail, cheerful, fair and courteous in their dealings with staff and colleagues, keep in control of things, loyal to the organization, achieve their targets, good time managers.

Adair suggests that a person can be a good manager but not necessarily a good leader unless they also have leadership attributes (considered in the next section). Mullins and Christy (2010: 425) give further consideration to this, stating that 'whereas leaders are not necessarily managers it could be argued that all managers should be leaders'. There remains a lack of agreement as to whether you can be a manager without being a leader and vice versa. Management is, however, an important aspect of nursing as nurses are expected to manage care, time and resources while maintaining high quality care. The overall aim is to have managers who are also good leaders and to begin developing management, leadership and teamworking skills throughout the educational process. This should help with the transition from student to RN.

Managing patient care and making decisions

From very early in your practice and academic education you will be considering the best available evidence for managing and treating conditions affecting patients within your field of practice. You will also need to have knowledge of other fields of practice to enable you to effectively, skillfully and holistically manage your patients' care. This should be done in collaboration with patients and their carers, as well as other members of the interprofessional team as treatment may only be a small part of caring for your patient. To develop your skills in caring it is important to gain an understanding of how and why decisions are made. Clinical decision-making is explored in more depth in Chapters 7 and 8 of this book, however, it is important to consider how this links to management. Banning (2008: 188) describes clinical decision-making as 'a process that nurses undertake on a daily basis when they make judgements about the care that they provide to patients and management issues'. As a student nurse you are in an ideal position to ask questions about this often complex cognitive activity which is linked to the management of care. Many of the staff you work with will be experts in their field and may appear to make care decisions intuitively (Benner 2001). Asking questions such as 'why did you decide to . . .' and 'how did you come to that decision' will help develop your understanding. It is good practice to also ask yourself these types of questions as it can help you reflect on your development and identify any gaps in your knowledge. The aim is to challenge you to develop while maintaining confidence in your own abilities. You should always speak with your mentor if you are concerned about any aspects of your development. This is a requirement identified in the NMC *Standards* (2010) and in the *Code* (NMC 2008).

Management of care and decision-making are inextricably linked at all levels. The role of a ward sister, for example, may not necessarily be directly providing care for patients, however, they will be expected to manage a clinical area and make decisions that can impact on the overall quality of care provided. You will be supported to develop management skills throughout your pre-registration programme. The NMC (2010) *Standards* emphasize the importance of being able to identify priorities and manage time and resources effectively while maintaining high standards of care. This may seem daunting when you start your first practice placement, however, your mentor and the team will help you on this developmental journey. As you progress you will begin to become more independent, under the supervision of your mentor, in making care decisions. Towards the end of your education you will be supported to 'take the lead in coordinating, delegating and supervising care safely, managing risk and remaining accountable for the care given as you begin to prepare for the transition to being a registered nurse' (NMC 2010). These steps can happen at different times for different people as team members try to ensure there is gradual exposure to increased responsibilities.

Key learning

- There is lack of consensus about an agreed definition for management.
- Management of quality patient care requires good decision-making skills, time management skills, resource management and planning skills.

Case study 9.1a: Mr Jones

Mr Jones, is an elderly man who is confused and has been found standing on the arms of a chair in the area of the ward where female patients are located. He is shouting very loudly. He has been incontinent of urine and is causing upset to the patients nearby. The health care assistant has been unable to persuade him to sit down and he is responding aggressively to patients trying to provide assistance. He is at risk of falling.

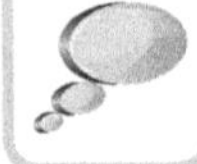

Activity 9.2

- How would you manage the situation described in the case study of Mr Jones?
- Write down your ideas on how best to intervene. Discuss these with a colleague.

There are many strategies that you might consider in relation to Mr Jones. But what did you identify as the main goal or priority in this situation? Was it related to managing the risk to Mr Jones? Did you consider what might go wrong? What skills did you draw on and how did you decide to proceed? Did you involve others?

Case study 9.1b: Mr Jones

The ward manager speaks quietly to Mr Jones suggesting they have a chat together, invites him to sit down and offers to make him a cup of tea. Mr Jones accepts the offer and sits down in the chair. However, when the ward manager goes to make the tea, the health care assistants start to drag the chair backwards towards Mr Jones' bed. Mr Jones starts to scream. When the ward manager returns she asks the health care assistants what is happening. They respond that they needed to get Mr Jones back to his bed to change him into clean clothes as he cannot be left in wet trousers and his family are due to visit and get cross if they find him wet. They also indicate that they are concerned to maintain Mr Jones' skin integrity.

 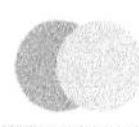

Sometimes health care staff may have different views about how to manage a situation, such as the one described in the case study above. The NMC states that as a student nurse you should: 'take the lead in coordinating, delegating and supervising care safely'. There will be times when you have to make a decision when there are conflicting views so it is important that you are able to provide a rationale for your decisions, justifying your actions, drawing on relevant guidelines and evidence and considering the patient's needs.

Activity 9.3

Think of a situation when you have encountered different ways to proceed.

- How did you account for the different approaches?
- How would you account for the management of Mr Jones that you suggested earlier?
- Is there only one best way to do anything?

Do you think the ward manager in the case study is an effective leader? Justify and explain your answer and then read the following section.

Leadership

What is leadership?

A clear definition of leadership is difficult to find. Mullins (2007: 363) suggests that leadership 'is a relationship through which one person influences the behavior or actions of other people'. This influencing relationship between the leader and their followers is noted by Curtis *et al.* (2011a) as a common theme of many definitions. Leadership is often associated with skills such as 'innovation', 'development', 'inspiration' and the ability to challenge the status quo; management on the other hand can be associated with administration, maintenance and control (Borrill *et al.* 2002; Mullins 2002; Curtis *et al.* 2011a). Consideration also needs to be given to the fact that the skills of both a leader and a manager may be inextricably linked.

Once you start to explore leadership it soon becomes apparent that it is a complex phenomenon. Historical and cultural perspectives have influenced the development of theoretical approaches to leadership and a selection of these different approaches is outlined below.

The traits approach to leadership

This is one of the earlier theories that 'leaders are born and not made'. This theory focuses on the qualities of the leader and early research suggested that there were a number of innate qualities that were inherited and could be measured (Bass and Stogdill 1990; Mullins and Christy 2010; Northouse 2010). Examples of such traits may be leaders who are confident, loyal and charming. This approach has been included for consideration as there do seem to be some people who are natural leaders. Can you think of some individuals you have encountered in nursing who appear to be natural leaders? The research, however, suggests that although attempts have been made to identify specific traits that are common to leaders there is too much subjectivity about what makes a good leader. Other potential influences such as environment, the situation and the leader's relationship with their followers also play a part (Mullins and Christy 2010; Northouse 2010).

The functional approach to leadership

The functional approach to leadership focuses on the behaviours of both the leader and the followers and recognizes the impact these can have on each other. Action-centred leadership (Adair 2003; Adair and Thomas 2004; Adair *et al.* 2008) outlines the functions of the leader in helping the group work effectively. This would involve the leader in interpreting what is going on and then motivating others in the team to ensure they act in a way that achieves the group goals. An example would be when a nurse in the community takes charge of a situation with which she is familiar, perhaps because she knows a patient well, and enlists all members of the interdisciplinary team to achieve an appropriate admission following an exacerbation of a long-term condition. The role of the leader is to behave in a way that enables other members of the team to work towards the patient's goal objectives. Any member of a team can behave in a functional leadership role.

The situational approach to leadership

This approach focuses on the situation as the influencing factor with different situations requiring different leadership styles. Leaders respond to the specific demands of the situation and their followers' characteristics and needs. Hersey *et al.* (2000) describe their contingency theory, associated with situational leadership, which assesses the readiness of the followers. For example, at the beginning of a new task a person may require a significant amount of direction and support, therefore the suggested leadership approach at this time would be *authoritarian or 'telling'*. As the person becomes more proficient the leader would change their style accordingly to be more *'permissive'*. You should be able to relate this to particular examples during your clinical placement when working with a mentor and recognize that as you became more experienced in a particular skill, the mentor's style altered. When followers are at their most proficient the leader would use a *'delegating'* style as minimal direction and support is required. No doubt as you move into your final year as a student you will experience more situations where you will delegate work to others as you practise leading a team. There may always be times, such as during a sudden emergency, when an *authoritarian* approach is needed by the leader who takes charge.

Another strategy used in the situational approach is 'participative'. This style may be used in learning groups in university when you work in a participative manner with peers.

Transformational leadership

Transformational leadership is described by Mullins and Christy (2010) as 'transforming performance'. This is done through the use of the leader's interpersonal skills to enable them to make links to their followers' values. Once this connection is made it generates an environment of trust, enabling people to develop and work cohesively together. Yukl (2006 cited in Mullins and Christy 2010: 391) states that to use a transformational approach the leader must:

- articulate a clear and appealing vision;
- explain how the vision can be attained;
- act confidently and be optimistic;
- express confidence in followers;
- use dramatic and symbolic actions to emphasize key values;
- lead by example.

From this list it is clear that the emphasis with this approach is the relationship between the leader and the followers. If you compare this to the NHS *Leadership Framework* (National Leadership Council 2012) you may see a number of similarities.

These are a few different approaches to leadership and it may be useful for you to explore them or others in more depth, particularly when you start to take on a more formal leadership role. Having an understanding of leadership and management theory early in your career will help you to more successfully develop practice. This will give you a framework to thoroughly think about how to plan, implement and evaluate any changes as well as consider appropriate leadership styles.

Key learning !

- There are numerous leadership theories that can offer insights into different styles of leadership and can help with your personal development.
- Leadership can occur at any level within an organization.

 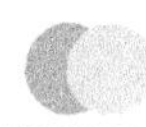

So far you have been provided with some background to what is meant by leadership from a nursing perspective and your role in developing leadership skills as a student nurse. It is appropriate to now look at what leadership means for you as a student in practice.

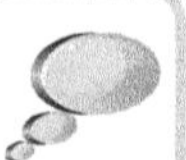

Activity 9.4

Take a few minutes to consider and reflect on the following questions:

- What is your leadership role as a student nurse?
- Who do you lead? Or put another way, who are your followers?

Once you have done this, compare your reflections to the ideas presented below.

Learning to lead as a student nurse

Curtis *et al.* (2011a) argue that student nurses are leaders to patients because they provide assistance to this group and patients are reliant on the expertise of the student nurse at the time they are providing care. As you progress through your education you may find yourself gradually leading more people by, for example, assisting the learning of other students or support staff. You may not have considered these important functions of leadership before because it is happening informally. Informal leadership is a legitimate and valuable form of leadership. Stanley (2008) suggests that people do not need to have positional power to lead and that many people influence care by demonstrating their personal values which influence their followers. Downey *et al.* (2011) state that informal leaders are 'hidden treasures' who are keen to share their knowledge in order to develop clinical care. If you think about these informal situations you may be surprised at how often you have the opportunity to provide leadership.

As you begin to influence others you need to be aware of the importance of continually enhancing your leadership skills. These skills will provide a foundation for you to not only provide high quality care but to influence future service development (NMC 2010). This is necessary when working in the rapidly changing environment of health to ensure that health care delivery is evidence-based and person-centred. Girvin (1998) found that nurses identified personal qualities, such as an ability to communicate well or inspire others, when they first described nursing leadership. This was of interest to her as she knew of people who had some of the personal qualities being described but they were not necessarily good leaders. This led her to explore the available literature and consider it within her experience as a nurse. Other authors have also found that nurses identify a number of different personal attributes in the people they value as leaders (Stanley 2008; Warriner 2009; Stanley and Sherratt 2010). These attributes will be considered after you have completed **Activity 9.5**.

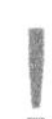

Key learning

- Leadership focuses on the development of relationships.
- Student nurses have a leadership role that develops as they become more experienced.

Personal qualities of good leaders

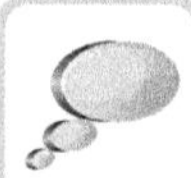

Activity 9.5

Think about someone you know who you think is an inspirational leader.

- Make a list of the personal qualities they possess that make them such a good leader.
- Compare this list to the one you made when considering management.
- What are the similarities and differences?

You may find that you can clearly categorize the differences and similarities between your chosen manager and leader, particularly if you have been able to think of people who clearly fit into each role. It would, however, not be at all surprising if you have found this task difficult, feeling that some people are both leaders and managers. Adair (2003) argues that this is because they have both leadership and management attributes. The confusion of terminology within the nursing literature may also increase the lack of clarity. It becomes apparent that what determines leaders are their actions and behaviours (Curtis *et al.* 2011a). Good leaders are described as being excellent communicators, their values and beliefs are clearly visible through their actions and they are both credible and knowledgeable role models (Girvin 1998; Warriner 2009; Stanley and Sherratt 2010; Curtis *et al.* 2011a; Downey *et al.* 2011). High quality communication skills in leadership behaviour enable relationships to develop with the people who follow. Kean and Haycock-Stuart (2011) suggest that leaders need to consider their relationship with the people who follow them because leadership cannot occur in isolation. They go on to argue that the leader–follower relationship is complex and that research has tended to focus on the actions of the leader rather that the people who follow. Peck and Dickinson (2009 cited in Kean and Haycock-Stuart 2011: 32) state that 'successful leadership in organisations is the result of the actions of many'. This means that leaders and followers need to work collaboratively to achieve the task, which in the context of health care should lead to high quality, person-centred care. Other attributes of leaders include integrity, confidence, trustworthiness, approachability and openness. Good leaders consider the 'bigger picture', have excellent communication skills, critically analyse situations and consider how to improve them to impact on patient care (Stanley 2008; Downey *et al.* 2011; National Leadership Council 2012).

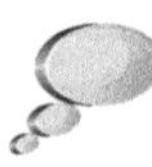

Activity 9.6

- How might Jess go about leading the change?
- What would she need to consider?
- She is trying to put patient priorities before ward routine and nursing practices and may find that she meets with resistance to change. How might she be encouraged to move forward with her ideas to improve patient care?
- What would you do?

It is essential that you consider your working relationships and how you develop these with the many different people around you. This is an important part of working as a student nurse within a team and will be considered in more depth in the next section exploring team working.

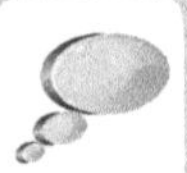

Activity 9.7

- Look at Domain 4 of the *Standards* (NMC 2010) and the National Leadership Council (2012) *Leadership Framework* which is available at: http://www.nhsleadership.org.uk/framework.asp.
- Use these to help you identify your developmental needs in relation to leadership and management and discuss them with your mentor, tutor or a colleague.

Case study 9.2: Jess

Jess, a student nurse, who had rotated over the full 24-hour shift in one ward, noticed that patients were often awake until as late as 2 a.m. because of late emergency admissions. Sometimes they were disturbed again during their sleep to change continence pads and were being woken at 6 a.m. when the drug round was carried out. During the day the patients were tired; too tired sometimes to engage in their planned therapies, and frequently aggressive. Jess wanted to try to change practice and see if the patients could be helped to sleep better with fewer disturbances and whether the drug round could be delayed until 8 a.m.

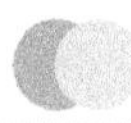

Team working

Teams are increasingly required to perform in complex and dynamic environments. This characteristic applies particularly to health care teams where interprofessional working and the need to work with patients and carers adds to the challenge of leadership.

What is a team?

The Royal College of Nursing (RCN 2007: 3) uses Katzenbach and Smith's definition to summarize what a team is. They define it as: 'A small number of people with complementary skills who are committed to a common purpose, performance goals and approach for which they hold themselves mutually accountable'. You are required to work effectively as part of a team throughout your career (NMC 2008, 2010). Teams can be structured in different ways and this varies from area to area. Even if you work in the same field of practice you will often find that every team can vary in the way it functions. You will have the opportunity to meet and work with many different people from many walks of life, both as a student and an RN. The NMC requires you to always treat people with respect including treating your colleagues fairly and without discrimination (NMC 2008).

Activity 9.8

Identify a patient from one of your practice experiences and make a spider diagram with the patient at the centre. Then add in all of the people your patient has been in contact with on their journey through the health care system (see **Figure 9.1** for an example).

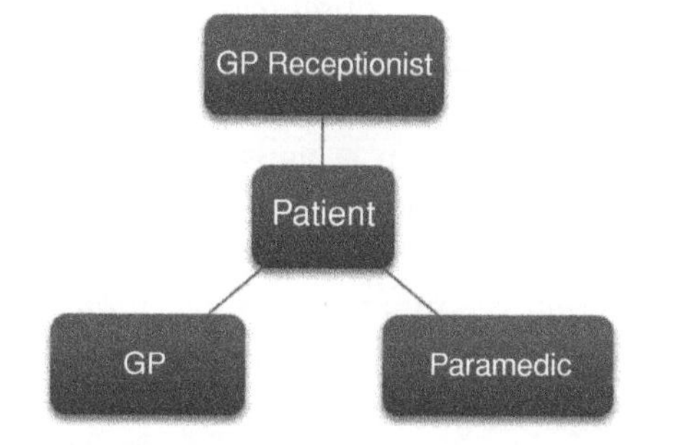

Figure 9.1 An example of a patient journey

When you start to consider the team from the patient's perspective, as you did in **Activity 9.8**, it is likely that your list of people who are involved will be quite large and potentially complex. There may be numerous other professionals involved in a person's care and all of these form part of the team of people who are helping the person on their journey. It is also important to consider carers and other people who the patient feels is significant to them. It may be that you had perceived some nurses as working more independently than others, but all health professionals are part of a large health care team. The reality is that no professional is truly independent; someone else is always needed to enable the smooth transition of the patient through services, regardless of where the services are located. It is important therefore that you consider the role of everyone involved so that any changes in the patient's care can be communicated and passed on to the appropriate people.

Activity 9.9

- Take a few minutes to reflect on a successful team you have been involved with (it does not necessarily need to be within health care), and list why you feel the team was successful. Then think of a less successful team and list why you feel this team was not successful.
- When you have read the section on team development and characteristics, compare the attributes you have identified to the discussion presented. Is the list for a successful team similar to the ideas presented below?
- Keep your list relating to a less successful team for **Activity 9.10**.

Stages of team development

Working as part of a team can be challenging, particularly when you are joining for only a transient period of time. Bruce Tuckman's (1965) stages of

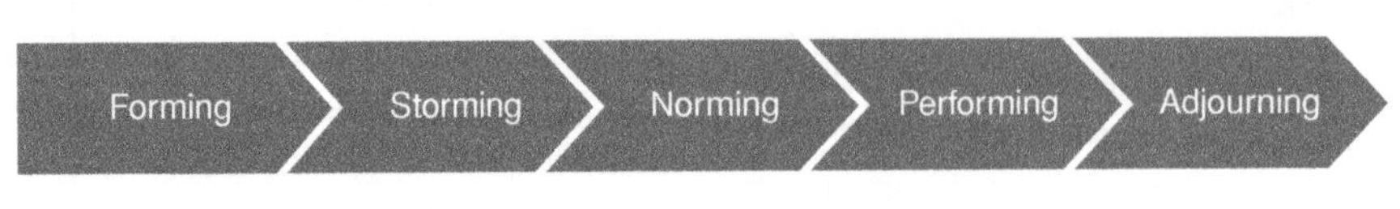

Figure 9.2 Bruce Tuckman's (1965) stages of team development

group development (see **Figure 9.2**) can be used when considering the different stages experienced by groups when new members join. Although this model is now over 45 years old it is a seminal piece of work and continues to be cited in texts discussing group development. The stages are known as *forming*, *storming*, *norming* and *performing*, and in later years a final stage, *adjourning*, was added for when teams have completed the task or are breaking up (Tuckman and Jensen 1977). According to Tuckman, groups need to go through the first four stages in order to reach maturity. It will depend on the experiences of the team you join as to where they are in their team development. If the team is in the 'performing' stage then you would expect to see a cohesive group working well together. If, however, they are in the 'storming' stage you may notice some tensions within the group. This is all a normal part of group development, and providing the group remains respectful to one another during the storming stage even if at times there appears to be conflict, positive developments can occur. It is a healthy stage as long as the team does not get 'stuck' within it. The inability to resolve conflict can impact on team cohesiveness, performance and the quality of care it provides (Borrill *et al.* 2002). This is when good leadership and excellent interpersonal skills can be used to help people move towards the team's shared objectives.

Characteristics of successful team work

Pearson *et al.* (2006) performed a systematic review of, among other things, the characteristics of nursing teams that contribute to a healthy working environment. They found that accountability, commitment, motivation, enthusiasm and communication were key components. Atwal and Caldwell (2006) also found that it is important to have an understanding of the roles of other professionals as well confidence and assertiveness. Pearson *et al.* (2006: 135) suggest that 'a multidisciplinary approach to the delivery of healthcare results in a number of improved outcomes' for both patients and staff. According to Borrill *et al.* (2002) the effectiveness of multidisciplinary team working impacts on effectiveness, innovation and mental health.

Another attribute identified in a cohesive team is the need for everyone to be aiming for the same goal (Adair and Thomas 2004; Atwal and Caldwell 2006). Belbin (2010: 98) describes a team as 'a group of players who have a reciprocal part to play and who are dynamically involved with each other'. This link with each other enables a group of people to become a cohesive team and highlights the importance of communication in building team relationships (Adair and Thomas 2004; Atwal and Caldwell 2006; Pearson *et al.* 2006; Kean and Haycock-Stuart 2011).

The optimum team number is an issue for debate, although between 8 and 12 people appears to be the general consensus (Acas 2007; RCN 2007; Mullins and Christy 2010). Belbin (2010) proposes that a team can consist of as few as four members, although it is worth noting that he suggests nine *team roles* for optimum functioning. Borrill *et al.* (2002) found that if you work in an area of the NHS that has more than 12 or 13 staff then subgroups naturally form. This is normal and if you think about a standard clinical area, of say 30 staff, as an 'organization within a larger organization', then you will see that splitting into three separate teams should enable optimum functioning. How does this compare with the numbers of people involved in the care of your patient in **Activity 9.8**? The key here is that the teams are working in

alignment with their objectives so that they all have the same focus: the patient and high quality care. They may, however, achieve the objectives differently. Although there is much debate in the literature about the difference between a group and a team, there is some agreement on some of the attributes needed for a well functioning team.

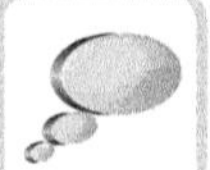

Activity 9.10

In **Activity 9.9** you were asked to identify some aspects of a less successful team.

- What would need to be done to make this team successful?
- Make an action plan for the first three aspects, outlining how you would address these issues if this team were a clinical team you were working with.
- What you would do in this situation once you are an RN?
- Are the actions for you as a student different from those you have identified as an RN?
- Identify any team working developmental needs and discuss these with your mentor, tutor or a colleague.

What skills do you need to work in a team?

Good communication skills are key to working in a team and even after years of experience you should continue to develop these as they are a complex but essential part of nursing practice. Failings in interprofessional communication can and do have devastating effects. This has been highlighted in high profile cases such as Victoria Climbié (Laming 2003), the Bristol Royal Infirmary (Kennedy 2000) and Baby P (Laming 2009). It is therefore important that you consider throughout your education how you are going to develop your communication and team working skills.The clinical placement staff will help identify appropriate developmental opportunities to improve your communication in relation to management, leadership and team working. It is, however, important to recognize that opportunities within your university to participate in presentations, seminar groups and lectures, all of which are excellent opportunities to gain confidence, ask questions and enhance your communication skills for the clinical setting (NMC 2010, 2011).

Patients and their families sharing their stories with you is one of the many privileges of being a nurse as well as an important aspect of being able to understand what patients want and need from their health care experiences. Patients and families are *part of the team* and should be treated with dignity and respect at all times, ensuring that a collaborative relationship is maintained. You need to ensure that you have this relationship to enable you to make appropriate clinical decisions, provide patient-focused care and advocate for your patient if required (NMC 2008, 2010). This is carefully outlined in the *Standards* and as a student nurse you are in an ideal position to spend time building a relationship with your patient. At first this may seem uncomfortable, but you will soon become experienced at meeting different people. Gaining an understanding of the person behind the condition is extremely important to help you build a rapport with the patient and their family. You need to ensure that it is a *collaborative* relationship where the patient is truly a partner in their care.

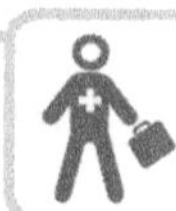

Case study 9.3: Moving and handling

An issue of poor practice in relation to moving and handling was raised when a student nurse was asked to assist with an episode of care in an area caring for older people with a diagnosis of dementia who required high levels of physical care. This involved staff moving a patient in a way which was not in alignment with the student's learning, resulting in the patient being physically lifted rather than using appropriate equipment. The student nurse declined to be involved in the move and mentioned it to the nurse in charge of the shift. The student also sought advice from their personal tutor who reported the situation to the link tutor for that area. The link tutor discussed this with the clinical manager who escalated the issue to the department's senior management team.

> **Activity 9.11**
>
> If you consider patients *within your own field of practice* who are vulnerable and need high levels of care then you should be able to reflect on the following questions:
>
> - How do you think you would feel in the situation outlined in the moving and handling case study?
> - How would you react if you saw something you considered to be inappropriate or poor practice?
> - What do you think might inhibit you from reporting this?
> - How do you think the clinical area received criticism in the case above?

In the case study the student was nervous about how they would be received and initially wanted to be moved to another area. They were supported by their personal tutor through the process of making a statement and meeting with the clinical manager. Both the clinical manager and the senior management team commended the student for highlighting the poor practice. The clinical manager also said that they would be keen to employ the student nurse once they were qualified as they needed staff who were willing to speak out to ensure high quality care.

This is an excellent example of how a student nurse can enhance patient care through both leadership and team working. It also highlights the fact that a team is much wider than those who provide the 'hands on' care. In this case there is the involvement of the student nurse, the teaching staff, the clinical team, the medical staff, the senior management team and moving and handling advisers. The team also involves the patient and their family or carers as these are the people services are provided for and therefore should always be at the centre of any care provision and decisions (DH 2006; National Leadership Council 2012). Although this is just one example, it reflects my overall experience when student nurses have highlighted concerns. Sometimes concerns can be the result of confusion or a misunderstanding. It is therefore really important to check with colleagues and ask them to explain their decision-making process so that you can develop your own decision-making skills in new ways. This allows you to learn from your experiences through reflection and evaluation (NMC 2010). The *Standards* also require you to learn through supervision and feedback. This can be done by discussing decisions with your mentor and asking for their view. Your mentor should not mind you asking for feedback or questioning their decision-making, as facilitating student nurses to develop their competence is a professional requirement (NMC 2008, 2010).

> **Activity 9.12**
>
> - Write down three things that you will do differently to enhance your practice as a result of reading this chapter. Discuss these with your mentor, tutor or a colleague.

Conclusion

This chapter has explored Domain 4 of the *Standards for Pre-registration Nursing Education* and considered the complexities of management, leadership and team working within the nursing context. Having in-depth knowledge, the ability to critically analyse situations, an understanding of how values, principles and assumptions affect the giving and receiving of care and having excellent interpersonal skills will enable you to develop as a practitioner. These are also important attributes for a good manager, leader and team worker and can assist nurses at all levels to provide high quality patient care. It is important to focus on leadership, management and team working early in nurse education as they are an integral part of the nurse's role, not an optional extra.

In summary:

- Leadership, management and team working skills are complex and inextricably linked in the provision of high quality health care.
- Student nurses are required to learn about leadership, management and team working and consider their contribution to this from the beginning of their education.
- Leadership, management and team working are an essential part of the role of nurses at all levels within organizations.

Further reading and resources

Curtis, E.A., De Vries, J. and Sheerin, F.K. (2011) Developing leadership in nursing: exploring core factors, *British Journal of Nursing*, 20(5): 306–9.

Mullins, L.J. (2007) *Management and Organisational Behaviour*, 8th edn. Harlow: Financial Times/Prentice Hall.

National Leadership Council (2012) *Leadership Framework*, available at: www.nhsleadership.org.uk/framework.asp.

Stanley, D. (2008) Congruent leadership: values in action, *Journal of Nursing Management*, 16(5): 519–24.

References

Acas (2007) *Teamwork: Success Through People*, available at: www.acas.gov.uk/CHttpHandler.ashx?id=349&p=0, accessed 6 August 2012.

Adair, J.E. (2003) *The Inspirational Leader: How to Motivate, Encourage & Achieve Success*. London: Kogan Page.

Adair, J.E. and Thomas, N. (2004) *The Concise Adair on Teambuilding and Motivation*. London: Thorogood.

Adair, J.E., Thomas, N. and Adair, J.E. (2008) *The Best of John Adair on Leadership and Management* (updated edition). London: Thorogood, available at: http://site.ebrary.com/lib/soton/Doc?id=10263887.

Atwal, A. and Caldwell, K. (2006) Nurses' perceptions of multidisciplinary team work in acute health-care, *International Journal of Nursing Practice*, 12(6): 359–65.

Banning, M. (2008) A review of clinical decision making: models and current research, *Journal of Clinical Nursing*, 17(2): 187–95.

Bass, B.M. and Stogdill, R.M. (1990) *Bass & Stogdill's Handbook of Leadership: Theory, Research, and Managerial Applications*, 3rd edn. New York: Free Press.

Belbin, R.M. (2010) *Team Roles at Work*, 2nd edn. Oxford: Butterworth-Heinemann.

Benner, P.E. (2001) *From Novice to Expert: Excellence and Power in Clinical Nursing Practice* (commemorative edition). Upper Saddle River, NJ: Prentice Hall Health.

Borrill, C.S., Carletta, J., Carter, A.J., Dawson, J.F., Garrod, S., Rees, A., Richards, A., Shapiro, D. and West, M.A. (2002) *The Effectiveness of Health Care Teams in the National Health Service*. Birmingham: Aston University.

Curtis, E.A., De Vries, J. and Sheerin, F.K. (2011a) Developing leadership in nursing: exploring core factors, *British Journal of Nursing*, 20(5): 306–9.

Curtis, E.A., Sheerin, F.K. and De Vries, J. (2011b) Developing leadership in nursing: the impact of education and training, *British Journal of Nursing*, 20(6): 344–52.

Darzi, A. (2008) *High Quality Care for all: NHS Next Stage Review, final report*. London: The Stationery Office.

DH (Department of Health) (2006) *A New Ambition for Old Age*. London: DH.

Downey, M., Parslow, S. and Smart, M. (2011) The hidden treasure in nursing leadership: informal leaders, *Journal of Nursing Management*, 19(4): 517–21.

Girvin, J. (1998) *Leadership and Nursing*. Basingstoke: Palgrave Macmillan.

Hersey, P., Blanchard, K.H. and Johnson, D.E. (2000) *Management of Organizational Behavior: Leading Human Resources*, 8th edn. Upper Saddle River, NJ: Prentice Hall.

Kean, S. and Haycock-Stuart, E. (2011) Understanding the relationship between followers and leaders, *Nursing Management*, 18(8): 31–5.

Kennedy, I. (2000) *The Inquiry into the Management of Care of Children Receiving Complex Heart Surgery at the Bristol Royal Infirmary*. Bristol: Central Office of Information.

Laming, W.H. (2003) *The Victoria Climbié Inquiry*. Norwich: The Stationery Office.

Laming, H. (2009) *The Protection of Children in England: A Progress Report*. London: The Stationery Office.

Mullins, L.J. (2002) *Management and Organisational Behaviour*, 6th edn. Harlow: Financial Times/Prentice Hall.

Mullins, L.J. (2007) *Management and Organisational Behaviour*, 8th edn. Harlow: Financial Times/Prentice Hall.

Mullins, L.J. and Christy, G. (2010) *Management and Organisational Behaviour*, 9th edn. Harlow: Financial Times/Prentice Hall.

National Leadership Council (2012) *Leadership Framework*, available at: www.nhsleadership.org.uk/framework.asp, accessed 2 April 2012.

NMC (Nursing and Midwifery Council) (2008) *The Code: Standards of Conduct, Performance and Ethics for Nurses and Midwives*. London: NMC.

NMC (Nursing and Midwifery Council) (2010) *Standards for Pre-registration Nursing Education*. London: NMC.

NMC (Nursing and Midwifery Council) (2011) *Guidance on Professional Conduct for Nursing and Midwifery Students.* London: NMC.

Northouse, P.G. (2010) *Leadership: Theory and Practice*, 5th edn. London: Sage.

Pearson, A., Porritt, K.A., Doran, D., Vincent, L., Craig, D., Tucker, D., Long, L. and Henstridge, V. (2006) A comprehensive systematic review of evidence on the structure, process, characteristics and composition of a nursing team that fosters a healthy work environment, *International Journal of Evidence-Based Healthcare*, 4(2): 118–59.

Peck, E. and Dickinson, H. (2009) *Performing Leadership.* Basingstoke: Palgrave Macmillan.

RCN (Royal College of Nursing) (2007) *Developing and Sustaining Effective Teams, Guide 1: What is a Team?* London: RCN.

Stanley, D. (2008) Congruent leadership: values in action, *Journal of Nursing Management*, 16(5): 519–24.

Stanley, D. and Sherratt, A. (2010) Lamplight on leadership: clinical leadership and Florence Nightingale, *Journal of Nursing Management*, 18(2): 115–21.

Sullivan, E.J. and Decker, P.J. (2009) *Effective Leadership and Management in Nursing*, 7th edn. Upper Saddle River, NJ: Harlow: Pearson Education.

Tuckman, B.W. (1965) Developmental sequence in small groups, *Psychological Bulletin,* 63(6): 384–99.

Tuckman, B.W. and Jensen, M.A.C (1977) Stages of small-group development revisited, *Group & Organizational Studies*, 2(4): 419–27.

Warriner, S. (2009) Midwifery and nursing leadership in the ever-changing NHS, *British Journal of Midwifery*, 17(12): 764.

10

Enhancing and developing leadership, management and team working skills in the community setting

Heather Bain and Mark Rawlinson

Chapter contents

Introduction

This chapter will explore the application of leadership and management skills when applied to community nursing. The content is primarily aimed at student nurses approaching 'sign off', however, the principles and application of knowledge are relevant to all students at any stage in their graduate programme, as well as in preceptorship and beyond.

As an adult learner you will have experienced in life a range of learning opportunities that have shaped your perception and understanding of what it is to lead and manage as well as what makes someone effective in this role; this may be from personal experience, observation or from what you might have read. As well as acquiring new knowledge, it is through acknowledging these life experiences and the application of thoughtful reflection that a deeper understanding of leadership and management can be developed (Bach and Ellis 2011).

The initial focus of the chapter will be on the importance of understanding the context of care, as well as highlighting the opportunities available to meet the Nursing and Midwifery Council (NMC) (2010) competencies presented in the list below.

NMC Domain 4: Leadership, management and teamworking

3 All nurses must be able to identify priorities and manage time and resources effectively to ensure the quality of care is maintained or enhanced.

4 All nurses must be self-aware and recognise how their own values, principles and assumptions may affect their practice. They

must maintain their own personal and professional development, learning from experience, through supervision, feedback, reflection and evaluation.

6 All nurses must work independently as well as in teams. They must be able to take the lead in coordinating, delegating and supervising care safely, managing risk and remaining accountable for the care given.

7 All nurses must work effectively across professional and agency boundaries, actively involving and respecting others' contributions to integrated person-centred care. They must know when and how to communicate with and refer to other professionals and agencies in order to respect the choice of service users and others, promoting shared decision making to deliver positive outcomes and to co-ordinate smooth, effective transition within and between services and agencies.

This chapter will also provide an opportunity to explore some key aspects of the management of care in the community, including care management, case management and caseload management. Aspects of team working will be integrated throughout the chapter. But first we will take a brief look at how as a student nurse you can start to develop your leadership and management capability by taking responsibility for your own personal and professional development, through managing your learning in your community placement.

Anticipating your learning needs

Building your leadership and management capacity does not begin when you start a placement. As an undergraduate student nurse you are not an empty vessel waiting to be filled. Taking personal responsibility for your own learning is an important part of qualifying as a graduate nurse and is an expected part of your professional role. One way of getting the most out of any placement is to pre-plan or investigate what the placement actually is, where it might be, and try and think about the scope of care and range of clinical challenges which you may encounter. A community placement will offer vast opportunities to meet the required competencies of the NMC (2010) and each placement will be different. So how can you go about getting to know your placement in advance?

- Ring the placement provider prior to your start date, introduce yourself and arrange an introductory visit to meet your mentor.
- Visit the placement provider's website or the Department of Health's (DH) website (countries specific). These portals will give you an indication of who works where and what they do. They may indicate what the clientele is and the population the placement serves.
- Identify relevant community focused journals and texts.

Figure 10.1 opposite is an illustration of how you might conceptualize a community placement from a user's perspective. The inner sphere represents the focus of your enquiry, for example, the patient and their family. Orbiting this might be a sphere populated by information about where they live. The next sphere might be their known health needs or personal targets to promote health and well-being; the next could be which health/ social care professionals (and non-professionals) are involved with them. Each orbiting sphere could have co-spheres, until you start to build up a matrix (or concept map) for that individual and their relationship to the community in which they live.

As can be seen from **Figure 10.1** and your undertaking of **Activity 10.1** it is possible to start to get an idea of the complexity of care delivery in the community. **Activity 10.1** could be repeated many times, for example putting the team you are working with at the centre and then creating a matrix that looks at the caseload management required for each day, each week, etc. Presenting your conceptualizations to your mentor is an ideal opportunity for reflection and discussion.

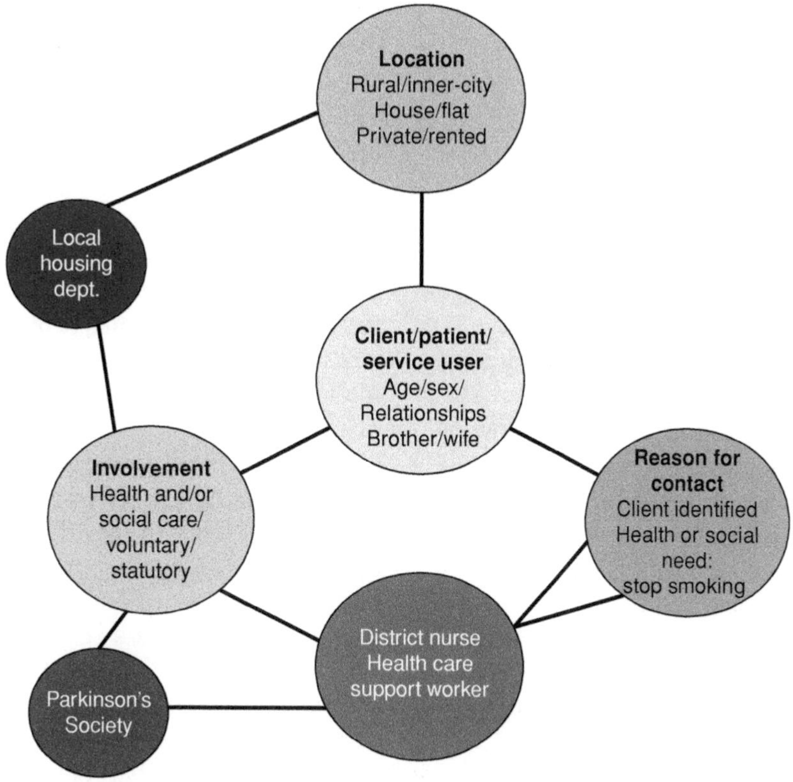

Figure 10.1 User-centred matrix

Activity 10.1

Now attempt to replicate **Figure 10.1** but put yourself in the centre sphere. Then put the NMC domain requirements for leadership in the separate orbiting spheres. Now build a matrix which utilizes the opportunities which you think might be available in your community placement.

The importance of leadership

According to the NHS Institute for Innovation and Improvement (2011) the development of leadership capability is an integral part of any clinician's (nurse's) training. Consequently a *Clinical Leadership Competency Framework* has been published (NHS Institute for Innovation and Improvement 2011). It is expected that all individuals operating in a clinical role will be able to demonstrate competence in the five identified domains:

- demonstrating personal qualities;
- working with others;
- managing services;
- improving services;
- setting direction.

Furthermore, each of the domains has four elements to it and each element has four competences to be attained. As a student nurse you are not required to demonstrate competence in the domains but they do serve as a useful framework to understand what being involved in shared or distributed leadership involves once you are qualified. These domains complement the NMC domains and will be threaded throughout the various activities and content in this chapter.

An attribute of strong professional leadership is to be able to look at yourself and your current capacity to lead and manage. This is a dynamic process and as you progress in your career the level of responsibility and scope of accountability also normally increases. As a student nurse on a community placement there are normally many opportunities for you to develop your leadership capacity. This will range from being involved in delivering one-to-one individualized care, to planning and managing a small caseload as well as working alongside the team leader to understand the management of the team's workload, for instance. What is, however, just as important to understand is the *context* in which you will be learning. The following sections provide you with a more detailed understanding of what leading and managing care in the community might involve, but we start with a brief exploration of what a 'community' might be: after all, this is what makes a community placement so different.

Nursing in the community

Developing an understanding of community, together with identifying health needs, is a prerequisite in order to plan effective health care for individuals, families and/or communities. The different settings for health care are more than just geographical or organizational variations and often require a different approach and philosophy to nursing care. The terms 'community' and 'community nursing' are ill defined in the literature, according to Chilton (2012). The differing perspectives on what a community is make it difficult to define, and it is therefore unsurprising that it is equally as difficult to define what community nursing might be, what or who a community nurse could be, and what that role entails.

Case study 10.1: John and Margaret

John and Margaret Sutherland are both 85 years old and living in a three-bedroomed detached country house in an affluent area. John is a retired teacher and Margaret has been a mother and housewife all of their married life. Financially they are struggling to maintain the house within their income and over the last few years they have used up their savings to put in central heating and replace their windows. With the current global economic situation their bills have escalated in the last year. However, they are reluctant to move as the house holds many happy memories.

Up until recently they have both kept good health but lately have been beginning to fail. John has developed maturity onset diabetes and Margaret's mobility has declined due to her rheumatoid arthritis and she is becoming increasingly confused. Last week she fell, causing a pre-tibial laceration. Jackie, their eldest daughter, a 60-year-old widow, has decided to retire and to relocate to be near her parents. Jackie is physically fit but overweight. Up until recently she has had a very stressful job and enjoys two or three large glasses of wine every evening to relax. Melissa, who has just turned 16, is the granddaughter of Jackie and has chosen to go and stay with her granny at her great grandparents' house for a week in the school holiday. Melissa has the potential to go to university and she is keen to study medicine. While she is at her great grandparents, she is being sick in the morning. She finally discloses to her granny that she is pregnant but is terrified to inform her mother.

Activity 10.2

- Try to define what you think a community might be. Consider what it might consist of, how it could be organized, what values and rules it may ascribe to, as well as where it might be and who could be considered to belong to any given community.
- Now consider Case Study 10.1, and for each individual (including the great granddaughter) develop a concept map (as in **Activity 10.1**).
- Try to identify which professionals or others could be involved with the family. What is important here is to start to think about why and in what capacity they may be involved and to remember that professionals often have multiple roles that occur simultaneously. The community nurse, for example, might be involved in the clinical care of Margaret regarding her rheumatoid arthritis and her leg laceration. That nurse would also be responsible for undertaking a risk assessment regarding prevention of falls, as part of promoting health and well-being.

Context of care

Communities are defined from many perspectives. If you accept that society in part is made up of various 'communities' and that some may be more visible than others, because they have certain characteristics or identifiable features (e.g. a demographic profile), then understanding the concept of a community becomes more accessible. At a very simplistic level, in health care, communities are often defined by a certain demographic characteristic (e.g. by age, sex or disease). We would suggest that as a student nurse, however, it is important to try not to limit your understanding of your patients and patient communities to these constrained definitions. Rather, it is pivotal to your understanding that you acknowledge the characteristics of differing cultures, expectations and needs.

It is important to understand the fundamental ethical principle at the heart of nursing: *that everyone is an individual and as such should be cared with due regard to this truth* (NMC 2008). According to the World Health Organization (WHO 1974), a community is: 'a social group determined by geographical boundaries and/or common values and interests. Its members know and interact with each other. It functions within a particular social structure and exhibits and creates certain norms, values and social institutions'. While this may be true of what a community *could* be, it could also be argued that this is not that representative of many of the communities which nurses often find themselves working in and with. For a district nursing team who are mainly involved with the housebound community (patients, carers and family) it would be unusual for *all* members (of that community) to *know* each other or interact with *each* other, let alone have a recognized social structure.

The communities the district nursing team normally serve will at one level be geographically orientated and comprise of a population of between 10,000 and 30,000 people. Working at this level requires the nurse to have strategic leadership and management skills and expertise based upon an understanding of epidemiology as well as local knowledge of social structures and networks if the intention is to understand/address need and actively promote health and well-being.

What emerges out of this brief discussion about the nature of communities is that a definitive definition is elusive if not illusive, a point well made elsewhere by Chilton (2012).

Despite this, for a student nurse or anyone new to community nursing, it is helpful to have a framework which allows a baseline of understanding to be developed. This ideally should address not just the *context* of care in the community but the *process* of care delivery. Laverack (2009) presents a framework that implies that communities can be understood through critical analysis of their key characteristics, these being:

- spatial dimensions – this refers to a place or locality;

- interests, issues or identities that heterogeneous groups of people share;
- social interactions that are often powerful in nature and often tie people into relationships or strong bonds with each other;
- shared needs or concerns that can be addressed by collective and collaborative actions (Chilton 2012).

However, the challenges facing nurses working in and with communities extend beyond the semantics of definitions, and extend to such influences as health inequalities, economic and employment opportunities, poverty and deprivation – in other words, the social determinants of health (Wilkinson and Marmot 2003). Addressing this type of need at a community level is primarily the responsibility of specialist community public health nurses, such as health visitors, school nurses, sexual health nurses and occupational health nurses, although local authorities have been charged with the responsibility to lead on public health in society (DH 2010).

For district nursing teams the same issues have to be recognized and addressed but often at an individual or group level (Rawlinson *et al.* 2012). Consequently, public health is also a central tenet of the practice of community nursing for other disciplines or, as Cowley (2007) so aptly puts it, public health is everybody's business. The central focus of this chapter is not public health per se, but it will be threaded throughout the various sections.

It should by now be possible to start to appreciate the complexity submerged within the concept of community nursing. We now consider the political context of community nursing, prior to looking in more depth at the delivery of care in the community. Community nursing is far more than just focusing on clinical care.

Political context and influences on community nursing

Policy is an integral component of community nursing and practitioners need to not only recognize the content of relevant health and social policy but appreciate policy is made as a consequence of decisions involving a wide range of people and organizations at local, national and international level. Within the UK, each of the four countries has its own health and social care policy, mainly due to the differing political stances since devolution (Bain and Adams 2011). While there is increasing divergence in terms of how health and social services are developed across the UK, all services have a shared approach that is 'shifting the balance of care'. Keeping people out of hospital is a priority (DH 2006; Scottish Government 2007), along with addressing health inequalities (Farrell *et al.* 2008; Scottish Government 2009a; Department of Health 2010; Welsh Assembly Government 2010). Then there are the challenges of an ageing population and workforce, with a greater number of people with multiple long-term conditions requiring complex health needs to be addressed in community settings (Welsh Assembly Government 2007; Scottish Government 2009b; Balanda *et al.* 2010; King's Fund 2010). Recent reports have suggested that the integration of health and social care has the potential to address some of these issues by improving services, resulting in better patient outcomes and better use of resources (Humphries and Curry 2011; Scottish Government 2012). Integration is well established in Northern Ireland, but is currently in its infancy in other areas of the UK, with some pilot sites now beginning to emerge. Unfortunately, like any period of significant change, there is the potential for a period of unrest. However, the consequence for community nurses of evolving policies has been the opportunity to influence local policy and increase their leadership and management capabilities in order to develop services to meet the policy agenda within the challenging context of the community (Dickson *et al.* 2011).

As a nurse you will have the opportunity on your community placement to explore how policy impacts on professional practice and understand the significance it has on quality improvement and service development to enhance people's well-being and experience of health care and its subsequent evaluation. Clearly nurses do engage

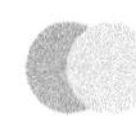

with policy at different levels to improve national and local services, and the National Occupational Standards for public health, mapped onto the Knowledge and Skills Framework, clearly outline how this can be achieved (Skills for Health 2009).

As a first-year student nurse it would be acceptable to have a broad awareness of policies that directly relate to yourself and to feed back any positive or negative comments relating to these policies to your mentor. However, as a nurse at the point of registration you would be expected to have knowledge of the major government policies relevant to health and inequalities, and to understand the implications for your practice. In addition you should be able to contribute to the development and implementation of specific policies, or identify the impact of policies and strategies on the population. Being actively involved in this would allow your mentor to assess your leadership potential.

Activity 10.3

Before commencing this activity, read it carefully and give some thought to how you might approach it – we would suggest you undertake this activity over a period of time.

- Access a local or national policy/strategy aimed at addressing health care needs in the community. You may find it useful to look again at Case Study 10.1 and consider policies relating to issues such as inequality, dementia, long-term conditions, nutrition, alcohol and teenage sexual health that may apply to this scenario.
- Consider the wider context of the selected policy/strategy and the local impact, then analyse it considering the implications for the role of nurses working in the community.

From examining both local and national policy you will recognize that there are many policies available aimed at improving health and well-being, and supporting people to live independently in the community. All provide vision and suggest strategies by which this might be achieved, and local policy is often developed to address national policy. Both national and local policy not only informs your practice in the community, but your practice helps to influence policy. Your contribution to issues such as quality, service design and the service user experience are all policy issues that are essential to nursing in the community (NHS Education for Scotland 2012).

Key learning

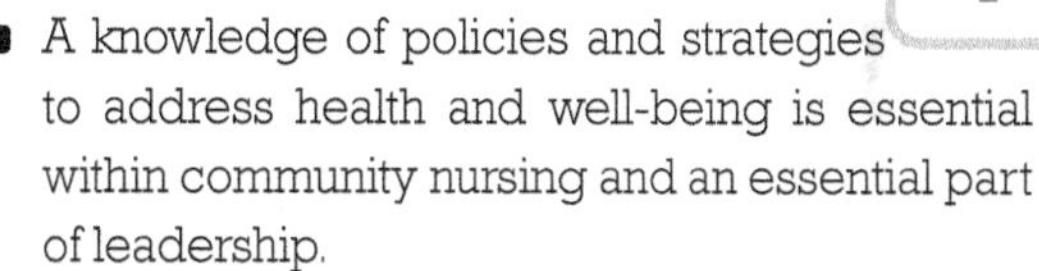

- A knowledge of policies and strategies to address health and well-being is essential within community nursing and an essential part of leadership.

Care at or close to home

Having a community experience grounded in the reality of care delivery in or close to someone's home environment provides a unique opportunity to see how care can be individualized and person-centred. Care-giving in the home environment is very different to hospital- or clinic-based care, because the home environment does not have the same structures, focus and equipment of a hospital-based setting. For example, there is no professional routine in a person's home, there are no hierarchical structures, such as those you find in a hospital, and most notably there is no continued presence of a health care professional. While all care is oriented around the patient's need whatever setting it is delivered in, factors such as how they live, where they live and with whom they live all have an impact on care-giving in the community context. That is not to say that a home is absent of resources and routines and not subject to policies and guidelines – it is – but they are in the background and the person(s) and their family network are usually more obviously the focus of the foreground.

As previously alluded to, delivering care in a wide variety of settings with variable facilities poses unique challenges (QNI 2010). In addition to having to comprehend and adjust to the environment in which the care is required, appreciating that often patients and families are much more involved in the negotiation of care and its subsequent management can be a challenge to existing ways of organizing, planning and monitoring care delivery.

Underpinning effective community nursing is the relationship that is established at the point of care delivery (Wilson and Miller 2012). Working with frail and vulnerable people across the life span will often require the community nurse (student) to demonstrate a range of effective and appropriate communication, management and leadership skills, because care in the home is nearly always associated with and dependent on a team or collective of practitioners. Empowering others is an ascribed aim of nursing care, and for this to be possible there needs to be clarity around responsibilities and management plans for empowering the patient and their family. This clarity needs to exist in order to promote health and well-being more broadly and not just revolve around the immediate task that is to be undertaken (Baker and Rawlinson 2012).

Consequently for the nurse (as illustrated in Case Study 10.1) this often involves undertaking a comprehensive assessment (sometimes jointly with other services) in order to coordinate a wide range of services and referrals to ensure a patient can manage at home (QNI 2010).

Patient-centred care in the home

A term often used in community nursing is that of being a 'guest' in someone's home (McGarry 2003). This approach to care clearly suggests that the patient is at the centre of the relationship with the health care professional, indicating that the power lies with the consumer and not the provider. This is a concept that is ideologically aligned with current government rhetoric, and can be put another way: 'No decision about me, without me' (DH 2010). However, maintaining this type of therapeutic relationship, where it is a fluent yet ill-defined concept, based on the idea of autonomy and choice (Wilson and Miller 2012), can be challenging, especially if patient/carer expectations are at odds with those of the nurse. Nurses need to take the position that optimal care is being patient-centred, based on the premise that all people want to be able (are able) to take decisions and responsibility for themselves (mental capacity withstanding), as opposed to the position that the nurse knows best.

Management of nursing care in the community: caseloads

In **Activity 10.2** you will have identified the variations in the approach to work organization, prioritization and delegation of nurses working in the community. However, all nurses in the community will commonly refer to their 'caseload'. Haycock-Stuart *et al.* (2008) describe the community nurse's caseload as a 'ward without walls'. Bain and Baguley (2012) define a caseload as the designated population in a practice or geographical area for which the community nurse is responsible. Caseload management is an organizational technique that involves individuals' and families' health care needs being met by the right person at the right time.

Activity 10.4

As a student, what experience have you had of caseload management? Have you identified any differences between how a district nurse, health visitor or school nurse manages their caseload? Do the processes you have observed manage the demand for the service? What skills are required to manage a caseload?

By doing **Activity 10.4**, combined with your practice learning experience to date, you will have recognized that caseload management is a complex process that involves a different set of skills from working in the acute sector and focusing on the care of individuals. There is little quality

 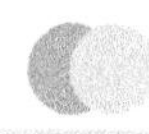

research in the literature on caseload management but there is literature offering professional opinion (Kolehmainen *et al.* 2010). Ervin (2008) identified three skills of caseload management:

- organization;
- prioritization;
- coordination.

However, considering the changing workforce in the UK, with an increasing number of support workers and assistant practitioners in the community, *delegation* also needs to be considered as an essential skill (Bain and Baguley 2012).

You now need to consider these skills in the context of community nursing and adopt an incremental approach to developing your competence in caseload management. As a student nurse you may have the opportunity to develop some of the following skills by starting with a small caseload.

1. *Organizational skills* provide the framework for caseload management. The approach taken depends on whether it is a corporate caseload as opposed to a single caseload being held and managed by an individual practitioner (Bain and Baguley 2012); or a GP-attached caseload where care is provided to all registered patients to a GP surgery; or a geographical caseload where care is provided to a whole population (Gould 2012); or an integration of different approaches. Understanding the approach taken to manage caseloads will help you to consider the structures utilized within the everyday planning of work. For example, clearly defined referral criteria will aid the management of the demand for the service and help achieve effective, efficient and equitable caseload management, and having a filing system (whether electronic or paper-based) will help to manage the workload.
2. The second identified skill for caseload management is *priority-setting*. However, setting priorities at an individual level is different from setting priorities for a caseload. Ervin (2008) describes priority-setting in the community on three levels. Firstly, it is a philisophy of care determined by the organization holding the caseload. Secondly, it is the scheduling of visits on a daily, weekly or monthly basis. And finally, it is the rescheduling of visits and also allowing capacity for new referrals to be admitted onto the caseload.
3. *Coordination* is the third skill required for caseload management, and involves effective communication between team members and among the multidisciplinary team (Ervin 2008). Coordination is a skill you will have developed throughout your undergraduate nursing course, and in the community you will be able to develop it further. Actively engaging in team meetings and case conferences will afford you this opportunity, as will participating in more recent concepts such as 'virtual wards'. A virtual ward is where the 'ward' mirrors a hospital ward but the patient remains in their own home, with the relevant services and professionals networking 'electronically' to manage the care (Ross *et al.* 2011).
4. Finally, *delegation* is important to consider. Delegation can be defined as the process of directing another person to perform tasks or activities. It involves a two-part responsibility. The one to whom authority is delegated becomes responsible to undertake the task, but the delegator remains responsible for getting the job done (Barr and Dowding 2008). The NMC *Code* (2008) states that:
   - you must establish that anyone you delegate to is able to carry out your instructions;
   - you must confirm that the outcome of any delegated task meets required standards.

It is acknowledged that delegation is a complex process, and even more so in the community

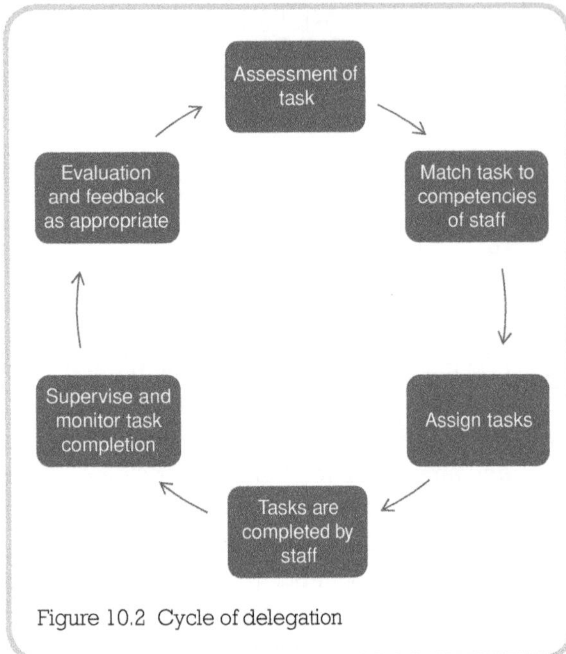

Figure 10.2 Cycle of delegation

when, often, people are lone workers and working in environments that are unpredictable. It is therefore essential that within teams there is an awareness of everyone's knowledge, skills and capabilities, there is familiarity with the evidence for risk management, and leaders need to be fully aware of the accountability, responsibility and authority issues that are interrelated. Gopee and Galloway (2009) suggest a six-stage linear process for effective delegation, and developing this into a cyclindrical process as illustrated in **Figure 10.2** could be seen to develop teamwork.

Activity 10.5

- Reflect on a day's activities from your community placement and the cycle of delegation in **Figure 10.2**. Was it clear what was delegated from the team leader? How did they make delegation decisions? Were the delegated decisions reasonable? You may wish to discuss this activity with your mentor.

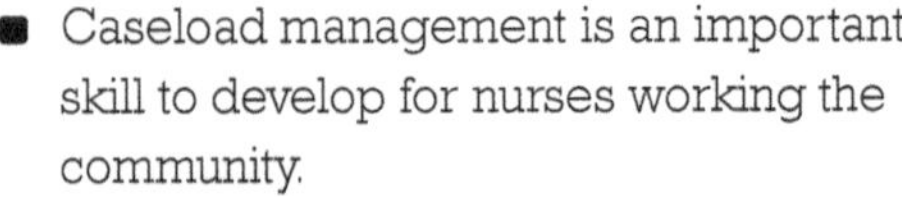

Key learning

- Caseload management is an important skill to develop for nurses working the community.
- Organization, priority-setting, coordination and delegation are key skills of caseload management.

When reading this section on caseload management you will have realized that the individuals within the caseloads are often referred to as 'cases' and all require different approaches to address their health care needs. In the literature this can be confusing as the term 'caseload management' is often confused with the terms 'care management' and 'case management', which are used interchangeably (Ervin 2008; DH 2010). The NHS has used these terms for many years in the areas of mental health and social care but now 'case management' is a term mainly used to address the management of long-term conditions.

The management of long-term conditions in the community

The management of long-term conditions is a key priority in all four countries of the UK. The Health and Social Care Model (DH 2005) illustrates the level of dependency of patients on health and social care professionals (see **Figure 10.3**).

You can see that there are three approaches to care according to need.

- **Level 1, self-care:** which encourages people to take an active role in managing their own health with support from health professionals. Some 70–80 per cent of people with long-term conditions are within this category.
- **Level 2, care management:** which is aimed at people with one long-term condition to allow them to manage their condition with the support from a multidisciplinary team.

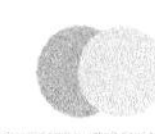

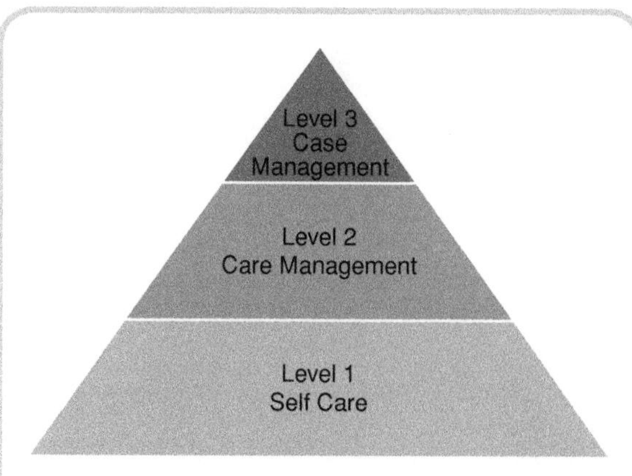

Figure 10.3 Health and social care model (DH 2005)

- **Level 3, case management:** aimed at people with two or more long-term conditions who have complex needs.

These approaches are not confined to one professional group and components will be integrated into your role as a nurse working in the community. The various health needs of the population allows for a diversity of approaches and interventions (Hutt *et al.* 2004). As a novice in the community you are more likely to be involved with self-care and care management but as you advance in your career case management will be an increasingly important concept. At this stage it is important that you have a broad understanding of the key principles of case management.

Case management

Case management is a generic term with no single definition which has led to confusion and uncertainty about what it involves. For example, in some contexts it refers to an intensive and time-limited intervention aimed at preventing an event such as a hospital admission. Others see it as ongoing individualized care aimed at keeping people well (Ross *et al.* 2011). Case management recognizes that the intensity of needs in people with long-term conditions varies and that care should be targeted accordingly. Ross *et al.* (2011), in their review of the literature, suggest that the key aims for case management remain unchanged and are:

- to reduce hospital utilization (avoid admission or promote earlier discharge);
- to improve care outcomes for patients;
- to enhance the patient experience.

Considering the aims of case management it is evident that it has the potential to be a significant element of the community nurse's role, and in particular the district nurse. Please note that in some areas of the UK terms such as 'community matron' or 'case manager' are used to define the role of community nurses undertaking work with this particular client group and this can cause confusion. However, for the purpose of this chapter it is more important that you understand what case management is.

Hutt *et al.* (2004) identified six core elements of case management:

- case-finding or screening;
- assessment;
- care planning;
- coordination and referral;
- monitoring;
- review.

More recently Ross *et al.* (2011) identified the same elements but redefined care coordination to include: medication management; self-care support; advocacy and negotiation; psychological support; and monitoring and review, followed by a final element – case closure for time-limited interventions (see **Figure 10.4**).

This approach mirrors the nursing process which you will be familiar with, however, Hutt *et al.* (2004) differentiate case management from similar approaches by the following features:

- intensity of involvement;
- breadth of services planned;
- duration of involvement.

There are many different models of case management used in the UK (Lewis 2008) such as Evercare, Kaizer and Pfzizer and the more recent virtual ward (Ross *et al.* 2011). The evidence of their effectiveness is mixed due partly to the complexity of

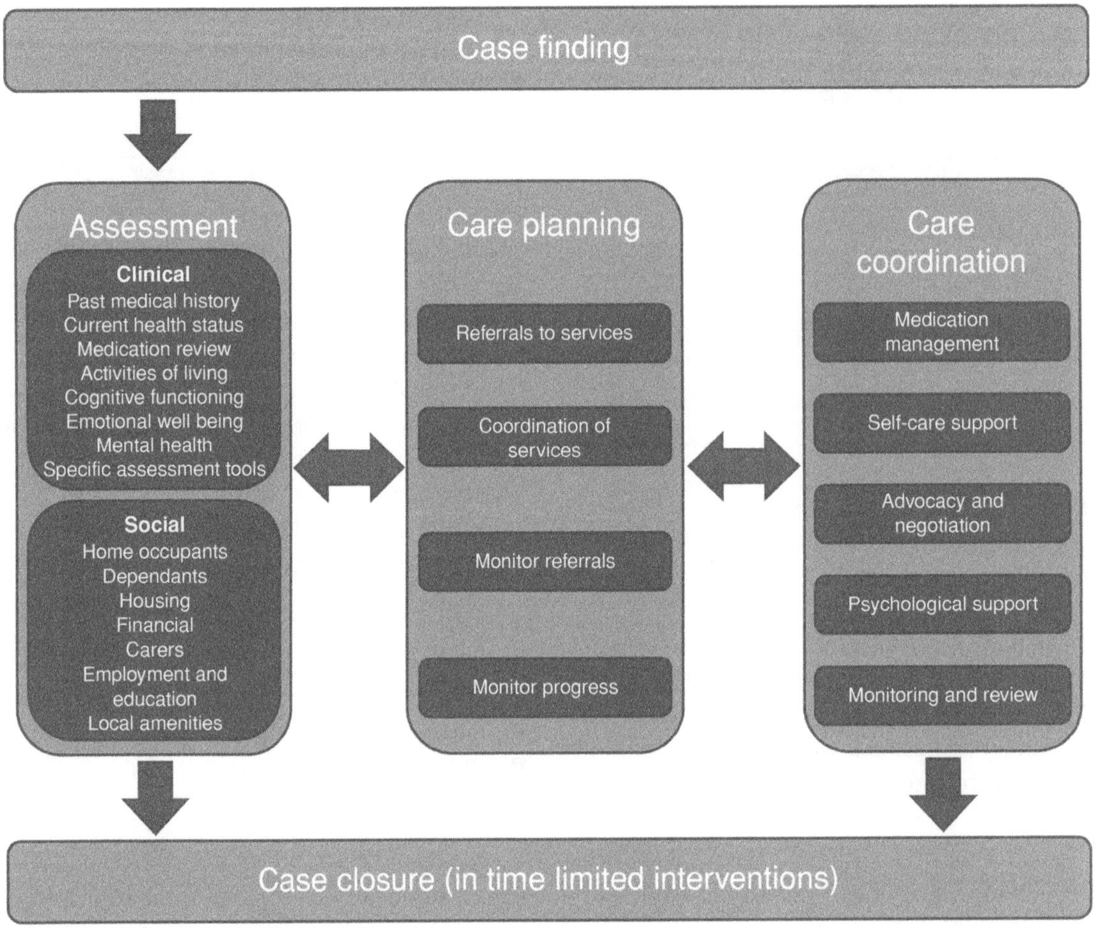

Figure 10.4 Components of case management

the factors involved, and not all case management models measure outcomes. However, it is acknowledged that case management is a valid approach for managing people with complex needs and long-term conditions in the community. Factors identified in the more successful examples range from the competencies of the individual case manager to the overall programme design and the context in which these operate (Ross *et al.* 2011).

There are different levels of responsibility for nurses within case management. However, it is clear that it requires practitioners to be working towards an advanced level in an autonomous role and that effective leadership is required for both its development and its delivery. The enabling factors that Ross *et al.* (2011) identified are:

- assigned accountability;
- clarity around roles;
- clinical and non-clinical skills:
  - interpersonal skills
  - problem-solving skills
  - negotiation and brokerage skills
  - prescribing qualification
  - access to adequate training;
- building relationships:
  - between case managers and their patients
  - between case managers and GPs
  - between case managers and hospital staff;

- programme design:
  - targeting and eligibility
  - caseload size
  - single point of access/assessment
  - continuity of care
  - effective use of data and communication processes;
- factors in the wider system:
  - shared vision and objectives
  - collaboration between health and social care
  - aligned financial flow and incentives
  - stakeholder engagement
  - resources and services available in the community.

It is identified that case management requires to be an approach that is supported by relevant policy and infrastructure that is well organized and delivered within an integrated care system (Ham 2009). This will then result in improving patient experiences and outcomes (Powell-Davies *et al.* 2008). Community nurses therefore need to embrace the case management approach to meet the changing demography of the population. Case study 10.2 provides one example of a case management approach.

Activity 10.6

In the light of Ian's case study, consider a client from your community placement who would have benefited from the principles of case management.

- What would be the advantages of this approach to the service, the primary health care team and the client?
- What key skills are required to undertake an assessment of the client?
- What resources are required to manage their care, including input from nurses and other members of the multidisciplinary team?

Case study 10.2: Ian

Ian is a 78-year-old man who has recently moved into a sheltered housing complex in a town after having given up his farm following several hospital admissions. He is a widow with two grown up children living 100 miles away and has a past medical history of chronic obstructive pulmonary disease (COPD), Parkinson's, type 1 diabetes and rheumatoid arthritis. He has had four hospital admissions in the previous six months for unstable blood sugars and exacerbations of his COPD. On his last hospital admission a care package was commenced with a daily visit from a formal carer to assist with personal hygiene and supervise medication. It also resulted in a referral to the district nurse to act as case manager.

The case management approach involved:

- development of anticipatory care plan – shared with Ian's GP and the out of hours service outlining his full range of needs;
- weekly visits from the district nurse;
- carers increased to twice daily to assist with evening meals and supervise medication;
- patient education programme about lifestyle advice in relation to diabetes, COPD, rheumatoid arthritis and Parkinson's;
- installation of a telehealth monitoring system to record a range of vital signs on a daily basis, to be transmitted to a monitoring centre;
- fortnightly meetings via the virtual ward to discuss and plan care with the multidisciplinary team;
- six-monthly medication review by the district nurse who is a non-medical prescriber;
- one exacerbation of COPD managed at home due to early intervention;
- one hospital admission where an early discharge was facilitated due to the support mechanisms in place.

Conclusion

This chapter has offered an insight into some of the management and leadership skills required in the context of community nursing and builds on the previous key points of Chapter 9. The importance of team work and collaborative working to meet health care needs is threaded throughout the chapter, and the concepts of caseload management and case management have been explored. It is hoped that having read this chapter you will have developed an understanding of management and leadership issues in the context of community nursing, and recognized that the development of effective leadership and management skills and expertise is considered to be a continuous and evolving process (RCN 2012).

Further reading and resources

Chilton, S., Bain, H., Claridge, A. and Melling, K. (eds) (2012) *The Textbook of Community Nursing*. London: Hodder Arnold.

NHS Education for Scotland (2012) *Modernising Nursing in the Community*, available at: www.mnic.nes.scot.nhs.uk.

Ross, S., Curry, N. and Goodwin, N. (2001) *Case Management: What is it and how it can be best implemented?* available at: www.kingsfund.org.uk/publications/case_management.html.

References

Bach, S. and Ellis, P. (2011) *Leadership, Management and Team Working in Nursing*. Exeter: Learning Matters.

Baker, D. and Rawlinson, M. (2012) *Student Nurses Have the Right to Appropriate Learning Opportunities in Practice. How Capable is Practice at Providing Them*? Harrogate: RCN Education Forum Conference.

Bain, H. and Adams, D. (2011) Strategic context of policy – a look at UK policy for the four nations, in E. Porter and L. Coles (eds) *Policy and Strategy for Improving Health and Wellbeing*. Exeter: Learning Matters.

Bain, H. and Baguley, F. (2012) The management of caseloads in district nursing services, *Primary Health Care*, 22(4): 31–7.

Balanda, K.P., Barron, S., Fahy, L. and McLaughlin, A. (2010) *Making Chronic Conditions Count: Hypertension, Stroke, Coronary Heart Disease, Diabetes. A Systematic Approach to Estimating and Forecasting Population Prevalence on the Island of Ireland*. Dublin: Institute of Public Health in Ireland.

Barr, J. and Dowding, L. (2008) *Leadership in Health Care*. London: Sage.

Chilton, S. (2012) Nursing in a community environment, in S. Chilton, H. Bain, A. Clarridge and K. Melling (eds) *The Textbook of Community Nursing*. London: Hodder Arnold.

Cowley, S. (2007) Foreword, in I. Coles and E. Porter (eds) *Public Health Skills: A Practical Guide for Nurses and Public Health Practitioners*. Oxford: Blackwell.

DH (Department of Health) (2005) *Supporting People with Long Term Conditions to Self Care*. London: DH.

DH (Department of Health) (2006) *Our Health, Our Care, Our Say: A New Direction for Community Services*. London: DH.

DH (Department of Health) (2010) *Equity and Excellence: Liberating the NHS*. London: DH.

Dickson, C., Gough, H. and Bain, H. (2011) Meeting the policy agenda, part 1: the role of the modern district nurse, *British Journal of Community Nursing*, 16(10): 495–500.

Ervin, N.E. (2008) Caseload management skills for improved efficiency, *The Journal of Continuing Education in Nursing*, 39(3): 127–32.

Farrell, C., McAvoy, H., Wilde, J. and Combat Poverty Agency (2008) *Tackling Health Inequalities – An All-Ireland Approach to Social Determinants*. Dublin: Combat Poverty Agency/Institute of Public Health in Ireland.

Gopee, N. and Galloway, J. (2009) *Leadership and Management in Health Care*. London: Sage.

Gould, J. (2012) Organisation and management of care, in S. Chilton, H. Bain, A. Clarridge and K. Melling (eds) *The Textbook of Community Nursing*. London: Hodder Arnold.

Ham, C. (2009) The ten charactersitics of a high performing chronic care system, *Health Economics, Policy and Law*, 5: 71–90.

Haycock-Stuart, E., Jarvis, A. and Daniel, K. (2008) A ward without walls? District nurses' perceptions of their workload management priorities and job satisfaction, *Journal of Clinical Nursing*, 17: 3012–20.

Humphries, R. and Curry, N. (2011) *Integrating Health and Social Care. Where next?* available at: http://bit.ly/fQ0hDl.

Hutt, R., Rosen, R. and Macauley, J. (2004) *Case Managing Long Term Conditions: What Impact Does it Have in the Treatment of Older People?* available at: http://bit.ly/ZpQj9W.

King's Fund (2010) *Long-term Conditions*, available at: www.kingsfund.org.uk/topics/longterm_conditions.

Kolehmainen, N., Francis, J., Duncan, E. and Fraser, C. (2010) Community professionals' management of client care: a mixed-methods systematic review, *Journal of Health Services Research and Policy*, 15: 47–55.

Laverack, G. (2009) *Public Health, Power, Empowerment and Professional Practice*. Basingstoke: Palgrave Macmillan.

Lewis, S. (2008) Case management, in R. Neno and D. Price (eds) *The Handbook for Advanced Primary Care Nurses*. Maidenhead: Open University Press.

McGarry, J. (2003) The essence of 'community' within community nursing: a district nursing perspective, *Health and Social Care in the Community*, 11: 423–30.

NHS Education for Scotland (2012) *Modernising Nursing in the Community*, available at: www.mnic.nes.scot.nhs.uk.

NHS Institute for Innovation and Improvement (2011) *The Clinical Leadership Competency Framework*. London: DH.

NMC (Nursing and Midwifery Council) (2008) *The Code: Standards of Conduct, Performance and Ethics for Nurses and Midwives*. London: NMC.

NMC (Nursing and Midwifery Council) (2010) *Standards for Pre-registration Nursing Education*. London: NMC.

Powell-Davies, G., Williams, A., Larsen, K., Perkins, D., Roland, M. and Harris, M. (2008) Co-ordinating primary health care: an analysis of the outcomes of a systematic review, *Medical Journal of Australia*, 188(8): S65–8.

QNI (Queen's Nursing Institute) (2010) *Position Statement – March: Nursing People in Their Own Homes – Key Issues for the Future of Care*. London: QNI Press.

Rawlinson, M., Baker, D. and Fergus, M. (2012) Public health – promoting health and wellbing, in S. Chilton, H. Bain, A. Clarridge and K. Melling (eds) *The Textbook of Community Nursing*. London: Hodder Arnold.

RCN (Royal College of Nursing) (2012) *The Principles of Nursing Practice*. London: RCN.

Ross, S., Curry, N. and Goodwin, N. (2011) Case management, what is it and how it can be best implemented, available at: www.kingsfund.org.uk/publications/case_management.html.

Scottish Government (2007) *Better Health, Better Care*. Edinburgh: Scottish Government.

Scottish Government (2009a) *Equally Well: Report of the Ministerial Task force on Health Inequalities*. Edinburgh: Scottish Government.

Scottish Government (2009b) *Improving the Health and Well-being of People with Long-term Conditions: An Action Plan*. Edinburgh: Scottish Government, available at: www.scotland.gov.uk/Publications/2009/12/03112054/11.

Scottish Government (2012) *Integration of Adult Health and Social Care in Scotland: Consultation on Proposals*. Edinburgh: Scottish Government.

Skills for Health (2009) *Public Health Skills and Career Framework*. Oxford: Public Health Resource Unit.

Welsh Assembly Government (2007) *Designed to Improve Health and the Management of Chronic Conditions in Wales*. Cardiff: Department for Health and Social Services/Welsh Assembly Government.

Welsh Assembly Government (2010) *Doing Well, Doing Better*. Cardiff: Wesh Assembly Government.

WHO (World Health Organization) (1974) *Expert Committee on Community Health Care Nursing, Report of the WHO Expert Committee* (Technical Report Series no. 558). Geneva: WHO.

Wilson, P. and Miller, S. (2012) Therapeutic relationship, in S. Chilton, H. Bain, A. Clarridge and K. Melling (eds) *The Textbook of Community Nursing*. London: Hodder Arnold.

Wilkinson, R. and Marmot, M. (2003) *Social Determinants of Health: The Solid Facts*, 2nd edn. Geneva: WHO Europe International Centre for Health and Society.

11

Leadership, management and team working in an acute care setting

Debbie Goode and Pauline Black

Chapter contents

Introduction

In the previous two chapters you were introduced to the concepts of leadership, management and team working. You were encouraged to identify the importance of leadership from the start of your student journey. Key questions were posed and you were encouraged to reflect upon leadership at different stages of your learning and development as a professional nurse. It is important to remember the attributes and attitudes required to make a good leader and the impact they have on patient care, team working and your career development. These qualities also require adaptation, depending on which practice learning setting you are working in.

In Chapter 10 you focused on leadership skills and styles required by nurses in a community setting. Leading a caseload of patients or a team of staff, along with case management and its complexities were discussed using examples from community and public health perspectives.

This chapter will focus on an exploration of the *skills* of leadership, management and team working required from an acute care perspective. It will explore the components required to build a safe and effective team and identify, using case studies, examples of poor teamwork and their potential negative impact on patient care and safety. In particular the chapter will facilitate and support you in understanding and interpreting evidence and the application of developing graduate attributes by using examples drawn from the different fields of nursing practice.

Domain 4: Leadership, management and team working, generic standard for competence

The Nursing and Midwifery Council (NMC) for all nurses (2010: 20) states that:

> All nurses must be professionally accountable and use clinical governance processes to maintain and improve nursing practice and standards

of healthcare. They must be able to respond autonomously and confidently to planned and uncertain situations, managing themselves and others effectively. They must create and maximise opportunities to improve services. They must also demonstrate the potential to develop further management and leadership skills during their period of preceptorship and beyond.

It is also important to be cognizant of the need to demonstrate your leadership abilities both in a team setting and as an individual practitioner. Many of the skills and principles already discussed in this book, such as professional values (Chapter 2) and decision-making skills (Chapters 7 and 8) are implicit in the way in which leadership is demonstrated and actioned in clinical practice.

Skills of leadership, management and team working required from an acute care perspective

In order to discuss the skills that a nurse requires to lead, manage and be an effective team member it is useful to revise or revisit your own personal and professional attitudes and attributes.

Required personal attributes

In order to achieve competency you must become self-aware and recognize how your own values, principles and assumptions may affect your practice, especially in relation to leadership, management and team working. Each one of us has differing personal beliefs and values and it is these that make us unique.

Caring is a crucial and pivotal requirement for all nurses as professionals (McCormack and McCance 2010). Nursing is a unique profession where the care of others, often in a time of stress, vulnerability or panic, is evident. It is therefore crucial to understand that the way we view ourselves influences the way we interact with others. Often, if we are encouraged and praised we will feel positive and strive to do our best, and as a personal attribute it is important that we can demonstrate this to others also. When you think about your personal beliefs and values around nursing it will hopefully reflect and help to enhance a person-centred approach to care.

Activity 11.1

Take some time to reflect on the reason why you wanted to be a nurse.

- Has it changed since your application to the course?
- Is the course what you expected, either in a good way or in a negative way?
- What impact has nursing had on your life as a student and what path do you think nursing will take you down in your future life?

Required professional attributes

The NMC (2011) has published *Guidance on Professional Conduct for Nursing and Midwifery Students*. Several of these guidelines relate specifically to working as part of a team. This guidance should help you begin to formulate how you develop as a nurse as well as a member of the health care team, no matter what area, speciality or branch you practise within. The guidelines relate to the competencies that you must achieve prior to registration. However, as part of your ongoing journey it is important that your use of this guidance moves from a position of knowledge to a demonstration of practice, as this is a fundamental requirement of professionalism.

As a student who is required to develop and demonstrate leadership and management skills, it is essential that you have the correct policy knowledge to support your practice. In each field of nursing practice there will be strategic differences. Through your course to date you will have been introduced to many theories, statements, procedures and evidence to support your practice. In becoming a team member the skill is to integrate the best of all of these aspects into your own personal style, which helps to shape you as a professional. This will not happen immediately but will grow with your confidence and ability.

When working as part of a team it is pivotal that you become familiar with the roles and responsibilities of other people involved in providing health and social care. Importantly you will recognize the need to:

- work cooperatively within teams and respect the skills, expertise and contributions from all people involved with your education;
- treat all colleagues, team members and those with whom you work and learn fairly and without discrimination;
- inform your mentor or tutor immediately if you believe that you, a colleague or anyone else may be putting someone at risk of harm.

The person-centred nursing framework

Now that you have thought about your own personal and professional attitudes and attributes you can begin to place them within the context of leadership, management and team working. This will assist you in developing a strategy to achieve competency. The person-centred nursing framework devised by McCormack and McCance (2006) is one way to help you plan your learning and development as a nurse. It is comprised of four key constructs.

The first element is described as the *prequisites* (the attributes of the nurse). These would align themselves to the four domains of professional values, communication and interpersonal skills, nursing practice and decision-making, and leadership, management and team working. These are important as they relate to the generic and field-specific competencies and progression points that you have to achieve to qualify as a registered nurse (RN). So, for you to achieve competency, you must demonstrate that you are professionally competent, that you have the interpersonal skills necessary to be an RN in your field of practice, that you are committed to the job of being a nurse, as well as showing clarity in your beliefs and values and being self-aware. These qualities will enable you to develop the skills required to be part of a safe and effective team in any field of nursing.

The second element in the model is the *care environment*. This component of the framework focuses on the context in which the care is provided. This includes appropriate skill mix, shared decision-making, effective staff relationships, supportive organizational systems, power-sharing, the potential for innovation and risk-taking, and the physical environment. For many of you, each care environment may be new and you should begin to recognize how the dynamics of the environment may influence the care you provide. The environment or culture can play a large part in how you achieve your competencies as there can be differences in interprofessional behaviour, leadership styles, team dynamics and mentor support (Pollard 2009). As a final-year student especially, you will begin to develop your own management skills in each care environment. You should have studied academic modules or units on leadership and management that will enable you to reflect upon the type of leader, manager or team member that you wish to become. Often, though, the care environment will influence your style. This can happen as a result of positive and negative influences. You may witness attributes in other nurses that you want to emulate, such as the way Nurse Green always speaks in an informative manner to patients and families. However, in an acute setting you may also witness team dynamics and personal management styles that you definitely do not wish to copy. This may be the way Nurse Brown likes to be in control and does not delegate any aspects of management to others for fear they would not be completed to the correct standard.

The third element of the framework is *care processes*. This component of the model focuses on the actual development of person-centred care through a range of activities. If your focus in care delivery takes account of working with the patient's beliefs and values, engagement, shared decision-making, having sympathetic presence and providing holistic care, then you are developing person-centred care processes. To ensure your progression at each stage of the programme you are expected to deliver care with a high degree of effective communication skills that require a therapeutic engagement with the person (please refer to Chapter 6). Communication in leadership, management and team work is essential. For you to achieve these competencies you should begin to consider the patient or client as a *partner* in care.

The final element of the framework is the *person-centred outcome*. If you have begun to achieve the first three elements the results should be satisfaction with care, involvement with care, feeling of well-being and the creation of a therapeutic culture. If you have achieved this you will be able to reflect on your development as a questioning and compassionate practitioner. You will also have a structure on which you can develop your leadership, management and team working skills in the acute setting. Expectations follow from experience and the exposure that you have had to leadership, management and team working. In the previous chapters you will have reviewed the qualities that make a good leader.

Key learning !

- An awareness of how personal attitudes influence your practice is essential to guide your skill development in leadership, management and team working.
- Professional guidance provides you with frameworks within which to work.
- Understanding the influence of your attitudes and attributes and the environment and processes of care is integral to achieving person-centred outcomes for those in your care.

Leadership and management skills and their impact in acute care settings

In Chapter 9 you were introduced to the concepts, skills and differences of leadership, management and team working. Key questions you have addressed related to the required attributes and attitudes of leadership and the impact they have on patient care, team working and career development. You should now recognize that leadership and management are not the same, but are often discussed as one skill within nursing and health care. In this section you will focus on the effects of these attributes and attitudes on the delivery of acute care.

Clarke and Ketchell (2011: 2) provide a helpful a definition of acute care:

> The care provided to patients experiencing serious acute illness, which is often accompanied by a rapid and progressive deterioration in their condition, and which requires urgent assessment to determine the level of care required. This will normally require frequent monitoring and reassessment of need. Acute illness can complicate existing chronic illness.

The NMC (2010: 39) states that: 'All nurses must work independently as well as in teams. They must be able to take the lead in coordinating, delegating and supervising care safely, managing risk and remaining accountable for the care given'. For the student nurse it is vital that you focus on developing:

- dependability;
- accountability;
- responsibility;
- collaboration;
- responding/presencing;
- delegation/supervision.

Leadership in acute care settings

Leadership skills are essential to encourage and develop teams in any setting but in the acute care setting the clinical situation can change very rapidly. Admissions and transfers can happen at any time of the day or night and clinical conditions can be unpredictable and deteriorate without prior indication. The nature of patient illness in this setting can really test, stretch and challenge the personal and professional attributes you possess, as identified earlier, as well as your leadership skills and style.

Activity 11.2

Think of examples from your practice learning where you have observed events suddenly changing around you, and reflect on the response of the health care team.

- Who led?
- Was it the person you expected?
- What was the outcome?
- Would you act differently if you were in the situation tomorrow?

Effective leadership is a key characteristic of an effective team (WHO 2011). Effective team leaders facilitate and coordinate the activities of other team members and use their skills to be:

- confident and willing to lead;
- aware of their strengths and weaknesses and when they require additional help and guidance;
- vigilant as to what is happening around them;
- competent to make clinical judgements in order to set priorities and make decisions;
- able to delegate activities to the team in a manner that encourages strengths and overcomes weakness of each individual member;
- logical and fair when negotiating resolutions to conflict;
- able to use available resources effectively;
- able to create a culture that welcomes questioning practitioners and encourages feedback;
- able to communicate openly in a way that ensures all team members know exactly what is expected of them at any given point in time.

Leadership in acute care is essential because of the nature of the environment and the requirements of the patients. So when leaders can demonstrate and apply the skills outlined above, the impact on the workplace can be positive and effective. If the nurse as a leader does not demonstrate these skills then the evidence suggests that problems may occur. Padilla *et al.* (2007: 179) describe the five features of destructive leadership:

- it is seldom wholly destructive: there are both good and bad results in most leadership situations;
- it involves dominance, coercion, and manipulation rather than influence, persuasion, and commitment;
- it is focused more on the leader's needs than the needs of the team;
- it produces results that compromise the quality of the working experience for the team and detract from the team's main purpose;
- it will continue to thrive where there are susceptible followers and conducive environments.

These features are also explained in the 'toxic triangle', where the destructive leader is placed in a situation with susceptible followers and an environment which is conducive to further development of their poor leadership behaviour (Padilla *et al.* 2007: 180) (see **Figure 11.1** on the next page).

As a student you may experience some of these elements while on placement or during your course within the university. You may feel that you may be a 'conformer' due to lack of experience and in that respect become a susceptible follower. However, the NMC (2006) states that all practice

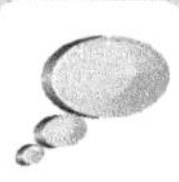

Activity 11.3

Have you had any experiences of bad leadership? If so:

- Think about the situation you were in at the time.
- How did your personal attributes help you deal with it?
- Did the environment have any impact on what was happening?
- What effect did this have on you?
- What have you learned from it?

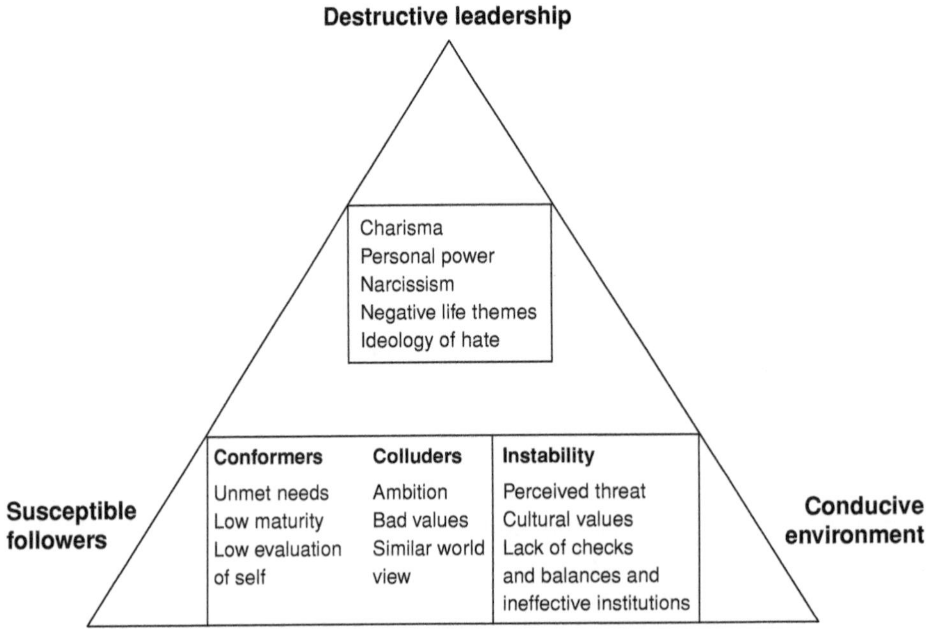

Destructive leadership

Charisma
Personal power
Narcissism
Negative life themes
Ideology of hate

Susceptible followers

Conformers
Unmet needs
Low maturity
Low evaluation of self

Colluders
Ambition
Bad values
Similar world view

Conducive environment

Instability
Perceived threat
Cultural values
Lack of checks and balances and ineffective institutions

Figure 11.1 The toxic triangle: elements in three domains related to destructive leadership

learning environments must be audited to ensure that they are conducive to learning for you; so this element should not occur. If it does there are 'checks and balances' in place within your university and the practice learning setting to ensure that action is taken to alleviate such problems. As you develop a set of skills to assist you in the acute care setting you will soon discover people who can help you. These people may be your lecturer, practice teacher, mentor or other staff member. You do not have to take this journey alone. If you are experiencing issues around leadership and/or management during your practice learning you need to address it before it becomes detrimental to your development.

Key learning !

- Effective leaders are facilitators who place the needs of the people in their team and in their care before their own status.
- Effective leaders need a team who are willing to commit to a shared purpose and goal. Destructive leaders have a need to force the team and those in their care to conform to the roles that have been set for them in order for the leader to feel successful.
- Destructive leaders often have team members who either submit to their authority without question or who try to imitate them – thus reinforcing their negative behaviour patterns.

Learning to lead and manage

Think about some activities that you have carried out with friends, colleagues, team-mates, groups, clients, professionals and other people. As you discovered in Chapter 9, leaders do not always have a management role and managers are sometimes not great leaders. As a student you should plan to observe and interact in as many team, leadership and managerial situations as possible. Your mentor will discuss this with you when you are developing your learning contracts and action plans for a particular period of practice learning placement, relating to your stage of training.

Skills of leadership and management in an acute setting

In acute care nursing managers have to develop many varied and skills. They have a physical environment to organize and maintain as well as a personal dimension to facilitate on many levels. Nurse managers must be the link to the organizational hierarchy as well as the ward leader in relation to staff, patients and families.

The government has encouraged support for ward managers as they have to develop skills to be able to cope with issues such as:

- conflict;
- apathy;
- stress;
- pressure and shortage of funds, staff and resources;
- personality clashes;
- bullying and harassment;
- delegation;
- cultural relationships/traditions;
- complaints;
- risk management.

Plus many more. What other issues do you think a manager will have to consider?

As a student who has to learn to manage a group of patients in the acute care setting, you will also be aware of many of these elements within your practice learning. You may wonder how you will be able to do this, but if you think about your transition from primary school to secondary education and the transition you have now made to university, you will realize that you have already managed many of the above situations.

When there is no clear leader in an acute setting the results can be disastrous (see **Activity 11.4**).

Activity 11.4

Martin Bromiley founded the Clinical Human Factors Group (CHFG) after the death of his wife in 2005. The website can be found here: www.chfg.org/about/background-to-chfg.

- Watch a reconstruction of what happened during that routine operation and have a look at 'Just a routine operation training video' at www.institute.nhs.uk/safer_care/general/human_factors.html. This highlights the issues of leadership, management and team working in acute care very clearly.

Team working

Lafasto and Larson (2001) believe that effective team members bring 'added value' to the group. These members contribute in a unique manner by, for example, building confidence and trust or by having a positive attitude to the work involved. Some of the issues of working in a team within the acute care area are exemplified in a survey of operating theatre surgical teams (Flin *et al.* 2006). Consultants, trainee surgeons and theatre nurses reported generally positive attitudes to behaviours that were associated with effective teamwork and safety. Some responses to the questionnaire demonstrated that there was a sense of personal invulnerability to stress and fatigue. Human factors of stress, poor communication and tiredness within teamwork are areas where teams can fail and patient safety can be compromised. The Patient Safety First campaign launched in response to the Department of Health's review of patient safety in England (DH 2006) is an example of how a focus on safety can improve outcomes for people requiring care. Further details can be found at www.patientsafetyfirst.nhs.uk.

The World Health Organization (WHO 2011) presents the qualities shown in **Figure 11.2** as timeless characteristics of teams that work well.

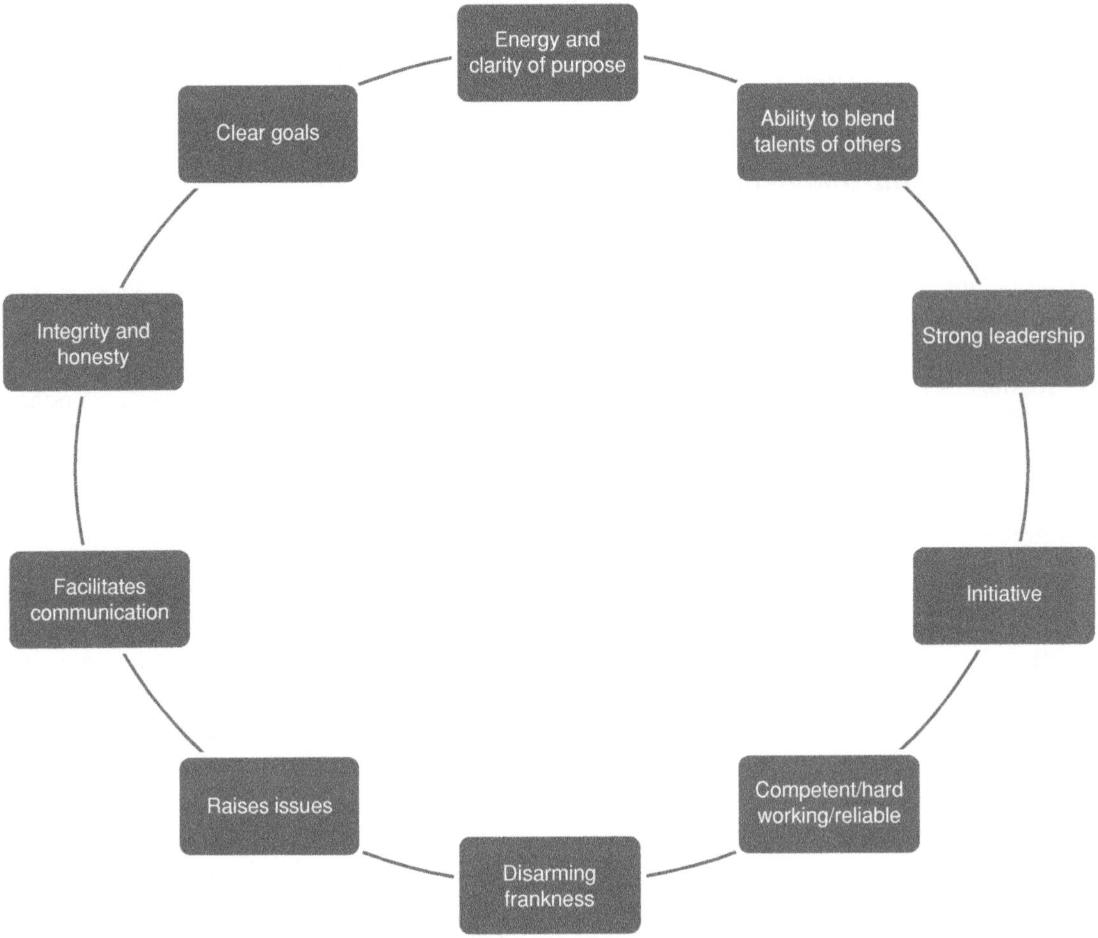

Figure 11.2 Qualities of an effective team member

Each of us has attributes that we can bring to a team, for added value. In health care settings such as acute care the ward manager of the clinical area may not have any say in the people allocated to the team, but the care delivery in the area will ultimately be their responsibility. One of the most important skills that you can learn to develop is to be able to manage *yourself*. You will have found that you have been able to develop different management skills during your course to date. When the course began you may have been hesitant in talking to patients and relatives but have now developed a method of managing this in a professional manner. For example, if you canot answer a relative's question you would respond by saying, 'I do not know the answer to that question, but I will find out for you.' Fear of questions can then be removed from an encounter because you have a method for managing the situation. You also may have been able to manage your time in the practice learning environment by developing learning contracts and making action plans in relation to specific skills you wanted more experience in. So by developing the skill of self-management you

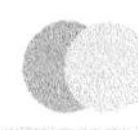

will already have become a person who can fit into a team.

Components of building a safe and effective team

Lafasto and Larson (2001) realized that each team has a goal to reach; something that they are trying to *do* rather than *be*. In order for the effective team to achieve that goal there needs to be an element of collaboration (working together with the multi-disciplinary team) and coordination (who is doing what, when and how?).

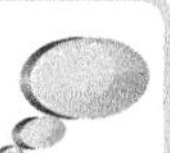

Activity 11.5

- As a student, what experiences have you had in teams in the clinical area?
- Do they all work in the same way?
- Have you felt included in the team?
- What are the reasons why you did/did not feel included?

Pollard (2009) believed that the student experience of practice learning within interprofessional settings varies considerably. There were several contributing factors to the success of interprofessional learning as described by Pollard, including the influence of doctors and differing professional cultures; mentors' support for student engagement in interprofessional working; and individual students' confidence levels. The clinical areas when Pollard was writing were largely managed by nurses and some senior nurses were proactive in involving students in the work of the interprofessional team. However, Pollard found that many students lacked systematic support for interprofessional engagement. You may have had experience of working and learning with other professionals as interprofessional learning and activities are a common aspect of your nursing education as well as an expected outcome of your development. This may have given you the confidence to work within an interprofessional team as well as voice your opinion on patient care. Suter *et al.* (2009) present a case for competent collaboration: knowing how your professional culture will impact upon patient care as well as the ability to find your place within the clinical team, recognizing each participant's strengths. This can only happen in an environment or culture that fosters mutual respect and collaborative practice and therefore there is inevitably a strong correlation between the culture in which you work clinically and your ability to demonstrate clear leadership and management skills. In nursing there is a vital clinical element in teamwork: you have to know what you are doing when collaborating towards a common objective.

In any area of nursing, teamwork is seen as a vital component to achieving the common objective, which is quality patient or client care. Each one of us has different experiences and we bring different problem-solving skills to each situation. Neumann *et al.* (2010) presented a special report on the importance of interdisciplinary team working within the speciality of physical and rehabilitation medicine. They believe that teams work best because they not only have a combination of skills, but also work towards agreed aims using an agreed strategy. What one person lacks, another has in abundance: this is the strength of teams (see **Figure 11.3**). We can then support and develop one another to ensure that our working knowledge is at its most efficient. So a student going into his or her management placement will be supported by the rest of the clinical team to achieve competency at the final progression point. The sign-off mentor will facilitate clinical experience along with the medical and other allied health professionals.

The problem with teams is exactly the same as their strength: they are made up of individuals who have different experiences and bring different problem-solving skills to a given situation. Each team member may believe *their* way is best and this can lead to conflict.

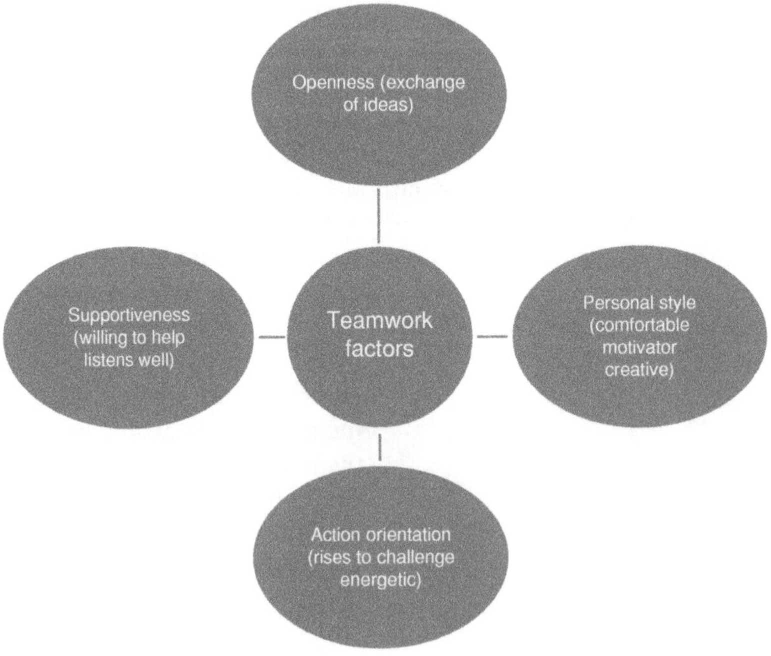

Openness (exchange of ideas)

Supportiveness (willing to help listens well)

Teamwork factors

Personal style (comfortable motivator creative)

Action orientation (rises to challenge energetic)

Figure 11.3 Factors that distinguish effective team members

Case study 11.1a: Nurse Blue

Student Nurse Blue is a Year 3 adult nurse in placement in the accident & emergency (A&E) department of a local hospital. It is week 6 of a 10-week experience. She has not had learning opportunities in this hospital area before. She has worked with her mentor on days and nights on a regular basis and has a good relationship with him. He is experienced in A&E nursing as he has worked in this area for over 10 years. He has mentored many students in A&E in the past.

On duty today is Consultant Able who is renowned for her high level of knowledge and expectations. She would say that 'she does not suffer fools gladly' and demands a high standard of care to be delivered. The next senior doctor on duty is Doctor New. He has only just begun his rotation into this clinical area and appears hesitant in his decision-making, often relying on nursing staff for guidance. The nurse in charge is dynamic A&E Sister Confident who has 15 years' emergency care experience. Her decision-making skills are rapid and responsive. The other senior nurse is Sister Duty; she is due to retire in three months' time. She has been allocated a heavy administrative role because the ward manager is on sick leave after surgery.

Also on the unit is Staff Nurse Element, who usually works nights but has been rotated onto days in order to undertake training. There is one agency nurse who has little A&E experience and can only care for trolley waits. She has been allocated this duty for the entire shift. The ward assistant is a mature student nurse who worked in A&E for 18 years prior to realizing her dream of getting a place at university to study nursing. She is in Year 2 of the same course as Student Nurse Blue. The ward assistant is working part time to help fund her place on the course. She has a daughter the same age as Student Nurse Blue. The ward clerk covers the whole of the emergency department, but is more familiar with the minor injury area, as this is where her desk is located.

Activity 11.6

- What are the skills, strengths and weaknesses of the members of the team outlined in **case study 11.2**?
- What questions would you ask about this team to help you work in this area? Think about their experience, skills and personal attributes but also consider the physical environment.

Poor teamwork and the potential impact on patient care and safety

Problems with teams can contribute negatively to the climate of communication within a team. Manser (2009) published a review of the literature on teamwork and patient safety in dynamic domains such as operating rooms, intensive care, emergency medicine and trauma and resuscitation teams. Flawed teamwork was shown as an important contributing factor in the analysis of incident reports or adverse events, usually in relation to communication issues. The issue of communication with different terms of reference (different clinical backgrounds) also caused breakdown in teamwork.

The WHO's multiprofessional *Patient Safety Curriculum Guide* (2011: 22) states:

> Patient safety skills and behaviours should begin as soon as a student enters a hospital, clinic or health service . . . Most health-care students have high aspirations when they enter into their chosen field, but the reality of health-care systems sometimes deflates their optimism. We want students to be able to maintain their optimism and believe that they can make a difference, both to the individual lives of patients and the health-care system.

The importance of patient safety

Patient safety within the acute care area has many elements. We previously outlined the person-centred framework in caring for our patients. Professional competency is one area that needs to be highlighted. As a student you should be working in a safe learning environment, one which places patient safety high on the agenda. Planning how you are going to achieve your learning outcomes in the practice learning area will assist you to develop management and team-building skills. A safe environment for you as a student is an area

Case study 11.2

It is 8.40 a.m. on a Friday morning and the A&E department is quite calm. There are a few patients awaiting transfer to wards and some waiting for minor interventions following triage.

Two patients arrive in the department at the same time, one via ambulance and the other by private car. The patient in the ambulance is Tom, a 56-year-old man complaining of chest pain. The second patient is Jane, a 9-year-old girl with learning disabilities who has had vomiting and diahorrea all night and has a pyrexia of 38.5°C.

Student Nurse Blue has been allocated Jane to admit to the department while her mentor admits Tom.

Suddenly, Tom has a cardiac arrest and everyone in the immediate care area runs to his cubicle. Student Nurse Blue has never seen an arrest and is keen to participate in resuscitation, having developed a learning contract for this in her portfolio. Consultant Able is off the floor at an audit meeting and Doctor New is the most senior doctor in the unit. Sister Duty is covering tea breaks and is at Tom's bedside. Student Nurse Blue is called into the arrest situation by her mentor.

Doctor New asks her to begin chest compressions, which she does effectively. In the meantime, Doctor New is trying to assess heart rhythm but does not instruct Student Nurse Blue to stop compressions while he does this. She continues as instructed but when Sister Duty observes this she shouts loudly at both Doctor New and Nurse Blue. Nurse Blue becomes very distressed at what she feels is a mistake in this acute episode and runs out of the cubicle. As she passes Jane she notices that her condition has deteriorated and her mum has fallen asleep with her head on the trolley.

Activity 11.7

Consider Student Nurse Blue's predicament in case study 11.2

- What actions would you take if you were in this situation?
- What happened in the few minutes that have just been described?
- Think about patient safety, communication and the learning environment.

that you may not have thought of before, but a safe nurse will ensure patient safety is maintained throughout an acute care episode.

Several suggestions are made on how to make your practice environment safer in the NHS document *Implementing Human Factors in Healthcare* (see http://bit.ly/YizsjA). It is recommended that safe and relevant communication can be achieved through the use of a structured framework to provide a systematic depth of information-sharing that will lead to timely action being taken. SBAR is an acronym for situation, background, assessment and recommendation, and is used as a technique for communicating critical information. It is intended to ensure that the correct information and level of concern is communicated in an exchange between health professionals (Haig *et al.* 2006). Thinking about the care provided in a systematic way can also influence practice safety. One way to achieve this is using the 'five Ws' approach (who, what, where, when, why). Keep on asking questions until you understand what is happening (see **Figure 11.4**).

Box 11.1 Using the SBAR tool

The Situation, Background, Assessment and Recommendation (SBAR) tool is systematic, logical and helpful and is often used by professional leaders in analysing a situation. Have a look at this link: http://bit.ly/10ilyGl.

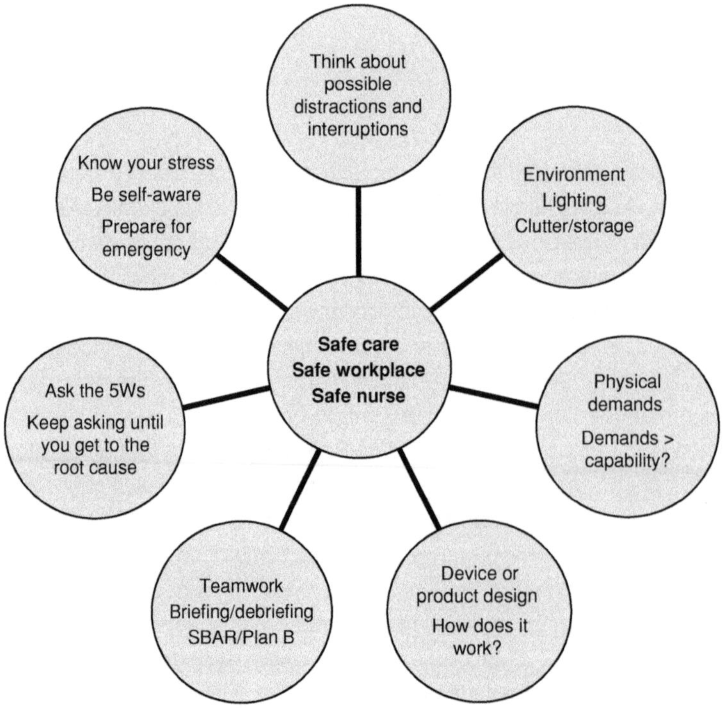

Safe care
Safe workplace
Safe nurse

Think about possible distractions and interruptions

Environment
Lighting
Clutter/storage

Physical demands
Demands > capability?

Device or product design
How does it work?

Teamwork
Briefing/debriefing
SBAR/Plan B

Ask the 5Ws
Keep asking until you get to the root cause

Know your stress
Be self-aware
Prepare for emergency

Figure 11.4 How to build a safe environment

Case study 11.3

Student Nurse Blue remembers what her mentor told her during her induction to the department. If there is an emergency she should push the emergency button and all staff will come to the area where the call has originated from. She hesitates for a moment, thinking that she will be shouted at again, but then looks at Jane and thinks to herself:

- Jane is deteriorating
- There are not enough staff on the department to deal with Tom's arrest and Jane's condition
- I do not have the knowledge, experience and skills to deal with this on my own
- I need help

So she pushes the emergency call bell.

Within seconds other staff arrive at her bedside. Sister Duty asks, 'What has happened?' Student Nurse Blue remembers a technique for team members to accurately share information and ensure that the focus is on the information being communicated. She reports using the SBAR tool (situation, background, assessment, recommendation).

Situation

What is going on with these patients?

There are two patients who need urgent attention. Tom has arrested in Cubicle 2. Doctor New and Sister Duty are in the cubicle performing CPR. They have the crash trolley. Nurse Blue has found her patient, Jane, unresponsive.

Background

What is the clinical background or context?

Tom, a 56-year-old man complaining of chest pain, was admitted 10 minutes ago. No family are here yet. Jane, a 9-year-old girl with learning disabilities, has had vomiting and diahorrea all night and has a pyrexia of 38.5°C.

Assessment

What is the problem?

Tom may have had a myocardial infarction. Jane has shallow, rapid breathing and is a very poor colour. Her mother is beside the trolley. Nurse Blue is concerned about the deterioration in her condition.

Recommendation

What should be done to correct the problem?

Having outlined the situation Student Nurse Blue asks Sister Duty's advice on how to proceed.

How did Student Nurse Blue deal with this situation?

She left Tom's cubicle distressed and annoyed, but then her observation skills overtook her own sense of injustice. She used her skills of recall from previous learning to apply the SBAR tool to provide a structured handover to Sister Duty.

She realized that as a team member she did not have the skills to act in Jane's best interests and knew when and how to call for help. There were several factors that impacted on her experience of teamwork. Look back at **Figure 11.4** and identify them.

After the situation in A&E has been resolved and both patients have been stabilized Student Nurse Blue is angry at the way Sister Duty spoke to her in the arrest situation and feels that there is now a bad relationship between herself and Sister Duty. She wants to resolve the issue and speak to Sister Duty.

Leading resolution in conflict situations

As nurses in a professional environment we have to respect the other person's viewpoint, even if we do not agree with them. It is sometimes very difficult to work alongside a person who completely disagrees with your view or assessment of a situation. When this happens it is often necessary to speak to the other person to resolve an area of conflict. Arnold and Boggs (2007) highlight several methods that could assist you in cases such as this. These have been integrated into a diagrammatic plan of action, shown in **Figure 11.5**.

A key demonstration of professional behaviour expected of all professionals, particularly leaders, is the ability to apply these strategies as part of your day-to-day practice. Pivotal to this is your ability to communicate appropriately. It is evident that the qualities of leadership in a professional are multifaceted and require a range of knowledge, approaches and skills. Learning to manage situations that you are uncomfortable with will assist you in developing a personal and professional portfolio of coping strategies that will stay with you for your whole life.

Case study 11.4

Student Nurse Blue is able to speak to Sister Duty with her mentor and explain that she felt angry and humiliated that she was shouted at during the arrest, even though she was conducting herself in a professional manner and doing as instructed by Doctor New. Sister Duty is able to understand this and apologizes for shouting. She explains that she felt under a lot of pressure at the time and should not have reacted in that manner. Student Nurse Blue is able to reflect on her A&E experience as one which clearly improved her communication and team working skills. She was able to demonstrate competency in these areas for her mentor.

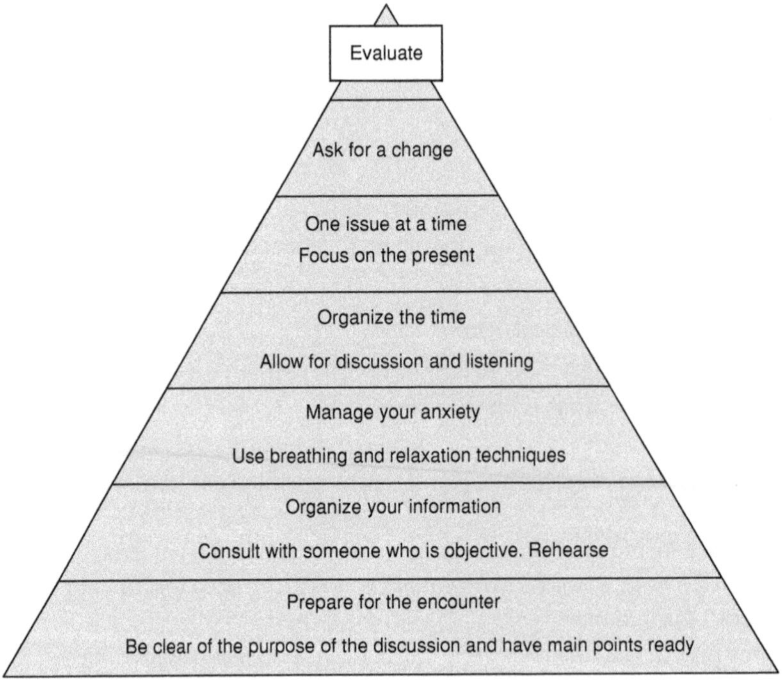

Figure 11.5 Developing a strategy to address conflict

 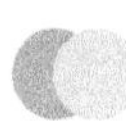

Conclusion

This chapter has focused on the skills of leadership, management and team working from an acute care perspective. The components needed in order to build a safe and effective team were highlighted through a case study. Examples of poor teamwork and their potential impact on patient care and safety were presented in relation to clinical evidence.

In summary:

- To become an effective practitioner you must be aware of your own personal and professional attitudes and attributes.
- Effective leadership is a key characteristic of an effective team. Lafasto and Larson (2001) believed that effective team members brought 'added value' to the group. These members contributed in a unique manner by, for example, building confidence and trust or by having a positive attitude to the work involved.
- Patient safety can be improved by good teamwork, especially communication.
- Reflection on your experiences will assist you in developing a plan to achieve competency.

Further reading and resources

http://bit.ly/10dWhvN. The NHS Institute has developed a leadership framework to provide guidance, available at this link.

http://www.institute.nhs.uk/. The NHS has developed leadership and management programmes and a suite of resources that can be accessed at this link.

You will also find the following links helpful:
http://www.nmc-uk.org/Students/
http://bit.ly/10PIAHb
http://www.patientsafetyfirst.nhs.uk/
http://nhsleadershipframework.rightmanagement.co.uk/website/default.aspx
http://www.nmc-uk.org/Students/
http://teamstepps.ahrq.gov/abouttoolsmaterials.htm
http://www.patientsafetyfirst.nhs.uk/ashx/Asset.ashx?path=/Intervention-support/Human%20Factors%20How-to%20Guide%20v1.2.pdf

References

Arnold, E. and Boggs, K.U. (2007) *Interpersonal Relationships: Professional Communication Skills for Nurses*, 5th edn. Philadelphia, PA: W.B. Saunders.

Clarke, D. and Ketchell, A. (eds) (2011) *Nursing the Acutely Ill Adult: Priorities in Assessment and Management*. Basingstoke: Palgrave Macmillan.

DH (Department of Health) (2006) *Safety First: A Report for Patients, Clinicians and Healthcare Managers*. London: DH.

Flin, R., Yule, S., McKenzie, L., Paterson-Brown, S. and Maran, N. (2006) Attitudes to teamwork and safety in the operating theatre, *Surgeon*, 4(3): 145–51.

Haig, K.M., Sutton, S. and Whittington, J. (2006) SBAR: a shared mental model for improving communication between clinicians, *The Journal on Quality and Patient Safety*, 32(3): 167–75.

Lafasto, F. and Larson, C. (2001) *When Teams Work Best*. Thousand Oaks, CA: Sage.

Manser, T. (2009) Teamwork and patient safety in dynamic domains of healthcare: a review of the literature, *Acta Anaesthesiol Scand*, 53: 143–51.

McCormack, B. and McCance, T.V. (2006) Development of a framework for person-centred nursing, *Journal of Advanced Nursing*, 56(5): 472–9.

McCormack, B. and McCance T.V. (2010) *Person-centred Nursing: Theory and Practice*. Chichester: Wiley/Blackwell.

Neumann, V., Gutenbrunner, C., Fialka-Moser, V., Christodoulou, N., Varela, E., Giustini, A. and Delarque, A. (2010) Interdisciplinary team working in physical and rehabilitation medicine, *Journal of Rehabilitation Medicine*, 42: 4–8.

NMC (Nursing and Midwifery Council) (2006) *Standards to Support Learning and Assessment in Practice*. London: NMC.

NMC (Nursing and Midwifery Council) (2010) *Standards for Pre-registration Nursing Education*. London: NMC.

NMC (Nursing and Midwifery Council) (2011) *Guidance on Professional Conduct for Nursing and Midwifery Students*. London: NMC.

Padilla, A., Hogan, R. and Kaiser, R.B. (2007) The toxic triangle: destructive leaders, susceptible followers, and conducive environments, *The Leadership Quarterly*, 18: 176–94.

Pollard, K. (2009) Student engagement in interprofessional working in practice placement settings, *Journal of Clinical Nursing*, 18: 2846–56.

Suter, E., Arndt, J., Arthur, N., Parboosingh, J., Taylor, E. and Deutschlander, S. (2009) Understanding and effective communication as core competencies for collaborative practice, *Journal of Interprofessional Care*, 23(1): 41–51.

WHO (World Health Organization) (2011) *Patient Safety Curriculum Guide*, multi-professional edition. Geneva: WHO, available at: http://tinyurl.com/c6lbcsm.

SECTION

5

Achieving competencies: simulation, working with mentors and learning when working abroad

Simulation: crafting your care

Eloise Monger and Kate Goodhand

12

Chapter contents

Introduction

This chapter provides an insight into the use of simulation as a means to learn the craft of caring. The complexities of learning a craft are acknowledged and a set of practical activities are suggested to help get the most out of your experiences. The chapter will demonstrate how students in all fields of practice can utilize simulated practice activities as part of their learning to achieve the Nursing and Midwifery Council (NMC) competencies. We will outline how simulation is built on learning theory and discuss the ways in which you can use simulated practice to link what you learn in lectures with what you do in your practice placements. The chapter will provide an insight into the underpinning thinking that you will need to engage with to get the most out of simulated practice and highlight how experiences in simulation contribute to the development of graduate attributes. The case studies from the University of Southampton and Robert Gordon University draw on research evidence to illustrate the sophisticated nature of this method of learning. By focusing on 'learning how to learn in practice placement' and 'making the most of feedback', the objective is to provide practical advice which students can use to capitalize on their simulated practice experiences in the real world.

This chapter is relevant to all of the NMC competencies in each of the four domains: professional values; communication and interpersonal skills; nursing practice and decision-making; and leadership, management and team working.

Simulation: enhancing professional skills and competence

Learning, rehearsing and perfecting the skills required to qualify as a nurse is a complex and challenging task. Most importantly, these skills extend well beyond the ability to perform physical tasks. In order to be prepared for the exciting and ever-changing world of health care, you will embark on a journey of personal, professional and academic discovery. A variety of strategies and techniques are used throughout your course to assist in the process of developing these professional and graduate attributes. The most obvious professional development strategy is the requirement for nurse education in the UK to incorporate learning not only in the university, but also in real health care environments. This helps students contextualize the knowledge required and recognize the practical competencies associated with that knowledge. The ability to apply the theoretical knowledge gained from academic study to clinical situations, and to do this well, is one of those essential attributes. Another is the ability to reflect on, and develop, one's professional skill set from experiences in practice. This means not just being able to undertake the physical task, but to demonstrate compassion, respect and sound decision-making while you are doing it. Being able to put theory into practice is not as easy as it sounds, nor is the development of the range of learning skills that are required in such different environments. Learning will occur in both theory and practice; however, for that learning to have added value, there needs to be a conduit between the two so that the 'understanding' does not get separated from the 'doing'.

Figure 12.1 depicts these learning relationships. Everyone begins their nurse education with a range of experiences of health care: personal episodes of ill health, and those of family and friends, being a carer, doing voluntary work, unpaid work experience or work as a health care assistant. These life experiences, both good and bad, will have been an important influence in your decision to pursue this career path and the experiences you will encounter throughout your career will continue to shape your learning. The combination of theory and practice during a nursing course builds on past experiences and provides the framework for the personal and emotional development which is necessary to support professional caring. Over the past decade, simulation and simulated practice have emerged as educational techniques to help students develop these relationships in learning.

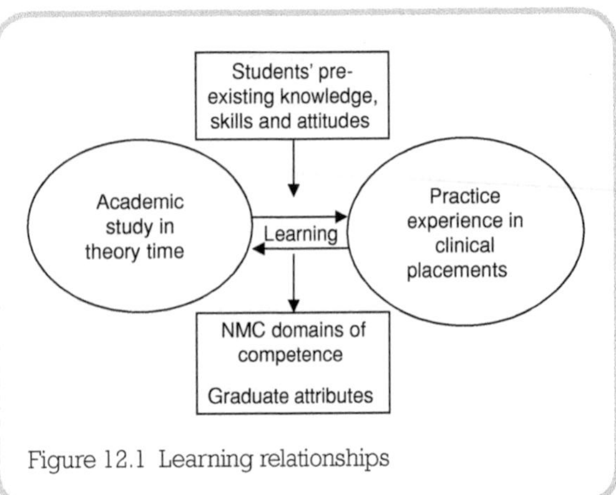

Figure 12.1 Learning relationships

What is simulation?

The NMC describe simulation as any simulated teaching and learning activity that is applied to teach and assess skill acquisition through an interactive experience (NMC 2007; Ricketts 2011). Gaba (2004: 126) describes it as a technique that may be used 'to replace or amplify real experiences with guided experiences that evoke or replicate substantial aspects of the real world in a fully interactive manner'. The majority of simulated activity in health care involves combinations of simulated ward environments, mannequins/equipment and/or simulated patients (which generally means actors) (O'Hagan *et al.* 1986) and the students' interactions with a set scenario (Kneebone *et al.* 2006; Scherer *et al.* 2007). These scenarios can be generic – i.e. relate to all fields of practice – or field specific – i.e. adult, child, mental health or learning disability. It is likely that students in the different fields will have exposure to a different balance of environment/equipment/actors depending on the aims of the sessions. Mental health and learning disability students may participate in more scenarios with actors, whereas adult and child field students are likely to have comparatively more exposure to sophisticated computer controlled mannequins, which can replicate physiological signs and symptoms.

An example of a generic scenario would be an initial patient/client assessment, which would include demonstration of communication skills, appropriate use of standard precautions (hand washing and infection prevention), history-taking and recording of observations, reporting of relevant facts to senior colleagues and documentation, all using actors as patients.

Adult and child field

Adult and child field student simulations often involve interaction with sophisticated computer controlled patient mannequins which are designed to demonstrate physiological changes. These mannequins can simulate breathing, blinking, speaking, bleeding and fitting, and they have pulses, heart sounds, lung sounds, reactive pupils, etc. They can be programmed to deteriorate or improve, depending on the student's actions. As an example students may be asked to care for a post-operative patient who starts to bleed internally and develops the signs of hypovolaemia.

Mental health and learning disability fields

The scenarios in the mental health and learning disability fields more commonly use real people as simulated patients in order to focus on therapeutic techniques, risk assessments, case presentation, etc. These activities involve a subtlety of communication which cannot be achieved with mannequins, and simulated patients generally require specific training to be able to accurately represent the behaviours required in the scenario.

> 'A simulation creates a scenario that mimics a real life situation. For this reason, simulations provide a way for students to gain experiences in problem solving and decision making without the realities and demands of an actual clinical situation.'
>
> (Gaberson and Oermann 1999: 135).

This quotation highlights two important issues:

- Simulation mimics reality but is not real. Equivalence to real practice is therefore dependent on the student's perception of how real the scenario is, and this may vary with the activity undertaken.
- Simulation is safe, for both patients and students. It is common practice for high-risk industries to use simulation when training staff – for example, pilots. In fact, many people would not be prepared to put their trust in a pilot who had not done simulator training, such is the value placed upon it.

Activity 12.1

- How would you feel about enaging in a simulated practice experience: about being watched, maybe even filmed, and about discussing your performance afterwards?
- Next consider the public's expectations of the care they receive. Ask a few friends and relatives who are not health care professionals what they think about nurses practising skills in simulation before they do them with real people.
- What are the differences in views or attitudes that this exercise highlights?
- Has thinking about the perceptions of others in terms of the work nurses do altered your initial thoughts?

Lastly we should consider what simulation is *not*:

- simulation is not a replacement for practice;
- unless you are specifically told to prepare for an exam, simulations are not tests: you will not be judged against your peers and you will not be told off for getting anything wrong.

Simulation and learning theory

To learn a practical task requires performance of that task. The ancient Chinese proverb, 'I hear I forget, I see I remember, I do I understand', is a simple way of thinking about the value of simulation, a method of learning reportedly practised since 800 BC (Wildman and Reeves 1997). Health care professionals in general, and student nurses in particular, are recognized as a distinct group of learners, striving to acquire the knowledge, skills and attributes needed for professional practice. It is recognized that the outcome of this type of learning is *competence*. The way in which learning, in order to achieve competence requires different components was first recognized by Aristotle who made a distinction between technical and practical knowledge. Ryle (1949) describes this distinction more accessibly as 'knowing that and knowing how'.

Eraut (1994) categorized these forms of knowledge further, as the building blocks of what he describes as *experiential learning*:

- knowledge of people;
- situational knowledge;
- knowledge of practice;
- conceptual knowledge;
- process knowledge or know-how;
- control knowledge – knowledge of the self, strengths and weaknesses, how to receive feedback, how to utilize knowledge from other sources and limit self-reliance.

Boud *et al.* (1993) assert that the essence of how people learn from experience is by a cycle of activity, reflecting on that activity, relating it first to what is known from past experiences, then to what it may be used for in the future, and finally validating it against the experience of others. Simulation works in that way: it provides the opportunity to perform an activity and then to debrief and reflect upon the experience in a structured way to identify the points of learning for individual students. Experiential learning theory also recognizes that individual students will learn different things from exposure to the same event, because of the personal nature of their learning journey.

As Frye (2000: 541) has suggested: 'There really can be no goal where taking the journey itself is the best thing to be done'. This means that you should expect that your experience in a simulation scenario will be completely personal to you. What you learn will be framed by your previous life experiences. Your learning may be about the tasks in the scenario, but may equally provide clearer insight into how you learn, what you think about certain issues, how you feel about certain situations, or how you handle your emotions. Your expectations of what will happen in a simulation may turn out to be very different from the reality, and what you learn may be different from what your colleagues learn, but this is perfectly normal. Whether in simulation or in clinical practice, you need to learn to take the journey and capitalize on whatever events occur along the way.

Key learning !

- Experiential learning in simulation allows you to identify and develop strategies of learning that you can use in clinical placement.

Preparing for simulation

Building on **Activity 12.1**, spending some time thinking about your expectations of a simulated practice experience is an excellent first step to prepare for such an experience. Developing your understanding of the use of simulation will also help. Learning in both simulation and practice is very definitely active. You therefore need to approach these experiences with an open mind, do any pre-reading or e-learning activities set by your tutors and familiarize yourself with the NMC competencies.

The purpose of this chapter is more than providing an overview of simulation in nurse education. The intention is to translate some of the research evidence and experience from two of the leading centres for simulation in the UK into practical advice that students can use. This provides an example of research evidence and will enable you to develop your skills in using evidence from two case studies to inform and enhance practice, as discussed in Chapter 1. We have therefore chosen two elements, situated within the domain of Eraut's 'control knowledge', which have very practical relevance for students. We now use two case studies to demonstrate simulation at work. The first (**12.1** opposite) is from the University of Southampton and focuses on how students can use simulation to develop understanding of their strengths and weaknesses, utilize knowledge from other sources to limit self-reliance and learn how to get the most out of practice.

The second case study (**12.2**, p. 182) is from Robert Gordon University and focuses on how to receive feedback, and how this enables students to gain knowledge of themselves.

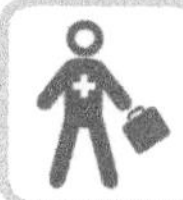

Case study 12.1: Learning how to learn in practice: lessons from the University of Southampton

Up until 2007, any simulated practice activity undertaken as part of a nursing programme was not considered as practice and therefore had to be accounted for in theory time. In 2006, with the growing acceptance that more universities were choosing to use simulated activities, the NMC commissioned work to assess the value of simulation in supporting student learning as part of their clinical hours. The results from the 13 participating universities were amalgamated to produce the NMCs final report which concluded that simulation enhanced students' practice learning and that up to 300 'clinical practice' hours could be used in simulated practice (NMC and Council of Deans for Health 2007). The University of Southampton was one of the participants and the research evidence provided data from 348 students' experiences of simulation in Year 2 of the programme. Year 2 nursing students (277 adult field, 53 child field and 18 mental health and learning disability), undertook field-specific simulated practice activities in groups of three to four students at a time.

This evaluation data was corroborated by the field notes of the researchers and reports of the mentors – practitioners who had not facilitated simulated practice before – who confirmed that the majority of students engaged in the scenario as if it were real. 90 per cent of students felt that the learning was valuable and relevant. It is interesting to note though that only 50 per cent felt that it helped them learn how to work in a team. This finding fits with experiential learning theory and demonstrates that this kind of learning is personal; the students state that they have learned but not all of them are considering other people working with them. This demonstrates normal student development, where in Year 1 you are completely focused on yourself and the learning of practical skills. In Year 2, you will begin to feel more confident with your role and recognize your place in the wider team, and by Year 3 the majority of students will have gained professional self-confidence. The research data shows that about 50 per cent of the Year 2 students were aware of the teamwork element which reflects this period of transition from selfish learner to self-confident professional learner.

What do students think?

The following student comments demonstrate the three main issues which were identified as important after the simulation.

1. The comparison of the students' expectations of the experience and the actuality.
   - 'OK once you got used to it.'
   - 'More real than I thought.'
   - 'I am on a medical ward – it's very like the patients on my ward.'
   - 'But it's like this every day in practice.'
2. The physical reality of the simulated environment.
   - 'It's dead quiet – would be easier if it were noisy.'
   - 'You don't stand around on the ward – other patients would make it more real.'
   - 'Not just one patient – [do] this job and another, other distractions would make it more real.'
3. Linking theory and practice.
   - 'Gets you really thinking, it puts things together.'
   - 'Here it's like placement, but I understand the processes.'
   - 'Theory – could think about it a bit, but didn't think I was practising. When I saw others doing it I thought "God, that's how its done, sounds more professional".'
   - 'The first couple of weeks on a placement you are determined to keep theory in the

> forefront, but after a couple of weeks you forget the theory and do it properly. Doing this once a week while in practice would keep it fresh in your mind. In practice – you do the same as everyone else which is not always the best practice.'

These quotes provide a clear insight into how experiences in simulation get students to think about their practice.

What the quotations above illustrate is that simulation is not about learning an individual task, like giving an injection. Although the simulations involved undertaking a number of tasks, the students do not describe those tasks when considering their learning. They do, however, appear to be thinking broadly about their performance, what they did well and what they needed to improve, and how. This is, of course, partly because of the way the facilitators led the debrief, but it is a good example of how simulation allows you to recognize your strengths and weaknesses. If you can do this, you are able to identify where you need to practise more, and if you cannot do it, your learning will be serendipitous and potentially much slower than if you actively worked at it.

Does reality matter?

Activity 12.2

At some point you will have been involved in a simulation, although you may not have thought about it that way: a mock exam, a rehearsal for a play or interview practice, for example. Think back to those activities. What did you think at the time? Was your expectation of the event different to the actuality? Did it help you when the real event occurred? Was it important for the practice to be 'real'?

Simulation provides the opportunity to practise a skill, in context, without the fear of making mistakes. It allows students to develop the arts of observation and building relationships while performing tasks. Counterintuitively, the use of mannequins can highlight the types of cues which are used in the observation of, and in relationship-building with, real patients because they are missing. Students often suddenly recognize that with a real patient they would be looking at the patient's body language or their colour and that it would be easier with a real person. The learning is about recognizing how we rely on these cues and how we can develop our skills of observation. In a similar way, the removal of some cues makes the assessment more focused on appropriate questioning, distillation of relevant facts and using frameworks for assessment. The removal of the subtle intuitive sense you get from a real patient focuses the mind on the objective physiological evidence presented. When the evidence is presented in this way, it is possible to begin to understand how to use theoretical knowledge to build the bigger picture of what is happening with the patient. This is what the students were saying when they talked about 'putting it all together'. It is not until this objective bigger picture can be seen that it is possible to communicate patients' problems professionally, or to hone decision-making skills. If you are interested in the reading more about the ways we have been researching some of the challenges posed by simulation, Gobbi *et al.* (2012) provides a useful summary.

The cumulative findings of these research studies have informed the 'stacking' approach to simulation at Southampton (see **Figure 12.2**).

'Skills stacking' means that simulation scenarios are embedded in the curriculum to provide sequential opportunities for learning. Skills are built up like a pyramid, adding a new layer each time. During the first few weeks of the course, the concept of professional values is introduced and linked to skills (see Chapter 2). This is then consolidated by the first simulation experience which focuses on practising communication with the patient to demonstrate compassion in a professional way and professional information-sharing with colleagues.

 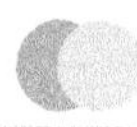

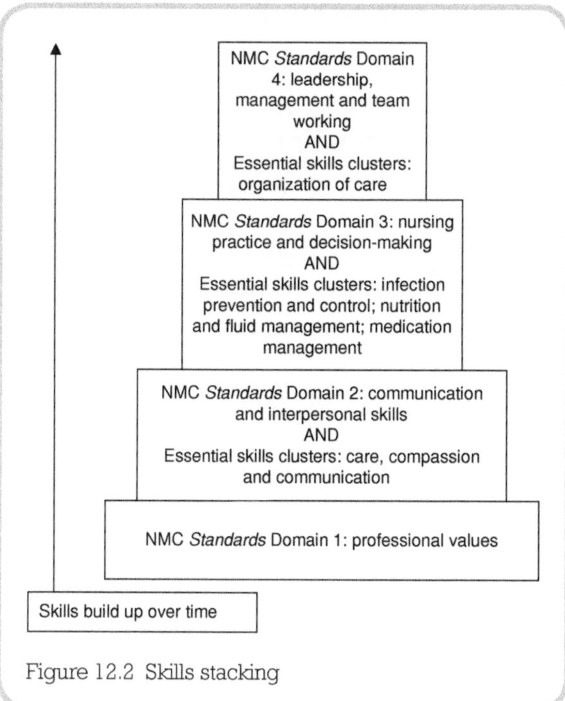

Figure 12.2 Skills stacking

In Year 2, students have had time in clinical practice, and we expect them to bring those experiences to simulation. The field-specific scenarios develop decision-making skills while students demonstrate their professional values and hone their communication and practice learning skills. The scenario design and debrief process highlight how essential skills (infection prevention, nutrition, fluid and medication management) and holistic care (psychological, social and spiritual well-being) are becoming embedded in the way students are working in practice. This provides direction to students to recognize personal progress which is essential for the transition from dependent to independent learner.

In Year 3, the scenarios challenge and extend students' developing decision-making skills. By this stage the students' range of practice experience will have firmly embedded professional values and communication skills, and allowed them to develop confidence in the identification of patient problems and the associated initial decision-making. The scenarios will focus on building evidence-based action plans to manage the identified problems in appropriate ways. The simulation is timetabled to occur prior to the final practice experience so that students can reflect on their learning needs, identify areas for development and use the last placement to complete their skills set.

Limiting self-reliance

The ability to develop professional relationships is fundamental, and one of the most important initial lessons to learn in simulation is how to get the best out of your mentor in practice – when to ask, how to ask, and how to act (you can explore working with your mentor in more detail in Chapter 13). In simulated practice, the environment is similar to the 'real world' which makes it easier to recognize different strategies to communicate most effectively with health care professionals. Your facilitators may 'act' or role-play both good and bad practice in order to help you develop sound strategies of communication. This will be followed by a debrief which is structured to help you learn from the discussion and feedback. Recognition of the pitfalls of communication between professionals in a busy environment forms the development of this theme in Year 2 and 3 scenarios. Developing strategies to 'park' certain pieces of information until later is extremely important as you begin to take a more senior role in clinical environments. As an example: taking a phone call, receiving information, and then being side-tracked by a pressing clinical problem. The loss of these seemingly trivial pieces of information is a huge problem for any health care environment, and the consequences can be extremely serious, even if they seem harmless at the time. Seeing other students' strategies and hearing facilitators', tried and tested techniques can help you find ways of dealing with these kinds of issues more quickly and efficiently. For further discussion on communication see Chapters 4, 5 and 6.

Simulation experiences also provide opportunities to try out different strategies that you may not have felt comfortable with attempting in practice. It can be a bit like trying on a different set of clothes; if you are normally shy and happy to take orders, try giving some orders and see how it feels, and likewise the other way around. In order to get the most out of simulation, students must be self-aware and open to constructive criticism. For some personality types this comes naturally; others will find it more difficult. The recognition of the personal challenges posed by this type of activity is fundamental to professional development. When we consider our development to adulthood, some of the most important lessons learned will have been by making mistakes: getting burned by something hot, trusting a 'friend' who lets you down, or failing a test because you didn't prepare. In simulation, we see students making mistakes, but we also see things being done well, and both will be referred to in the debrief. Highlighting events in this way is a really powerful way to learn, but it is not unusual to see students feeling embarrassed or even upset. When someone cares about what they are doing, or feels that attention is focused on them, that is to be expected. To manage this very human emotional response, we talk through the practical lessons that the whole group can take away for the future. Where an error has been made we also point out that we know that because of the power of the learning, they will never make that mistake again, which is a really positive message to take away. The other students in the group also gain a real insight into the personal impact of making an error, which is equally valuable. Getting it right in real life is the part that matters.

Key learning

!

- Simulation is a learning opportunity; no one can get hurt.
- Learning by doing, both by doing well and by making mistakes, is very powerful.

Receiving feedback

Case study 12.2: Lessons from Robert Gordon University

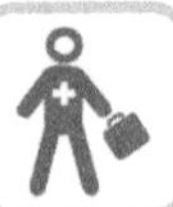

At Robert Gordon University School of Nursing and Midwifery, there is an established 'volunteer patient programme' facilitated by staff from the clinical skills centre. The volunteers are members of the public who simulate real patients by playing specific roles in the ward and in community settings; sometimes this involves complex scenarios, other times it means simply allowing students to practise non-invasive clinical skills such as manual blood pressure. The volunteers receive an induction after they have been accepted onto the programme and about two-thirds of them have also received training in how to give feedback to students.

Involved third-year student nurses participate in a ward simulation and then receive verbal face-to-face feedback from volunteer patients (Webster *et al.* 2012). Yin's (2009) six case study steps were followed and focus groups were used to collect data from the volunteers, from which four distinct topics were defined which will be of interest to you. The volunteer patients recognized that unless they played their role of patient authentically, the learning experience of the student may be compromised. They also recognized the importance of constructive critical feedback from staff to enable them to feel supported to carry out their role in order to meet the needs of academic staff and students.

In the clinical simulations, volunteer patients were requested to provide feedback on communication and interpersonal skills. The volunteers suggested they would prefer to do this in a one-to-one, face-to-face situation so that it could be done in an honest and open way without causing embarrassment to the student.

A very strong sense of empathy for the student situation was evident and the volunteers realized how nervous the student nurses became.

For this reason the volunteer patients did not like giving negative feedback and were keen to encourage and support the student nurses. This support mirrored what occurred in clinical environments when the volunteers had been service users. The volunteer patients said that motivation to become a volunteer patient came from having been a patient and experiencing health care provision first hand. The need to 'give back' was strong and they felt that their ability to play the role of patients was enhanced as they had first-hand experiences to draw on. They felt knowing what to expect gave them authority to give feedback to students.

Feedback is critical in facilitating learning and a very powerful tool (Hattie and Timperley 2007; Norcini 2010). The NMC values the role of feedback in the learning process as students make the transition to being a registered nurse (RN). Under Domain 4 (leadership, management and team working), the importance of real patients giving student nurses feedback is highlighted under Competency 4:

> All nurses must be self-aware and recognise how their own values, principles and assumptions may affect their practice. They must maintain their own personal and professional development, learning from experience, through supervision, feedback, reflection and evaluation.
>
> (NMC 2010)

The benefit to you as a learner of getting feedback from others, including patients, is that you can start to see yourself as others see you, which is crucial because patients are receiving their care from you. As simulations that occur in the clinical skills centre should be as authentic as possible, it makes sense to include the volunteers in giving feedback to students. For further discussion of receiving feedback in practice, see Chapter 14.

What does this mean for you as a student nurse?

Simulation affords you as a student with the opportunity to receive specific feedback on how you performed as a nurse and delivered care. Volunteer patients take their role very seriously and request feedback on their own performance from staff and students. It is important, therefore, that any dialogue between you and the volunteer is based on mutual respect and that you value their contribution. Without them, simulation scenarios would often not be as real.

Volunteers want to encourage you in your chosen profession and prefer to give face-to-face feedback in a one-to-one situation so that the feedback can be individual, honest and constructive. This will enable you to start to see yourself as others see you. Remember, volunteer patients have a great deal of empathy with you and want to help you, so any comments are well intended. If something is raised that worries you or is not explained fully, then please raise this with your simulation facilitator. Finally, remember that as past, current and future service users, volunteers are well placed to provide you with valuable feedback.

Making the most of feedback

It is important that you make the most of any feedback received and continue your development while on clinical placements. As student nurses and developing professionals, it is critical that we learn to listen to feedback, reflect on it and move forward. The person giving the feedback should be aware that in order for it to be effective, it should be facilitative – a two-way interaction between the student and the educator, more like a dialogue or conversation. It should focus on the task rather than the individual, be specific and be linked to personal goals or the learning outcomes for the simulation activity (Archer 2010). It is important that as the receiver of feedback, you are open to suggestions and prepared to think about the comments made to you. Then you can engage in a period of reflection where you can consider the feedback in detail. Reflection is the process through which you look at yourself and your practice objectively. It is not about being overly critical of yourself or being superficial or dishonest. Sitiver suggests that through reflection we can develop a deeper self-awareness (2008: 163). Being self-aware is defined by Bulman and Schutz (2008: 30) as being 'conscious of one's character, including beliefs, values, qualities, strengths and limitations'. The process of using reflection to develop self-awareness is a continual one, and the method by which you continue to develop, even when you are a qualified nurse. Using a reflective model can help you by providing a structure for your thoughts. There are many models available in the literature for you to have a look at. A really simple one is Borton's (1970) framework (cited in Jasper 2006: 73). He suggests that in order to reflect, you should ask yourself three very simple questions:

- What?
- So what?
- Now what?

Activity 12.3

Think about a recent event on placement or in your workplace that you felt you dealt with well and ask yourself:

- What? Describe the event as it happened.
- So what? What was the significance of this event to you?
- Now what? What does this mean for the future?

As pointed out right at the beginning of this chapter, learning how to craft your care is not easy. It is a process that you need to engage with and understand, and the final part of simulation, the debrief, is where this starts to happen. In general, simulated activities are relatively short – 30–45 minutes is about average. However, the debrief is generally as long, if not longer than the activity itself. This is where you will be guided by your lecturers to pull out the learning points for you. One method that can be used to structure the debriefing activity is to use the ABCD of effective feedback (Student Participation in Quality Scotland 2011) and this may be employed by the facilitators or used as a tool to get students to provide feedback to each other:

- **Accurate:** try and give specific comments rather than generalizations; as evidence you might cite examples or numbers.
- **Balanced:** positives as well as negatives.
- **Constructive.** Try to offer solutions for negative points.
- **Depersonalized:** rather than mention names of individuals, describe the experience and the impact it had on you.

This structure provides a framework for *effective* feedback.

Activity 12.4

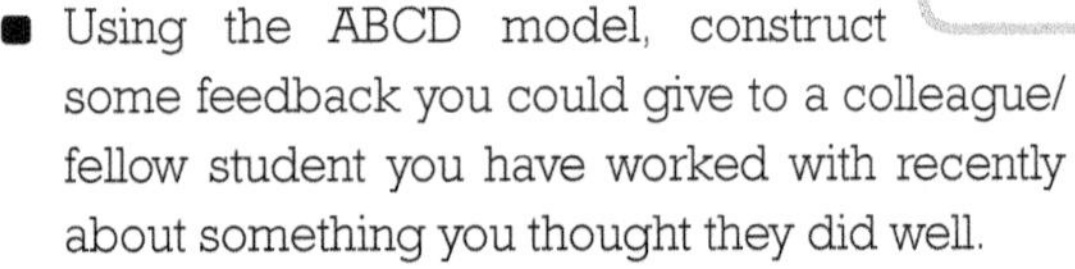

- Using the ABCD model, construct some feedback you could give to a colleague/fellow student you have worked with recently about something you thought they did well.
- How easy/difficult was it to do this?

The debrief as a 'reflection on action' (Schön 1983) is likely to encourage you to work through what you did, identify the important issues, explore what you know, or what find out would help you learn from the experience. Your facilitator will point out some of the links to the theory which you should examine further. Practising this process will enable you to develop the skills to be able to do this for yourself when reflecting on practice in the future. When you are on practice placement, the time to reflect on an episode with your mentor will be limited because of the pressures of working in the real world. The ability to develop the skills to identify significant episodes and to reflect on them, both with your mentor when you have the chance, and on your own when you don't, will help you get

the most out of your placement experiences. One of the benefits of simulation is that the time to do this is built in, but in order to get the most out of the experience you will need to reflect further on your own, and explore the theoretical links which were pointed out to you. Listening to feedback and then reflecting on what others think can help you gain knowledge about yourself and enable you to learn from your actions and even mistakes. This will build your 'control knowledge' as we described earlier in the chapter (Eraut 1994). The whole process of engaging in a simulation activity, receiving feedback and then reflecting on it will enable you to make the most of any simulation experience, making your student journey a valuable one and ultimately assisting you in the transition to becoming a qualified practitioner.

Key learning !

The debrief after the session and the personal reflection you undertake afterwards is where the learning happens.

Conclusion

In conclusion, simulation is used in nurse education for a number of reasons. It is used as a tool to provide students with opportunities to develop strategies to link theory with practice, making the most of learning from experience, and is based on established theoretical underpinnings. By describing two case studies where research has positively influenced the incorporation of simulated practice into nursing programmes, it is hoped that we have been able to provide practical examples of how you can capitalize on these opportunities in your journey to professional registration. Even if you do not have the opportunity to engage in simulated activities during your course, it is hoped that we have provided some useful tips which will help you learn the craft of caring.

In summary:

- Experiential learning in simulation allows you to identify and develop strategies of learning that you can use in clinical placements.
- Simulation is a learning opportunity; no one can get hurt.
- Learning by doing, both by doing well and by making mistakes, is very powerful.
- The debrief after the session and the personal reflection you undertake later are where the learning happens.

Further reading and resources

Gobbi, M.O., Monger, E.J., Weal, M.J., McDonald, J., Michaelides, D. and DeRoure, D. (2012) The challenges of developing and evaluating complex care scenarios using simulation in nursing education, *Journal of Research in Nursing,* 17(4): 329–45.

Jasper, M. (2006) *Professional Development, Reflection and Decision Making*. Oxford: Blackwell.

Watkinson, G., Spencer, A., Monger, E., Weaver, M. and Gobbi, M. (2006) Case study 17a: using technology to teach clinical skills, in C.A. Weaver, C. White Delaney, P. Weber and R.L. Carr (eds) *Nursing and Informatics for the 21st Century*. Chicago: HIMMS.

References

Archer, J.C. (2010) State of the science in health professional education: effective feedback, *Medical Education*, 44: 101–8.

Boud, D., Cohen, R. and Walker, D. (eds) (1993) *Using Experience for Learning*. Buckingham: Open University Press.

Bulman, C. and Schutz, S. (eds) (2008) *Reflective Practice in Nursing*, 4th edn. Oxford: Blackwell.

Eraut, M. (1994) *Developing Professional Knowledge and Competence*. London: Falmer Press.

Frye, N. (2000) *Northrop Frye's Writings on Education*, edited by J. O'Grady and G. French. Toronto: University of Toronto Press.

Gaba, D.M. (2004) The future vision of simulation in Health Care, *Quality Safety Health Care*, 13(S1): i2–i10, available at: http://1.usa.gov/14vpklG.

Gaberson, K.B. and Oermann, M.H. (1999) *Clinical Teaching Strategies in Nursing*. New York. Springer.

Gobbi, M.O., Monger, E.J., Weal, M.J., McDonald, J., Michaelides, D. and DeRoure, D. (2012) The challenges of developing and evaluating complex care scenarios using simulation in nursing education, *Journal of Research in Nursing*, 17(4): 329–45.

Hattie, J. and Timperley, H. (2007) The power of feedback, *Review of Educational Research*, 77: 81.

Jasper, M. (2006) *Professional Development, Reflection and Decision Making*. Oxford: Blackwell.

Kneebone, R., Nestel, D., Yadollahi, F., Brown, R., Nolan, C., Durack, J., Brenton, H., Moulton, C., Archer, J. and Darzi, A. (2006) Assessing procedural skills in context: exploring the feasibility of an Integrated Procedural Performance Instrument (IPPI), *Medical Education*, 40: 1105–14.

NMC (Nursing and Midwifery Council) and Council of Deans for Health (2007) *Simulation and Practice Learning Project: Outcome of a Pilot Study to Test the Principles for Auditing Simulated Practice Learning Environments in the Pre-registration Nursing Programme: Final Report*. London: NMC, available at: www.nmc.org.

NMC (Nursing and Midwifery Council) (2010) *Standards for Pre-registration Nursing Education*. London: NMC.

Norcini, J. (2010) The power of feedback, *Medical Education*, 44: 16–17.

O'Hagan, J.J., Davis, L.J. and Pears, R.K. (1986) The use of simulated patients in the assessment of actual clinical performance in general practice, *The New Zealand Medical Journal*, 99(815): 948–51.

Ricketts, B. (2011) The role of simulation for learning within pre-registration nursing education – a literature review, *Nurse Education Today*, 31: 650–4, available at: www.elsevier.com.

Ryle, G. (1949) *The Concept of Mind*. Chicago: University of Chicago Press.

Scherer, Y.K., Bruce, S.A. and Runkawatt, V. (2007) A comparison of clinical simulation and case study presentation on nurse practitioner students' knowledge and confidence in managing a cardiac event, *International Journal of Nurse Education Scholarship*, 4, Article 22, epub 21 November.

Schön, D.A. (1983) *The Reflective Practitioner*. New York: Basic Books.

Siviter, B. (2008) *The Student Nurse Handbook*, 2nd edn. Edinburgh: Elsevier Health Sciences.

Student Participation in Quality Scotland (2011) Introductory Course Rep Training, available at: www.sparqs.ac.uk/reps/section.php?cat=78.

Webster, B.J., Goodhand, K., Haith, M. and Unwin, R. (2012) The development of service users in the provision of verbal feedback to student nurses in a clinical simulation environment, *Nurse Education Today*, 32(2): 133–8.

Wildman, S. and Reeves, M. (1997) The value of simulations in the management education of nurses: students' perceptions, *Journal of Nurse Management*, 5(4): 207–15.

Yin, R. (2009) *Case Study Research Design and Methods*, 4th edn. London: Sage.

13

Working with mentors: how to get the most from working with your mentors in practice

Sheila Reading, Alison Trenerry and Cathy Sullivan

Chapter contents

Introduction

This chapter aims to prompt you to think about, and prepare for, your practice experiences. Good preparation is essential for success. If you can get the preparation right it will help to make your practice experience rewarding and provide you with valuable learning opportunities. Practice is where you will achieve much of your learning and is often the most rewarding part of your programme. While part of good preparation requires you to consider the need to take responsibility for your own learning, remember your mentors will facilitate it for you and help you to identify particular opportunities which are available to meet your learning needs. It is important that you reflect on how to optimize your working relationship with your mentors.

The importance of learning in practice

As a student nurse you will learn much about health care and your specific professional field by working within the reality of practice settings. Neary (2000) indicates that in nursing you learn by doing, and Midgley (2006) highlights that placements are where you can link theory and practice, the 'knowing what' with the 'knowing how' of nursing. You will not only gain and enhance clinical knowledge and skills – practice experiences will enable you to learn 'how to be' a qualified health care professional (Egan and Jaye 2009).

Learning within the practice setting is a fundamental process by which you will get to know what it is to be a competent practitioner in your chosen field and by which you will eventually become a registered nurse (RN) and graduate. Clinical practice gives you a unique opportunity to explore all aspects of a patient's care pathway. Understanding the wishes of an individual in relation to their specific physical, mental and other health needs is the basis to being able to deliver seamless and safe patient care. As the Department of Health (DH) White Paper on *Equity and Excellence: Liberating the NHS* (2010) emphasizes, the focus of all nursing care must be on promoting the quality of a person's care and experiences.

During your programme, you will spend 50 per cent of your time in different practice environments, including community settings, voluntary organizations, clients' homes, acute care areas, nurseries, primary health care, public health care, highly complex care settings and many others. You will have supernumerary status while working in practice. This means that while you are undertaking practice experiences as part of your programme of study you are in addition to the established numbers of nurses working in any given location. You will be allocated a negotiated workload that is within your scope of practice and that meets your learning needs. Your allocated practice placements will be exciting, rewarding and dynamic but on occasions may prove challenging, uncomfortable and potentially stressful as you learn how to work with others and care for clients. That is the nature of contemporary health care practice. However, each placement has the potential to offer you a rich learning experience and, importantly, you will always have a mentor, and other staff, available to support and facilitate your learning.

Allocation of practice learning experiences

The practice learning circuit is usually extensive and may be geographically spread across a large area. Your university will work in partnership with a number of trusts and many independent and voluntary sector providers to provide you with the required experiences to qualify as a safe practitioner. Be aware that you may be expected to travel to a placement or move into accommodation near your placement if it is situated a long way from your university or the transport links are poor.

Sharing personal information with the practice area

Your university works in partnership with their practice learning providers and as such it is required to share some of your personal information with them as you will be providing care within their organization. This usually includes:

- your name and student number – this will be used for allocating you a mentor, roistering you shifts, etc.;
- verification of good health and good character as required by the professional bodies;
- verification of statutory and mandatory skills that have been undertaken before commencing practice.

Key learning !

- To become a competent practitioner 50 per cent of your programme time is undertaken in practice where you will have supernumerary status and be supported by a mentor.

Competence in practice

Practice experience offers the opportunity to learn more about nursing care and working with others; however, it takes time to become competent. An experienced nurse is able to undertake many complex skills but may not easily be able to explain

UNCONSCIOUS INCOMPETENT
At this stage you are not aware of your own inabilities and may do something wrong without knowing it
Your mentor can help you to recognize areas which you need to learn more about and offer opportunites to observe and practise in order to develop your competence
CONSCIOUS INCOMPETENT
At this stage you are aware of your deficits and not sure how to do the task. You may give it a go and make mistakes. Although we all learn from our mistakes it does not always help our confidence or self esteem
The mentor can support you in refining your skills and perhaps demonstrate, or model how to do things and observe you while giving guidance
CONSCIOUS COMPETENCE
Now you are becoming competent. But you are a little hesitant and slow and have to concentrate hard on what you are doing. You may need to break the task down into stages or steps
Your mentor encourages practice and can provide feedback to support your further improvement
UNCONSCIOUS COMPETENCE
You are now able to practise without having to think much about it and you feel confident
Your mentor will encourage you and hopefully you will receive praise and recognition for your achievement.
It is importnat to ensure poor habits do not emerge at this point

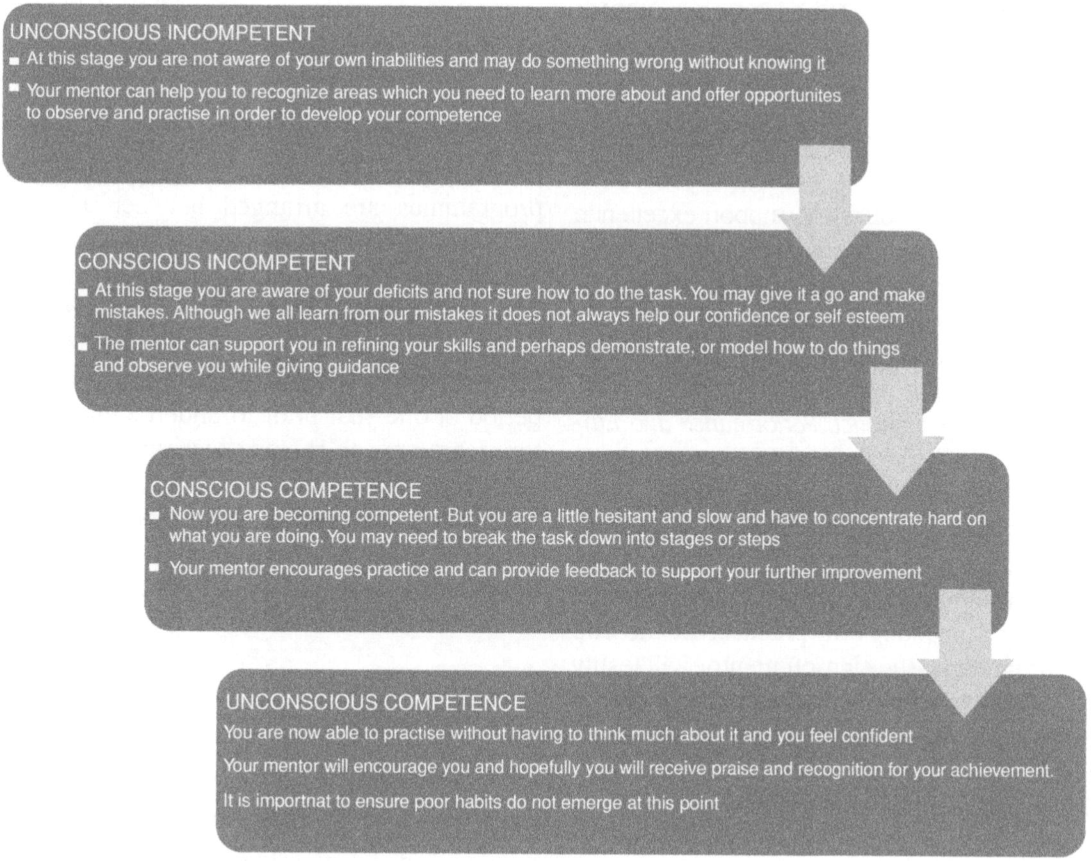

Figure 13.1 Conscious competence model diagram adapted from Howell 1982

how this is done as it has become almost automatic, like riding a bike or driving a car.

Howell (1982) has described a four-stage model to explain the processes involved in learning new skills, known as the *conscious competence* model (see **Figure 13.1** above). You may find this helpful when discussing your development, learning goals and achievements with your mentor.

It is important to recognize that you will be performing at different stages of the model depending on what it is you are learning to achieve competence in. For example, you may be unconsciously competent in some aspects of communicating with patients but unconsciously incompetent when starting to lead a team in practice. There are always areas of practice in which you will be strong and others where you are only beginning to learn.

Key learning !

- Practice experiences are rich learning environments where you will become consciously competent.

Mentors: gatekeepers to the profession

> Mentorship is pivotal to students' clinical experiences and is instrumental in preparing them for their role as confident and competent practitioners.
>
> (Myall *et al.* 2008)

The Nursing and Midwifery Council (NMC) *Standards for Pre-registration Nursing Education* (2010) consists of two distinct elements:

- standards for education;
- standards for competence.

The standards for education support excellence in student learning and assessment in practice placements, and define the principles and professional scope of standards required of your programme providers to ensure good mentorship for students. RNs are professionally required by *The Code: Standards of Conduct, Performance and Ethics for Nurses and Midwives* to 'facilitate students and others to develop their competence' (NMC 2008b). Ultimately, it is the mentors you work with in practice who make the day-to-day judgements on whether you are achieving the required standard for competence in practice. At the end of your programme the sign-off mentor will testify as to whether you have achieved the competencies required to register as a nurse in your chosen field. Remember, the NMC register exists to protect the public and maintain and promote professional standards. The role of the sign-off mentor therefore has considerable responsibility.

There are many people other than mentors who support learning in practice. Link teachers, practice educators, the providers of clinical placements, the university and others, such as commissioners of nurse education and the NMC, all collaborate to ensure mentors are supported in their role and that the optimum learning environment is provided for students.

Mentors, associate mentors and buddies

There are many staff that can support your learning in clinical practice to achieve the required competencies. You should always ask your mentor about working with other people who can offer specific learning opportunities as it is important to have exposure to different perspectives and sources of expertise in clinical practice. You may find you have a named 'associate mentor' or 'buddy' to work with. This is a strategy for ensuring you have support from another member of staff, for example when your mentor is busy or off duty.

Mentor preparation

One day you too will be a mentor. Mentorship programmes are arranged between placement providers (NHS, private and voluntary sectors) and universities. All registered mentors will have undertaken a programme of study and assessment to achieve the mentor standards (NMC 2008a). A mentor must have been registered for a minimum period of one year prior to undertaking the mentor programme and being successfully assessed as able to facilitate student learning, supervise and assess in practice. To become a sign-off mentor requires the mentor to be experienced and registered on the same part, or sub-part, of the register as the one you are aiming to register on.

Activity 13.1

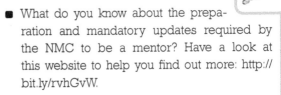

- What do you know about the preparation and mandatory updates required by the NMC to be a mentor? Have a look at this website to help you find out more: http://bit.ly/rvhGvW.

Having looked at the website can you answer the following questions?

- How much time are you required to spend with your mentor?
- What shifts do the *Standards* require that you work?
- What is the minimum length of time required for you to spend in your final practice experience?

To support the work of mentors, all placements are audited to ensure they are suitable learning environments for students, and annually mentors must demonstrate evidence of mandatory updating

'to maintain and develop their competence and performance' (NMC 2008a).

> **Key learning**
>
> - Mentors are gatekeepers to the profession and are required to undertake a programme of preparation for the role and thereafter annual updates.

Mentor and student expectations

> **Activity 13.2**
>
> - What do you think mentors expect you to do as a student to enhance your learning? List 5 to 10 things and then review them with your peers.
> - What do you expect from your mentors to support and enhance your learning? List 5 to 10 things and again review them with your peers.
> - Compare and contrast the answers on your lists.

Talking to some second-year students revealed that they expect mentors to be:

- enthusiastic;
- generous with praise;
- able to give feedback constructively and in private rather than shout or yell at them in front of others;
- polite: to call them by name, and not just 'student';
- willing to say thank you.

According to the literature a good mentor from the student perspective is someone who is supportive, and acts as a good role model, teacher, guide and assessor; someone who has a genuine concern and the student's interests at heart (Andrews and Chilton 2000; Gray and Smith 2000; Neary 2000). Mentors will monitor your progress and, as well as providing you with feedback, will help you to identify further learning goals and possible strategies for successful achievement in practice.

> **Activity 13.3**
>
> - Think of people you have worked alongside who have helped you learn new skills, increased your knowledge and insight, changed your attitudes to something or have given you confidence in what you were doing.
> - Make a list of these people and identify what they did that most helped your learning. This will help you when you talk to your mentor to outline specific approaches that encourage your learning in practice.

Preparing for going into practice placements

Starting a new clinical experience can cause a number of emotional responses. Students normally experience some excitement, tinged with a little anxiety, about starting a new practice placement but get some comfort in knowing their mentor is able to provide guidance and support (Gray and Smith 2000). Research confirms that all students feel like novices in very unfamiliar settings when they start a new placement (Spouse 2001).

Here are some examples of second-year students' views on starting new placements:

- 'You really do not have any confidence when you first start your placement.'
- 'You worry about working with your mentor.'
- 'It is not always easy to integrate into a team in a relatively short time.'

Sometimes disappointment or annoyance can be experienced when you are allocated a placement that is not to your liking or is not where you see yourself working when qualified. There are a number of ways to manage these emotions.

Activity 13.4

How do you feel before starting a new practice experience? It will help if you write down your feelings and thoughts about going into a new clinical area and take this document with you on your first day to discuss with your mentor. Try to include some positive feelings and emotions in your list. This will give you and your mentor a basis to start from when planning your placement to ensure that you are able to overcome any fears or anxieties, while at the same time building on areas that you feel more confident with. Doing this each time you go to a new placement can help you manage the situation more positively and confidently.

Before starting a new practice experience you will find it helpful to do the following.

1. **Make sure you know where you're going.** This may seem obvious, but knowing the placement name and location clearly means this is one less thing to be concerned about. You will not be looking for the placement location at 7 a.m. on the morning you are due to commence and therefore can confidently walk onto the ward or department. Find out about the best travel options and costs, and leave adequate time to get there. Car parking, meal availability, and any accommodation requirements should be planned for in advance to reduce last-minute anxieties.
2. **Contact the ward or department by phone.** This enables you to speak to a member of staff, get your off duty and maybe arrange a visit before you officially start. It demonstrates that you are organized and keen to attend the placement while also enabling you to ask if there is any 'pre-placement' work that would benefit you when you start.
3. **Investigate the clinical area you will be working in and the experience you are likely to gain.** Having an understanding of the nursing care that is offered in the practice setting and undertaking some 'revision' is helpful. For example, checking on the law regarding lone working and other social, ethical and legal frameworks relevant to working in mental health care settings, learning disabilities care, child health, family situations or community care is always worth doing. This will enable you to start forming a 'picture' of the care you will be involved in giving and is key in enabling you to 'hit the ground running'. Looking at the organization's website will also give you some insight into how the whole service is run.
4. **Find out about your practice area and the type of client group you are likely to meet.** Is there any reading you could undertake before you commence your placement that would help you understand the client group you will be caring for? Reading about client experiences will enhance the knowledge, skills, values and attitudes needed for safe and effective nursing practice. Doing this will help you feel more confident and empowered to build initial rapport with clients by demonstrating a sincere interest in their condition and an understanding of their potential needs.
5. **Ensure that you adhere to professional expectations.** Wear your uniform as required by the organizational policy (e.g. hairs off the collar, nothing below the elbow, reduce jewellery, etc.). This is essential, not only in giving a professional impression but in ensuring patient safety and reducing infection risks.
6. **Make sure you are punctual and ready to start work at the beginning of your shift.** You should try as much as possible to mirror the off duty of your mentor or buddy mentor. Be prepared to undertake all shifts (including weekends and nights). Remember you will be doing unsocial hours when you qualify.
7. **Overall, the main message is to be proactive and positive.** That means talking initiative for your learning. You may feel that the experience is not for you, but there

is learning to be had in all experiences. Remember, do not always wait to be told what to do e.g. if phone rings answer it.

The Royal College of Nursing (RCN) has published an excellent resource for students starting placements entitled *Helping Students Get the Best From Their Practice Placements* (2006). Access a copy of this online and read it prior to starting your placement.

Key learning

!

- It is important to consider a range of practical matters about a new practice experience in advance to ensure you plan and are well prepared for it.

Your first day in a new placement

The first day in placement is when you start to find your feet. You will of course be nervous – this will be expected by the new team you will be working with and who will be supporting you in your learning and gaining of new experiences.

Mentors and other staff are used to new students arriving. You will, however, need to work to integrate yourself into the new environment as quickly as possible so that you are able to spend time developing your clinical skills and knowledge. Undertaking the activities suggested above should give you a firm foundation but you are also going to need to make an effort at becoming a member of the team. The following are useful ways forward.

1. Introduce yourself to as many members of the team as possible. Do not restrict this to the nursing staff, as many other staff will be involved in the care of the patient/clients. The quicker you become familiar with the roles staff have in the care of patients, the quicker you will be able to expand your learning, through observing staff at work and undertaking visits with them (e.g. with occupational therapists on home visits). These interactions will enable you to gain insight into the roles and responsibilities within the immediate and less immediate team – all of which contribute to individual patient pathways and the seamless transition between services.
2. Develop your relationship with your mentor and buddy. This is central to your learning and progress in clinical practice. Having a positive attitude is important and demonstrating that you are keen to learn is always beneficial. Understanding that every activity you are involved in is a learning opportunity is important, and this does not end when you have registered.
3. Be prepared – ensure that you have your assessment of practice document with you and that you have completed all the necessary paperwork required.
4. Complete any induction paperwork that you have been given. An orientation to the placement is very important in gaining an overview of your practice base.
5. Ask questions and follow them up if you feel that you have not got a full answer or that you don't understand it. Mentors will show you how to do something if you don't know or understand, but don't forget they have other work to do as well.
6. Be honest about any lack of capability you have in terms of either your knowledge or previous clinical experience. An open discussion will enable you and your mentor to gain an insight into areas that you need to develop and which can be offered in that placement area. Remember, it does not all need to be clinical: it may be that you are working in the community and need to understand how the acute service and community services work together, or how clinical specialists work across the health care sector to provide mental health care provision.
7. Become familiar with your preferred learning style and discuss it with your mentor – this will help you plan learning opportunities.

8 If you have any learning needs or a disability that you require an adjustment for, you will need to discuss this with your mentor.

> **Key learning**
>
> !
>
> - It is important to acknowledge and deal with any emotional feeling about the practice placement that may impact on your learning and share this with your mentor. Be proactive, ask questions and start getting to know your mentor and others as soon as possible.

Learning to give quality care

After undertaking the above, it is time to focus on learning as much as possible within the time you have. Caring for patients and clients in whatever environment you find yourself means you are in a privileged position. You will be involved in the life of others, sometimes for only a short time, others for longer. Key to this is the establishment of productive relationships with patients and their families. Over the course of your programme, one area that you should concentrate on is your role and your responsibility in the delivery of quality nursing care. As you go through the placement and observe and take part in delivering quality care, write down your experiences and record what you have learned. Use your portfolio for this. Check your learning about quality care with your mentor to get their perspective and to invite feedback. By the end of your programme you will have developed insight into quality nursing care and be able to articulate this, regardless of where you are working.

Developing a learning contract

It is important to develop the ability to identify your learning outcomes or goals and learn how to write an action plan or learning contract (see **Table 13.1**). This process will allow you to be more active in your learning and to identify a wide range of resources that are available to support your learning. Developing a learning contract is a creative activity and can be used to positively promote your relationship with mentors. It will also encourage you to evaluate your achievements and reflect on your progress in achieving your goals.

Table 13.1 An example of a learning contract

Learning need: what am I planning to learn?	**Goal/aim Why?**	**Resource or learning activity How?**	**Date for achievement When?**	**Evaluation and review How well completed? Any further learning?**
To understand the processes involved and demonstrate competence in the successful discharge of patients from hospital care	To gain experience of successfully preparing and supporting four patients being discharged from hospital care to community care	Work alongside mentor and become familiar with discharge planning and liaison with relatives, carers and other health care professionals		
Mentor signature		Student signature Date:		

Activity 13.5

- Think about your present or next practice placement. Review your learning needs and make a list of learning activities you might need to undertake.
- Once you have a list you can talk to your mentor and agree on an action plan or learning contract. This should include the activities you will need to undertake to achieve your goals.

Hint: a good reference for this is Elcock (2006).

Making progress in practice settings

In his theoretical exploration of how people learn, Wenger (1999: 74) indicates that it is a student's participation in the activity of the placement with others that provides the basis of the learning experience:

> Practice does not reside in books . . . it resides in a community of people . . . it exists because people are engaged in actions whose meanings they negotiate with one another . . . Being included in what matters is a requirement for being engaged in a community's practice, just as being engaged defines belonging. What it takes for a community of practice to cohere enough to function can be very subtle and delicate.

Activity 13.6

The quote from Wenger offers several points to consider when working with a mentor. Think about the following.

- How do you negotiate with your mentor?
- How do you demonstrate being willing to engage in nursing care?
- What helps you to feel 'included' in the practice activities of any particular placement?

Developing your insight and self-awareness of these things can improve your self-confidence as a student nurse and help you to learn and achieve new skills and competence in practice.

Working with your mentor and other members of the multidisciplinary team

You need to consider your responsibilities for your own learning during placement. The RCN (2007: 16) states that: 'It is important to understand that students have a central role in maximising their learning experience during placement, taking responsibility in directing their own education through interaction with relevant staff and the creation of learning experiences'.

As you will have read at the beginning of this chapter, mentors undertake the support of students following the successful completion of their mentorship programme. Your relationship with your mentor is central to your achievements while in clinical practice and therefore this relationship needs to be built on a firm footing. Mentors help you in planning your learning. It is very important that you make yourself aware of the variety of learning opportunities available in a practice placement as you may find that your practice experience is not in one place and may follow a patient journey or pathway.

For your part, as a student nurse with an assessment of practice document to complete, you must be fully aware of the NMC requirements and have considered how these can be met, particularly after the completion of your first placement. You should become increasingly aware of the areas that you need to be working on, whether it be undertaking a specific clinical skill (e.g. undertaking simple dressings before moving on to more complex ones), or improving your confidence when advocating for a patient on a ward round.

It is important to understand that each practice experience is not a hundred-yard dash where you achieve everything, have it signed off and then forget it as you move to your next experience and the next race. Each experience is part of a relay race with the feedback from one mentor being the 'baton' for future learning and development. The NMC requires an ongoing record of achievement that demonstrates continual and stepped progress across your entire programme with all feedback documented.

Being proactive is important throughout your practice experience. The more self-motivated you are, the more learning you will achieve, whether it be managing a patient's care, supporting other students or team working. Taking up all opportunities to learn about the patient's condition, the organization in which you are working and the political landscape of the NHS will all contribute to your development as a nurse who is able to manage the complexities of clinical care within the context of the ever-changing health care environment. Being adaptable is fundamental to maintaining high quality care within the reality of resource restrictions and political change.

Engaging with others to support your learning in practice

Although practice placements are where you learn and develop your competence, each placement environment is part of a particular social world (Goffman 1961) and as such you will need to understand the specific, and often hidden, subtle or unspoken cultural practice of each of your placements. Your mentor will be crucial in supporting you in doing this. Consider another quote from Wenger (1999: 75):

> Mutual engagement involves not only our own competence, but also the competence of others. It draws on what we do and what we know, as well as our ability to connect meaningfully to what we don't do and what we don't know – that is, to the contributions and knowledge of others.

Wenger is highlighting the importance of observing and learning from others. It is always interesting to ask questions of others about what they are doing and why, and how they do what they do. You will need to be sufficiently self-aware to recognize your own strengths and also which areas you need to develop further. It is important to be honest with others about what you really *do* know, recognizing your capabilities, potential *and* limitations. If you have a learning need you will of course need to make your mentor aware so that you get appropriate support. It is important always to be honest with your mentor. Often you will be able to complete many of the activities asked of you in practice. However, in order to become more experienced or skilled at carrying out certain procedures you will need the support of your mentor. Frequently mentors will work with you to instruct you in how to engage in more complex and subtle activities that may seem to you to be performed automatically. By working together you can learn more about these subtle aspects of practice. This could include how to talk to different patients, how to assess their condition and how to identify their actual and potential problems.

As Spouse (2001: 519) states, if students are left to roam about talking to patients or carrying out mundane activities which keep them busy and out of the way, then they will miss out on: 'learning the artistry and the science of caring for . . . patients that mentor(s) could teach . . . The key element is the collaborative nature of the interaction between practitioner and student'. Spouse goes on to emphasize the importance of dialogue between mentors and students. You may want to use certain learning experiences to debrief with your mentor and help you plan for future opportunities. You can link this to any previous learning while in the university setting or identify any further learning you might want to follow up independently or possibly linked to a written assignment.

Learning from your patient care experiences

When working in clinical practice, consider the patient holistically: not just the condition or diagnosis they may have, but all the information you have about them as a person. Make links to the initial assessment, the ongoing care and all mental, spiritual, emotional and physical needs. To support your development and understanding of all aspects of caring for a patient or client, you should do the following.

- **Make the initial assessment of the patient/client.** Make sure that you record everything that is important to the care of the patient's condition but also other factors, such as spiritual beliefs, family and carers, any specific patient requests about their stay. You should consider the patient's interests/hobbies and how they may be able to maintain these while away from their normal surroundings (e.g. books to read, listening to music, links to the chaplaincy department).

- **Care for the patient/client during their episode of care.** This may be just for a clinic appointment or longer if the patient is in an acute setting or in their own home.

After the episode of care, you should reflect on what you have learned and ask yourself the following questions.

- Did you fully understand the patient's presenting condition? Did you know how this impacted on the signs and symptoms that the patient described and could you relate this to all the aspects of clinical care that the patient received?
- Where you had gaps in theoretical or practical knowledge or skills, what did you do?
- Did you fully understand the impact on the patient's life and family? What is your role in minimizing stress and anxiety for patients in the setting?
- Did you communicate with the patient in an appropriate way?
- What health advice/promotion did you give?
- Was the patient safe under your care at all times?
- Did you feel confident in the activities you undertook in caring for the patient?
- Did you challenge any aspects of care delivery?

These questions and the care that you deliver will contribute to your wider understanding of care delivery plus your ability to be an advocate for patients and clients.

Being reflective about your practice

Undertaking reflection on your clinical practice and linking it with theory will enable you to consider, creatively, different ways and methods of managing situations. Remember, all patients are different even if a situation is the same. Reflective practice will help you understand and manage your emotions and those of others. Using a reflective model (for an example see Chapter 7) will help identify your learning needs, motivate you to achieve goals and deal with challenges and setbacks, maintain your physical and emotional well-being, enable you to feel confident in your decisions and actions, and help you to have clarity of thinking when adapting to new situations.

Skills and competencies

You will have practice documentation developed by your university which you should share with your mentor throughout the practice experience. This comprises a set of learning outcomes that you are required to achieve, based on competencies and skills set by the NMC. The competencies have four domains which are:

- professional and ethical practice;
- care delivery;
- care management;
- personal and professional development (NMC 2010).

To support these domains the NMC (2010) has also identified Essential Skills Clusters (ESCs) to ensure you will develop the skills required for entry to the register. These are generic skills statements that are applicable to all fields of nursing and all fields of practice. However, the ESCs do not include all the skills and behaviours required of an RN and your university will include additional skills applicable to your field of nursing.

There are five ESCs:

- care, compassion and communication;
- organizational aspects of care;
- infection prevention and control;
- nutrition and fluid management;
- medicines management.

You and your mentor will need to sign each as you achieve them. Your mentor will then sign your paperwork at the end of the placement to show that you have passed the placement. It is therefore important that achieving these learning outcomes forms the basis of regular discussions of your learning needs and that records of achievement are completed regularly to help you successfully pass your placement.

When things don't go as planned

Not everything that happens in clinical practice will go as planned. This is the nature of supporting and caring for patients and their relatives who are in unfamiliar and stressful situations, and working in teams (both immediate nursing teams and interprofessional teams). It is good practice at the beginning of a placement for the student and mentor to clarify and discuss each other's expectations to ensure these are realistic. This will help to avoid any uncertainties or misunderstandings (Wilkes 2006). You will probably already be familiar with establishing ground rules. Understanding that the clinical area is going to challenge you on many levels is essential. Developing skills of reflection is crucial in enabling you to understand situations that you may find yourself in. You should reflect on the way that you and others responded and consider how the situation could have been managed differently, and from this will come learning. While situations may be similar, they will never be the same because of the individuals involved, and your reflection can support you to manage these differences. It is also worth noting that you should always reflect on what went particularly *well*. You may want to consider keeping a reflective diary (ensuring data protection is adhered to), or engaging in reflection with your mentor as ways of learning from the challenges of clinical practice.

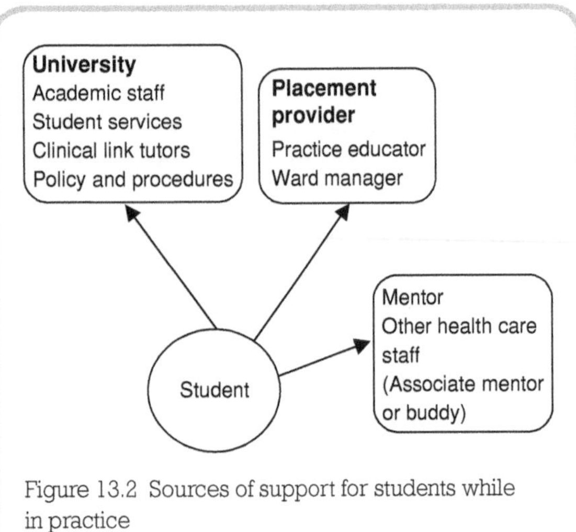

Figure 13.2 Sources of support for students while in practice

Activity 13.7

- Find out about your local policies and procedures for asking for support for your learning during your practice experience (see also **Figure 13.2**).
- Identify everyone you can ask for support when you are working in practice.

Failure to achieve in practice

Most students will be able to demonstrate competence in practice appropriate to their stage on the programme, but occasionally you may fail to achieve a competence at the first attempt, or fail a placement and have to repeat it. Duffy and Hardicre (2007) explored the reasons why students fail to achieve in practice and identified the following:

- poor interpersonal and communication skills;
- poor professional behaviour;
- lack of insight into own performance;
- not responding to feedback from mentors;
- personal issues, poor health, tiredness and lack of motivation or commitment;
- inconsistency in performance.

Mentors will be responsible for giving you feedback on your progress and will provide details of successes as well as highlighting areas for further development. The NMC considers it important that you have 'an ongoing record of achievement and that mentors have an audit trail to support their decisions' (NMC 2008b: 33).

Most students are aware of their weaknesses and it can be helpful to have a discussion with your mentor about this – perhaps documenting it and making a plan for action during a placement. Do not forget the role your personal tutor can play, or the clinical link tutor. They are there to support your learning in practice. Feedback is of little value if it is not responded to or if no action results from it. Remember, feedback from mentors, associate mentors and other members of the practice team will help you to identify your strengths and achievements as well as flagging up areas for further development and improvement.

Key learning

!

- There are times when you may find it difficult to achieve competencies in practice, but all feedback is helpful and needs to be responded to.

Activity 13.8

!

- If you felt uncomfortable about something your mentor was doing or saying such as calling you 'student' rather than by your name or criticizing you in front of others, what would you do about it?
- Consider this comment: 'My mentor had agreed earlier that day I could do the drug round with her but when I went to ask her about it she told me we were short of staff and I needed to help a patient eat his lunch. I had already helped this patient during the last week to eat his meals and was concerned as I needed to be signed off as competent in drug administration. But I could see no point in saying this to her again.' What would you do in this situation?

Challenges while working in practice

In the 1980s Melia (1987) explored how nurses were socialized into the profession, and described how students in placement spoke about 'getting the work done' and 'fitting in'. As a learner it is likely that you will want to fit in and feel like you belong. We all need to belong and feel very uncomfortable if we are excluded from a group. Naturally when you start in a placement you will quickly want to respond to the norms of the location in order to feel that you belong. In a research study carried out in Australia and the UK, Levett-Jones and Lathlean (2009) reported on how student nurses tend to conform and comply with situations in the practice setting. Sometimes it is easier to accept the values of the placement rather than challenge them:

> students related how they complied with unacceptable nursing practices because they were reticent to endanger their precarious sense of belonging. This was particularly true of students who felt less secure of their place in the nursing team
>
> (Levett-Jones and Lathlean 2009: 348).

Be prepared to question aspects of practice. As a student you are in the environment to learn and can ask for explanations or evidence underpinning practice. With developing confidence and knowledge you may become more able to speak up. Sometimes it is just about saying 'No' assertively. You may want to prepare yourself in advance and plan a time to meet with your mentor to discuss the situation. Be clear about what you want to say. You may want to refer to some evidence such as guidelines or policy and research to help you state your view. An important part of your learning is about empowering others, so make sure you can demonstrate that you are empowered to stand by your principles and values.

Mentors are people too

McKenzie (1991) found that when mentors effectively support students they found it easier to adapt and settle in to learn within a practice placement. Of course mentors are people too; they have their own work pressures and professional and personal concerns which can impact on how they respond to and support your learning (Cowan

2000). Here are two comments about mentors from students:

- 'I had a mentor who looked bored. Later I discovered she was actually preoccupied with some personal difficulties. Now I always remember that mentors are people too. More than that, they have been students too!'
- 'I have learned that my attitude impacts on the mentor and on our relationship. Despite sometimes hearing others say that X is a poor mentor I try to keep an open mind.'

There will always be people you do not get on with. One of these might be your mentor. However, remember you cannot always work with 'friends' and you must always behave professionally. This is an important aspect of personal and professional learning, both for your future career and for life. Consider what personal attributes you possess that would help you to build on past experiences and deal with more challenging individuals, rather than feeling frustrated, upset or possibly even about to give up. If you need help, do discuss the matter with another member of staff on the ward, or with your academic tutor or link lecturer.

Conclusion

You do not carry out practice experiences in a vacuum. You will be engaging with a range of people, from patients and their relatives to your mentor and other health care staff. You will bring your own values and cultural assumptions to your development as a nurse. However, as discussed in Chapter 2, it is critical that you have an awareness of these values and cultural assumptions and be open to learning from and respecting the different values and cultural diversity of others, be they patients, your mentor or other staff. At the heart of effective nursing is an ethos which respects the integrity and dignity of the other, whoever they may be.

In this and all that you may learn, the role of the mentor is fundamental to your learning in practice placements. While it cannot be guaranteed that you will not have any negative experiences, the research evidence indicates that most students are effectively supported by mentors in practice (Myall *et al.* 2008). Getting the most from working with your mentor will be helped by you being self-aware, self-motivated and self-confident. This chapter has highlighted some of the ways you can achieve this during the varying placements you will encounter in your programme.

Acknowledgements

We would like to acknowledge and thank Claire Millard, Liz Pearson and Chloe MacArthur, student nurses in the Faculty of Health Sciences at the University of Southampton and Kathryn. Reading for sharing their experiences of working with mentors and how they developed good working relationships with them.

Further reading and resources

Arkell, S. (2007) How nursing students can make the most of placements, *Nursing Times*, 103(20): 26–8.

RCN (Royal College of Nursing) (2006) *Helping Students Get the Best From Their Practice Placements: A Royal College of Nursing Toolkit*, available at: www.rcn.org.uk/publications/pdf/helpingstudents.pdf.

References

Andrews, M. and Chilton, F. (2000) Student and mentor perceptions of mentoring effectiveness, *Nurse Education Today*, 20: 555–62.

Cowan, L. (2000) Lessons of experience: working with students in community midwifery practice, in J. Spouse and L. Redfern (eds) *Successful Supervision in Health Care Practice: Promoting Professional Development*. Oxford: Blackwell Science.

DH (Department of Health) (2010) *Equity and Excellence: Liberating the NHS*. London: DH.

Duffy, K. and Hardicre, J. (2007) Supporting failing students in practice, 1: assessment, *Nursing Times*, 103(47): 28–9.

Egan, T. and Jaye, C. (2009) Communities of clinical practice: the social organisation of clinical learning, *Health: An Interdisciplinary Journal for the Social Study of Health, Illness and Medicine*, 13(1): 107–25.

Elcock, K. (2006) Wake up and learn, *Nursing Standard*, 20(49): 61.

Goffman, E. (1961) *Asylums: Essays on the Social Situation of Mental Patients and Other Inmates*. Oxford: Anchor Books.

Gray, M.A. and Smith, L.N. (2000) The qualities of an effective mentor from the student nurse's perspective: findings from a longitudinal qualitative study, *Journal of Advanced Nursing*, 32(6): 1542–9.

Howell, W.S. (1982) *The Empathic Communicator*. Belmont, CA: Wadsworth Publishing Company.

Levett-Jones, T. and Lathlean, J. (2009) 'Don't rock the boat': nursing students' experiences of conformity and compliance, *Nurse Education Today*, 29(3): 342–9.

McKenzie, K.M. (1991) A study of the perceptions of support among student nurses with a mentor and student nurses without a mentor in the clinical area. Unpublished MEd thesis, University of Aberdeen.

Melia, K. (1987) *Learning and Working: The Occupational Socialization of Nursing*. London: Tavistock.

Midgley, K. (2006) Pre-registration student nurses' perception of the hospital learning environment during clinical placements, *Nurse Education Today*, 26(4): 338–45.

Myall, M., Levett-Jones, T. and Lathlean, J. (2008) Mentorship in contemporary practice: the experiences of nursing students and practice mentors, *Journal of Clinical Nursing*, 17(14): 1834–42.

Neary, M. (2000) Responsive assessment: assessing student nurses' clinical competence, *Nurse Education Today*, 21: 3.

NMC (Nursing and Midwifery Council) (2008a) *Standards to Support Learning and Assessment in Practice: NMC Standards for Mentors, Practice Teachers and Teachers*. London: NMC.

NMC (Nursing and Midwifery Council) (2008b) *The Code: Standards of Conduct, Performance and Ethics for Nurses and Midwives*. London: NMC.

NMC (Nursing and Midwifery Council) (2010) *Standards for Pre-registration Nursing Education*. London: NMC.

RCN (Royal College of Nursing) (2006) *Helping Students Get the Best From Their Practice Placements: A Royal College of Nursing Toolkit*, available at: www.rcn.org.uk/publications/pdf/helpingstudents.pdf.

RCN (Royal College of Nursing) (2007) *Guidance for Mentors of Nursing Students and Midwives: An RCN Toolkit*. London: RCN.

Spouse, J. (2001) Bridging theory and practice in the supervisory relationship: a sociocultural perspective, *Journal of Advanced Nursing*, 33(4): 512–22.

Wenger, E. (1999) *Communities of Practice: Learning, Meaning, and Identity*. Cambridge: Cambridge University Press.

Wilkes, Z. (2006) The student-mentor relationship: a review of the literature, *Nursing Standard*, 20(37): 42–7.

Learning abroad: the student experience of nursing in a European or international context

14

Avril Milne, Jean Cowie and Brian Webster

Chapter contents

Introduction

This chapter will provide you with an overview of some of the benefits and challenges of working abroad. It will draw on the experience, expertise and knowledge of staff and students from one school of nursing and midwifery in the UK, the Robert Gordon University, Aberdeen, where a number of highly successful Erasmus and international student exchanges have been offered and embedded as a successful pre-registration student learning experience for some time. It will offer you a theoretical understanding of the benefits and learning opportunities that such exchanges can bring from a global perspective and stretch your understanding of cultural competence and the application of clinical practice in a range of varied health care delivery systems, as well as provide you with practical advice and considerations from years of experience. The chapter also provides you with some reflective analysis of our student nurses' experiences of learning abroad as well as useful tips for you, mentors and other academics in nursing departments across the UK.

The role of health care organizations in nurturing the development of a culturally sensitive workforce is essential to meet the expectations of increasingly diverse staff and patient populations (Papadopoulos *et al.* 2004). In recognition of these changing health care dynamics, the Nursing and Midwifery Council (NMC) *Standards for Pre-registration Nursing Education* (2010) have been aligned to the European Directive 2005/36/EC to promote mutual recognition of qualifications (European Commission 2005). This provides you, the student nurse, with an increased scope to undertake diverse learning opportunities outside the UK for a period of up to six months. Student nurses expanding their international profile via learning abroad experiences will be able to evidence key graduate attributes and qualities to prospective employers, thereby increasing the possibility of employment success (European Commission 2010; British Council 2012).

Gaining a theoretical understanding

The literature indicates that learning abroad enables you as a student nurse to go beyond the level of cultural knowledge gained through theoretical learning and develop a greater awareness of how your own cultural values impact on your professional practice (Greatrex-White 2008). In fact, Greatrex-White highlights the potential for you as a student to experience an obvious cognitive change as a result of a learning abroad experience and an increased awareness of different cultures. Learning abroad can provide you with a unique intercultural experience and exposure to foreign nursing cultures that can enrich your professional skills repertoire (Lee *et al.* 2007). We believe that the need for providers of nurse education, in collaboration with their practice learning partners, to develop valuable learning abroad opportunities for student nurses is an essential component of pre-registration nurse education today. The increasing multicultural nature of societies across the globe requires the registered nurse (RN) of tomorrow to be personally and professionally confident in their ability to respectfully care for diverse patient populations and effectively lead a multicultural nursing and health care workforce (Lee 2004).

Global demographics have changed significantly over recent years, with societies becoming increasingly multicultural and ethnically diverse. Across the globe, there is a demand for nurses to be able to deliver a quality health care service to people of differing cultures and to be effective members of a multicultural health care workforce (Lee *et al.* 2007). Within the context of your learning the responsibility for you to be prepared for professional practice in a culturally diverse health care environment, nationally and internationally, is crucial (European Commission 2009a; WHO 2009). The new NMC *Standards* provide you as a student with an opportunity to obtain a comparative experience of health and nursing in a different country and to build your personal and professional confidence and ability to provide culturally sensitive care (Lee 2004). Clinical learning abroad, whether it is observational or direct participation in health care, facilitates an opportunity to equip you with a versatile professional knowledge base and a preparedness for culturally competent nursing practice following graduation (Kokko 2011).

Activity 14.1

Try to identify why you think you might benefit from a learning experience in another country.

- What challenges would this pose for you?
- What personal attributes could be enhanced by this experience?

Global citizenship

The notion of global citizenship or global competency has gained popularity in education in recent years (Oxfam 2006; Diamond *et al.* 2011a, 2011b; Hounsell 2011). Oxfam has been a key player in promoting global citizenship in primary and secondary education; however, the principles and concepts are equally applicable in higher education. According to Oxfam (2006) a global citizen:

- is aware of the wider world and has a sense of their own role as a world citizen;
- respects and values diversity;
- has an understanding of how the world works economically, politically, socially, culturally, technologically and environmentally;
- is outraged by social injustice;

- participates in, and contributes to, the community at a range of levels from local to global;
- is willing to act to make the world a more sustainable place;
- takes responsibility for their actions.

Clearly, Oxfam's ethos of global citizenship has an integral place within higher education, and this is supported by Hounsell (2011) who identified global citizenship as one of the key graduate attributes for the twenty-first century. The Council for Industry in Higher Education (CIHE) (Diamond *et al.* 2011a, 2011b) refers to the concept of 'global graduates' and highlights their critical competencies as follows.

- **A global mindset:** to have an awareness of different cultures and values, and how one's own culture and values differ.
- **Global knowledge:** knowledge of the economics, history and culture of different countries.
- **Cultural agility:** the ability to understand the perspectives of individuals from different cultures and backgrounds and to empathize with these views and respond to them; the ability to cope with and adapt to living in different environments.
- **Advanced communication skills:** the ability to communicate effectively with others from around the world.
- **Management of complex interpersonal relationships:** the ability to manage relationships with diverse teams and clients from across the globe and deal with inherent challenges.
- **Team working and collaboration:** the ability to work collaboratively and empathetically with diverse teams from across the globe.
- **Learning agility:** the ability to rapidly assimilate knowledge and develop understanding in order to rapidly respond and adapt to new challenges, circumstances and cultures.
- **Adaptability, flexibility, resilience, drive and self-awareness:** these attributes underpin the above global competencies and are essential, enabling qualities.

Activity 14.2

- In what way can global citizenship impact on you and your clinical practice?
- What impact will global citizenship have on nursing in 10 years' time?

Take time to think these questions through and reflect on your answers.

Although the CIHE discusses the global graduate and global competencies in relation to industry and business, we believe that the concepts are equally applicable to the nursing profession. The global employee may also be the global patient or indeed the global colleague of the future. An understanding and respect of cultural diversity, inequity and social injustice, economics and politics is, therefore, essential for the graduate nurse of the twenty-first century.

With regard to the course and curriculum requirement for the NMC, the principles underpinning the philosophy of the global graduate and global citizen marry well with the four generic standards for competence set out in the new *Standards for Pre-registration Nursing Education* (NMC 2010). For example, fundamental concepts such as respect, dignity, compassion, culture, socio-economics, politics, social justice, inequity, partnership, team working, leadership, accountability and autonomy are just some of the shared values (Oxfam 2006; NMC 2010; Diamond *et al.* 2011a, 2011b; Hounsell 2011).

The benefits of learning abroad: exploring the evidence

According to Fielden *et al.* (2007), learning abroad has many benefits for you as a student. In addition to the opportunity to learn and develop language and linguistic skills, the learning abroad experience helps you to broaden your academic experience and to clarify your understanding within your field of study. It can also strengthen your commitment to your current studies and perhaps inspire you for further studies or for work overseas. We have personally witnessed this in our student nurses who have returned from a European or international learning experience, with some being rejuvenated and invigorated for an active career in nursing within the UK or overseas, while others have developed a better appreciation of the benefits and shortcomings of the health care system in the UK.

Table 14.1 highlights the benefits of learning abroad based on the evaluations of our students who participated in learning opportunities there.

Table 14.1 The benefits of learning abroad: student evaluations

Personal advantages to learning abroad	■ An independence that will benefit you for years to come ■ A self-belief and confidence beyond anything you can imagine ■ A greater awareness of who you are and what you believe in
Social advantages to learning abroad	■ Lifelong friendships with many people from across the world ■ Opportunity for future travel to visit new friends ■ An appreciation of different cultural beliefs, traditions and lifestyles ■ Increased social skills
Professional advantages to learning abroad	■ Professional confidence and assertiveness ■ Ability to communicate with people from different cultures ■ Ability to provide nursing care to culturally diverse populations ■ Ability to draw on a comparative knowledge of other health care organizations and nursing practices ■ Ability to establish a network of professional colleagues to share best practice ■ An understanding of different styles of health care delivery (e.g. NHS services free at point of delivery, whereas there are insurance and cost implications in other countries) ■ A fuller appreciation of the value of the role of the NMC in protecting the public and safeguarding patients (e.g. practitioner accountability in the safe administration of medicines) ■ Innovative alternative approaches to infection control that could be adopted in the UK (e.g. the routine autoclaving of hospital beds between patient use)
Impact on patient care	■ An appreciation of how patients may feel when they don't understand nursing jargon ■ Improved communication skills with patients and colleagues ■ Ability to recognize and value wider issues impacting on patient admission, health care delivery and discharge options ■ Increased understanding of need to practise person-centred nursing care
Impact on future nursing career	■ Raises the international profile of your CV ■ An advantage to gaining employment as an RN as employers increasingly value the outcomes of a learning abroad experience to their organization ■ Recognized internationally as a key graduate attribute ■ Adds value to your application for studies at masters and doctoral level

Fielden *et al.* (2007) also highlight that the experience of living, working and studying in another country facilitates personal growth and development that can enable you to confidently adapt to a new environment and country and in the process become more culturally perceptive and tolerant. The need for you to be able to integrate socially with local students and residents, as well as visiting international students from elsewhere, necessitates the development of enhanced communication and social skills to maximize the learning abroad experience. The personal and professional maturity and independence alluded to here has been frequently cited by returning student nurses as a key outcome of the learning abroad experience.

Learning abroad, therefore, promotes the development of graduate nurses who are confident as well as independent and autonomous beings who can face the many challenges that a career in nursing may present. Indeed, several nursing students who have participated in the learning abroad programme at the Robert Gordon University have opted to work overseas on completion of their nurse education. Others have reported a keen interest in the learning abroad programme from prospective employers and believe that the formal recognition of the academic credit gained from the experience has strengthened their CVs and been a key factor in their employment success (European Commission 2010; British Council 2012). This supports the notion offered by the CIHE (Diamond *et al.* 2011a, 2011b) that the experience of working abroad and being immersed in a different culture and lifestyle is invaluable and can propel graduates into being considered for rewarding and challenging roles.

From our experience, we believe that the student nurse of today will witness a growth in the amount of opportunities available to the nursing profession to become increasingly internationally aware from a professional perspective. For example, the World Health Organization (WHO), the International Council of Nurses (ICN), the British Council, the European Commission and the Voluntary Services Organization (VSO) are all key promoters of the internationalization agenda and provide valuable advice, guidance and resources about global health and nursing to individuals, private and voluntary organizations and the public. Each of the key organizations can be easily accessed via the internet and provide a rich resource for students and RNs and facilitate a greater international awareness about profession-specific topics.

Learning abroad in Europe

The Bologna Declaration, commonly referred to as the 'Bologna Agreement', is a key document in the European higher education arena (CRE 2000). Essentially the Declaration aims to converge or draw higher education institutions together so that there is greater understanding of the education systems and frameworks used in different countries. Within the Declaration it is clear that the intention is not to impose standards or uniformity among higher education institutions in Europe, but rather to promote a system of compatibility whereby academic qualifications obtained in one European country are recognized, accepted and transferred accordingly to a higher education institution in another European country. The Declaration, therefore, has established a European Higher Education Area (EHEA) that is able to provide world-class higher education that is attractive to you as a student as well as qualified staff, and is also competitive within the global economy. The overarching qualification framework developed by the EHEA consists of three cycles: bachelor, masters and doctorate. All countries of the EHEA are committed to developing national qualification frameworks that are compatible with the EHEA framework (Gobbi 2005; European Commission 2009b, 2011a) and the promotion of the EHEA is expected to strengthen student and staff mobility and employability within Europe and across the globe (European Commission 2009a).

Erasmus+

The Erasmus Lifelong Learning Programme (ELLP to be renamed erasmus+ as of January 2014) is funded by the European Commission and is directed at higher education institutions with the aim of promoting student and staff mobility within Europe. The European Commission, via the British Council, provides grants for you as students as well as staff activities within the ELLP (British Council 2012). Armed with the knowledge about ELLP activities and resources, the School of Nursing and Midwifery at the Robert Gordon University targeted new and existing European partners to create a centre of excellence for student nurse exchanges and collaborative staff activities. The School has established a strong presence in Europe with eight European partners in five different countries (Belgium, Finland, the Netherlands, Norway and Spain) and has successfully been engaging in pre-registration accredited student nurse exchanges for over 10 years. The number of student nurses and staff participating annually in an exchange programme has grown exponentially from three student nurses and two staff to 32 student nurses and eight staff per year.

Case study 14.1: Reflections of a third-year student nurse (ELLP)

The opportunity to participate in the ELLP has been an absolutely amazing experience. I was very excited about the exchange opportunity and also had some anxieties prior to departure. However my worries were needless as I found I was very well supported by staff at the university, on clinical placements and also by fellow students. Not only was I making friends with Finns but I was meeting students from other countries and other university courses who were also participating in the ELLP.

Although I was concerned about the language barrier I found that most students and many of the staff both in the hospital and university had a good command of English. In situations where the language barrier was an issue I had to resort to non-verbal means of communication. Although this could be hilarious at times it also made me realize the many challenges faced by minority groups and immigrants at home who have limited understanding of English.

During my time in Finland I had the opportunity to visit several places of cultural interest. I also had the opportunity to try skiing, go to the Arctic Circle and to visit a Snow Hotel with the other students. I was also invited into Finnish homes by my new friends and colleagues and able to experience Finnish life at first hand. Finnish people like to have a sauna and most have a sauna in their home. Where I stayed the sauna was available for girls two evenings per week or it could be booked for use privately. Myself and the two other girls from my university booked the sauna for us to use on our own. It was really nice.

On my practice placements I worked alongside an English-speaking mentor who ensured that I got to see lots of procedures and to go to theatre to see operations. It was interesting to see the similarities and differences in nursing practices. For example, the focus of nursing in Scotland is on caring and maintaining dignity, whereas in Finland more emphasis is placed on technical skills. I think my experience in Finland has given me a better understanding of health care systems and provision and also of the valuable role of the NMC. I've almost finished my course now and went for an interview for a nursing job. The interviewers were very interested in my ELLP experience and I'm sure it was this that gave me the advantage over the other candidates to secure the position as a staff nurse.

Taking part in the ELLP and living in Finland for three months has been an absolutely fantastic experience. I learned a lot about myself and my ability to cope in a new and strange environment and also to deal with any unforeseen challenges. I think I have grown as a person as a result of the exchange experience. I feel I have greater self-awareness and developed valuable transferable skills such as improved communication skills, the ability to adapt quickly to change and to use my initiative. I feel I have more confidence – certainly people have commented that I am more confident. The ELLP experience has been amazing and I feel very privileged to have had the opportunity to go to Finland. I would advise anyone thinking about taking part in the ELLP to just go for it – you'll have the experience of a lifetime.

Activity 14.3

- In what way do you think a learning abroad experience will influence your future career in nursing?
- How would you best prepare for a valuable learning abroad experience?

Making it work: our experience

The School's European Exchange Module supports the 'Study Mobility' element of the ELLP, which the Robert Gordon University actively chose to invest in rather than the 'Training Mobility' element (British Council 2012), in order to maintain the quality assurance role it has for all its practice learning partners. Student nurses exchange 13 weeks of their programmed practice learning during the third year of their course with an equivalent practice learning experience at one of the European partners. On successful completion of the practice learning experience, our student nurses receive 20 European Credit and Accumulation Transfer System (ECTS) credits from the European partner providing the exchange opportunity. In keeping with the ethos of the Bologna Declaration the ECTS credits are transferable between institutions (European Commission 2011b) and this is acknowledged as such in the student graduation transcript. The School provides a reciprocal arrangement for student nurses from the European partner institutions to undertake an equivalent practice learning experience and obtain the same ECTS credits, which in turn enriches not only the students learning but that of our NHS practice partners and academic staff alike.

The student nurse accepted for a learning abroad experience in Europe is encouraged to engage in fundraising activities to complement the grant they will receive from the British Council, in order to minimize the impact of the costs involved, and they are advised to contact the Royal College of Nursing (RCN) to determine the availability of professional indemnity insurance required for practice learning in Europe (RCN 2012).

We recommend that student nurses develop a study plan for outstanding coursework and assessments to reduce the workload during the learning abroad experience. Although each practice placement partner has a well stocked library of nursing texts and journals in English, student nurses are encouraged to creatively plan access to the library materials they require from the UK in advance of the exchange.

Activity 14.4

- Try to imagine you have been accepted for an Erasmus exchange in one of our European partner countries. Try to identify what you might need to explore about nursing and health care in that country before you leave.

Learning abroad in the USA

The opportunity for you as a student nurse to cross international boundaries to learn about nursing and health care in different countries is of growing global interest. The WHO has developed global standards for the initial education of nurses and midwives (WHO 2009) and the EHEA has announced a significant advance in cooperation between European and international partners to mutually recognize qualifications and support student and staff exchanges (Bologna Process 2007).

Within the context of the USA there is a wealth of literature available in relation to the value of transcultural nursing care and global nursing education (Leininger 2002; Siantz and Meleis 2007; GANES 2011). Although the culture of nursing within the USA differs from that of the UK, much can be learned about the ways in which the US nursing profession has faced the challenge of being able to provide culturally congruent nursing and health care to diverse patient population groups. It is anticipated that UK student nurses and RNs seeking to develop their cultural competence in professional practice will find a plethora of useful material via the internet to increase their cultural knowledge and ability to provide quality nursing care to culturally diverse groups in the USA.

Within the School of Nursing and Midwifery at the Robert Gordon University, we have specifically appointed a link teacher for the USA, who has devolved management responsibility for the student nurse exchanges to and from that country and maintains collaborative relationships with the partner institutions and key stakeholders. The US link teacher is responsible for maintaining a live audit trail of partner institutions, indicating their suitability as practice learning environments to support student learning. Furthermore, they are also central to the effective management of the UK student nurse selection process and provide academic and pastoral support to the UK and US student nurses throughout their learning abroad exchange experience.

Practice learning through observation is available to our third-year student nurses to experience nursing and health care in the USA by participating in a two-week observational learning experience. The student selection process is competitive and results in two student nurses being selected by each university (USA and the UK) to participate in the exchange programme and to act as 'buddies' to the visiting students. They jointly attend and present at civic events, visit university learning environments, observe clinical practice in a variety of health care settings and participate in a range of cultural activities (an important part of the learning experience). This learning abroad experience does not involve an exchange of academic credit as there is no formal assessment attached to the exchange programme at this moment in time.

Case Study 14.2: Reflections of a third-year student nurse (USA)

Participation in the American exchange programme provided me with an incredibly valuable experience, way beyond anything I had imagined. From day one, when I first applied for the opportunity, I found the whole experience to be very beneficial to me personally and professionally. Writing a supporting statement about why I should be chosen for the opportunity and promoting my personal and professional attributes at the selection interview was challenging and character building. I was delighted to be selected and felt proud that I was recognized as someone who could be an ambassador for the nursing profession, the School of Nursing and Midwifery and my country.

Prior to my visit to the USA, I shared the responsibility of 'hosting' the American exchange students during their two-week observational experience in Aberdeen. It was a fantastic experience for me to show off our beautiful country, and to explain how our health care systems works and how nurses are educated to provide person-centred care. I had never done this kind of thing before and it made me really appreciate my own culture, my nursing knowledge, and how this all fitted into the patient care I provided.

My experience in the USA was incredible. The private hospitals look like high-class office buildings and patients receive every service you can imagine, despite the cost. The public hospitals are different, less spacious with a greater demand for limited services in comparison to the private hospitals. It made me really appreciate the National Health Service we have in the UK.

My communication skills and confidence have improved immensely, particularly because of my ambassador role. I was able to hold conversations with so many new people who held a variety of senior professional or civic roles, which I executed with professionalism and dignity. I am confident that this experience will enhance my patient care, professional development and future career as a nurse. I am proud of my achievements and feel that I have proved that I was indeed worthy of this opportunity and responsibility. Maybe, one day, I will return to the USA to work there as a nurse.

Challenges of undertaking nursing practice in the USA

In our experience, student nurses often ask about the possibility of extending their observational experience to one that involves 'hands-on' direct patient care. Practice learning through direct participation in health care is an innovative endeavour to provide a student nurse exchange that facilitates a deeper learning and understanding of the professional and cultural differences of health care provision in the USA. The School undertook audits of selected US practice learning environments, which clearly indicated a wealth of opportunity available to UK student nurses to obtain valuable observational learning experiences. Within selected health care organizations there is also scope for UK student nurses to access dedicated educational units that provide appropriate mentorship and assessment to facilitate practice learning through direct participation in nursing and health care. However, the current US immigration rules and requirements are complex in relation to which visa you as a student nurse would require, including the purpose and duration of the exchange, and whether or not enrolment at the partner university is necessary. It is therefore imperative that UK universities and student nurses seek guidance and confirmation from an appropriate professional source about these issues before considering an opportunity to observe or directly participate in health care in the USA.

Professional and personal indemnity insurance is another prerequisite to being able to participate in a practice learning experience in the USA. As a student you must purchase this for practice learning, and it is available at a reasonable cost from US insurance providers. We recommend that consultation between the participating UK university and an appropriate professional source is recommended to ensure that you have the correct insurance protection required prior to observing or directly participating in health care in the USA. Although membership of the RCN provides professional indemnity for your work in the UK and Europe, it doesn't currently extend to the USA or Canada (RCN 2012).

Figure 14.1 shows the support networks in place to enrich the learning abroad experience.

Preparation for a learning abroad experience

Theoretical preparation for a learning abroad experience is an essential component of any exchange. At Robert Gordon University a specific credited theoretical module is a compulsory aspect of the learning experience to ensure that our student nurses are prepared for the multifaceted benefits and challenges that any such exchange can bring. Preparation includes the student nurses exploring key health and social care issues in a global context and comparing the nurse education and practice, health issues, and policy drivers impacting on health care provision in the UK and in the country selected for their learning abroad exchange. The summative assessment for the module includes a reflective analysis of the student nurse's learning abroad experience and the impact on their personal and professional development. It is our belief that you as a student are expected to be an ambassador for your profession, school, university, and indeed the UK.

Preparation for learning abroad includes meeting the admission requirements for each partner institution. For example, various vaccinations and screening for methicillin-resistant staphylococcus aureus (MRSA) and salmonella are required by some northern European countries and the UK. At Robert Gordon University our link teachers liaise with the relevant occupational health provider and each institution to ensure all exchange nurses meet the necessary requirements. In addition they are also responsible for ensuring that students comply with the required health screening process and application requirements referred to earlier and that they obtain approval from the Protecting Vulnerable Groups Scheme (Scottish Government 2011).

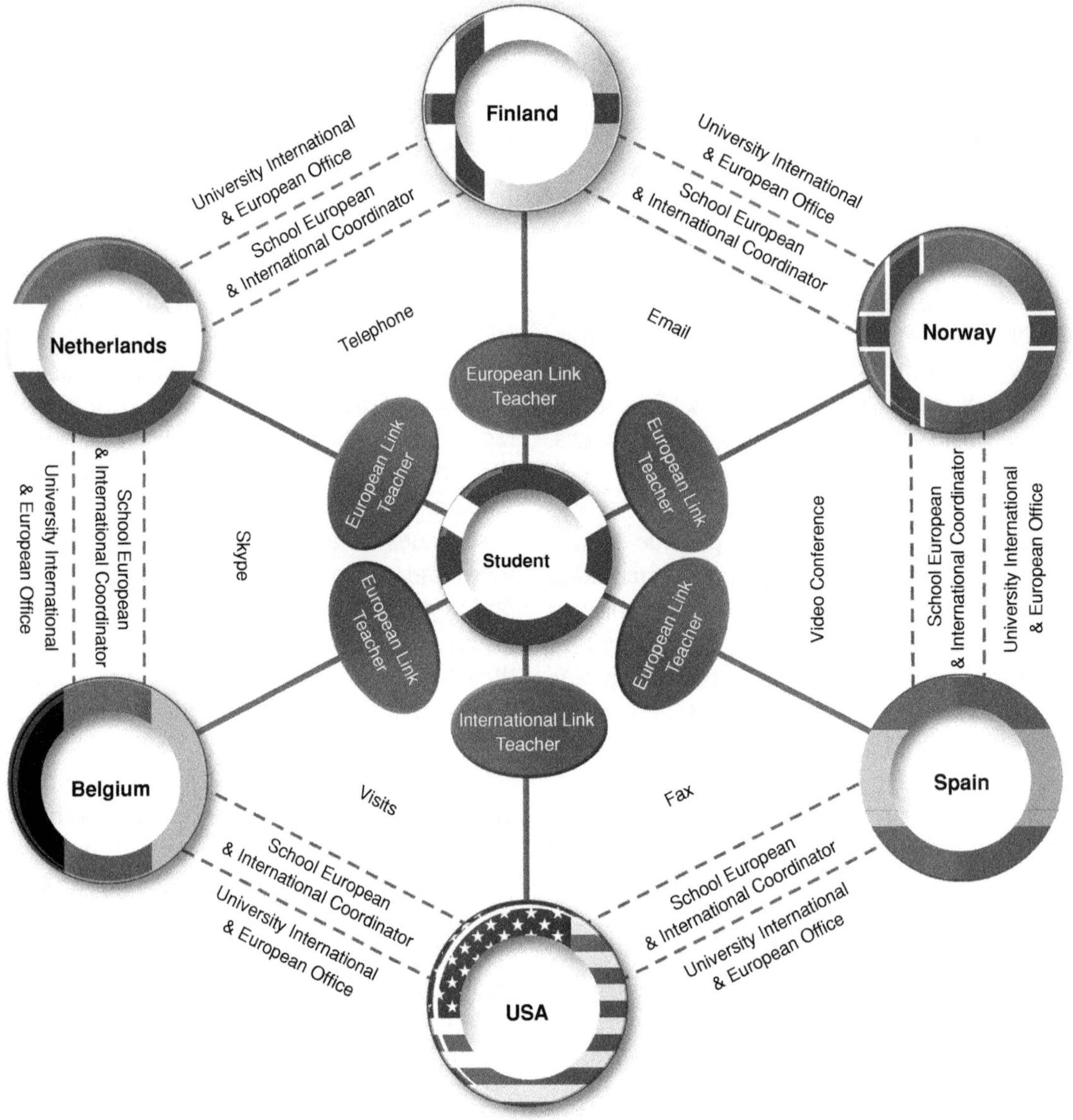

Figure 14.1 The support networks in place for students studying abroad

Table 14.2 provides you with some key considerations regarding general prerequisites for a learning abroad experience.

Understanding cultural contexts

In many countries across Europe, and in the USA, nurse education differs from that in the UK by being generic in principle with specialist options available following initial registration. In this respect it differs from the UK. Our exchange students often report that they were overwhelmed by the impact the different cultural contexts had on their own cultural views, but that this subsided as they adjusted to their new environment. Greatrex-White (2008: 537) makes reference to similar encounters experienced by the participants in her research and describes the process

Table 14.2 Key personal and professional prerequisites for a learning abroad experience

Insurances	**Health screening and immunizations**
• You will need to consider obtaining the professional liability insurance you require for clinical learning in Europe; make sure you are familiar with the insurance cover provided • You will need to consider obtaining the personal and professional liability insurance you require for clinical learning outside Europe (the host organization may be able to provide you with the details of insurance providers); make sure you are familiar with the insurance cover provided	• You will need to comply with the health screening requirements of the country you are visiting as well as the health care organization(s) providing you with clinical learning opportunities • Consult with your GP to determine if you require any vaccinations or other preventative measures prior to booking your trip
Criminal record status and protecting vulnerable groups	**Immigration rules and visa requirements**
• You may be required to provide evidence that you are safe to enter the country you plan to visit *and* to be able to access the health care organizations providing you with clinical learning opportunities. As this evidence is also required by the UK for you to be a student nurse, your university will be able to guide you through this process	• You will need to comply with the immigration rules and visa requirements of the country you will be visiting • Information is available via the internet and the international department (usually) at the host organization you are planning to visit, and your own university

as a 'disturbance that profoundly affects cultural perspectives'. Nevertheless, she seems to suggest that such a culture shock may be just what is required to develop culturally competent nurses. Wimpenny *et al.* (2005) also advocate the value of such personal confrontations to facilitate a greater awareness and understanding of the cultural values and practices influencing self and others, in order to prepare student nurses and RNs for work in an increasingly international workplace and multicultural society.

However, there are several key aspects to your preparation that will facilitate a good learning experience. **Table 14.3** highlights some key tips from a cultural, social, professional and personal perspective, suggested by our students and academic staff who have participated in learning opportunities abroad.

The future

The job market for graduates is predicted to become increasingly more international in the years to come. The CIHE (Diamond *et al.* 2011a) highlights that the business and industry sector already recruit from around the globe. Fielden *et al.* (2007) suggest that prospective employers want to recruit graduates who have experience of living and working in another culture or country, have an understanding of global issues, economies and cultures, and can manage complex international and intercultural relationships. Although Fielden *et al.* and the CIHE are discussing globalization and the international workforce in relation to business and industry, these concepts are also relevant to health professionals. Indeed, the current economic situation in some parts of the UK has led to limited job opportunities for nurses with a resultant increase in the migration of nurses to other parts of the UK or overseas. As with other professions, we believe that you as a nurse need to become more globally aware and to develop the attributes and competencies that not only reflect your graduate status but also demonstrate that you are truly a global citizen. Learning abroad

Table 14.3 Key tips for a learning abroad experience

Cultural	**Social**
• Learn the language of the country you will be visiting, especially the basics: please, thank you, good morning, etc. • Check the weather forecast so that you pack the clothes you will need • Find out the cost of food, etc. so you can budget appropriately • Make sure you know the full cost of your accommodation (you may need to buy bedding, crockery, electricity) • Find out bus fare/train costs and timetables • Know where to find the nearest food shop/24-hour supermarket • Identify the tourist attractions you want to see during your visit and build the costs into your budget • Know where the safe areas to visit are and where you should not go • Know what the time difference is and inform your friends and family • Be familiar with the laws and customs of the country you are visiting (e.g. you may be arrested in the USA for photographing federal buildings) • Know if the public transport systems are safe for you to use	• You can meet students from all over the world, so be prepared to embrace different cultures and learn as much as you can about others and yourself • You can make lifelong friendships with the people you meet because you are in a new situation and will need to build trusting relationships very quickly • Remember you are not on holiday. You will need to be independent and adventurous to pursue the social activities available during your visit • You may be unusually tired because of the adjustments you need to make to living and working in a new country, so planning your social activities is essential for maximum enjoyment • Always let someone know where you are
Personal	**Professional**
• Be open-minded • Don't worry about going on your own as you will soon learn to be confident and independent in a foreign country, but be wary of doing so at night • Be adventurous but stay safe • Check how best to access the internet and the costs involved • There will always be costs you didn't expect. Be prepared by saving more than you think you will need • Make sure friends and family know where you are and who to contact if unable to reach you • Register your visit with the British Embassy • Know how to access the police, the British Embassy, staff from host institutions and at home should you require any assistance • Ensure you have adequate medical and travel insurance (obtain the European Health Insurance Card, free online, for travel within Europe) • Don't book your flights until your learning abroad placement has been confirmed and all the paperwork has been approved (e.g. health screening, criminal record check) • Be mindful of customs regulations and baggage allowances	• Be prepared to clarify and negotiate your specific learning needs with your mentor abroad and to ensure there is a clear understanding about the completion of the documentation required for your nurse education programme • Be assertive and put yourself forward to learn as much as you can about nursing in another country • Remember, the patients are vulnerable and you are a professional student nurse • You will be amazed at how quickly you learn to communicate in different ways with patients and staff in another country • You will quickly learn to confidently speak the language spoken in the country you are visiting, if it is different to your own • Remember to access your own university for academic, professional and pastoral guidance if required • Finish all the coursework that you can prior to your visit to ensure maximum enjoyment of your learning abroad experience • Make sure you have access to any learning resources you require to support your learning abroad experience

experiences such as that offered by the ELLP and funded by the British Council enable you to realize your potential in the global job market in a safe learning environment. As noted earlier, the NMC recognizes the benefits of a learning abroad experience and has provided scope for student nurses to undertake a learning opportunity of up to six months outside the UK. In doing this it is acknowledging the forces of change and the need to educate and develop an internationally aware nursing workforce that is fit to work, lead and deliver health care in the globally diverse world of the future.

Conclusion

The opportunity to live, work and study overseas as part of your education provides an invaluable and life-changing experience that can be an asset to your personal and professional growth and which offers many benefits as you journey through life and a career in nursing. An overseas experience can add a new dimension to your education, taking your learning to a higher plane. You may learn about the *theory* underpinning concepts such as culture, politics, economics, injustice and inequity in the classroom, however, an overseas experience can synthesize this learning and make these subjects meaningful and relevant in so many ways within and outwith nursing. It is our belief that you as a student nurse will not only learn about the new culture and factors influencing health care and health care delivery in the overseas country, but that you will be able to reflect on your own culture and beliefs as well as the political influences that may impact on health, wellbeing and quality of life. The learning from such an experience is immense and difficult to fully articulate in words alone.

A note of caution: learning abroad experiences should not be embarked upon lightly. They require meticulous planning in order to ensure your safety, as well as that of patients and mentors. Furthermore, the actual learning environment needs to be audited to determine the suitability of the learning experiences and mentor support available for you as a student. In addition to this, practical issues such as vaccinations, health screening, visas and work permits, personal and professional indemnity, accommodation and living conditions, and in some instances the equivalent of the Protecting Vulnerable Groups Scheme, all need to be considered and addressed well in advance of any proposed learning abroad experience.

As the global economy evolves, technology advances and travelling becomes increasingly easier, the need for you as a nurse to develop global as well as graduate competence has never been so important. Opportunities for nurses to travel and work abroad are increasing and nurses, therefore, need to be culturally aware and tolerant as not only may they be working alongside colleagues from other nationalities, they will also be required to sensitively care for patients from other cultures, whether working in the UK or overseas. In addition to developing core graduate attributes, you as a student nurse will need to embrace the concept of global competence and demonstrate your leadership to become a fully fledged global citizen and international leader in nursing.

In summary:

- Learning abroad offers a unique opportunity to enhance your awareness of cultural competence as well as refine specific graduate attributes.
- Careful attention to planning both academically and practically is required to ensure a successful experience.
- Nursing is becoming an increasingly global profession and the future will hold opportunities for a more mobile workforce.

Further reading and resources

www.britishcouncil.org/erasmus-about-erasmus.htm. The webiste for the British Council.
http://uk.embassyhomepage.com. The website for the British Embassy, London.

http://bit.ly/wAISY. The website for the British Foreign and Commonwealth Office (FCO). There is a section here on travelling abroad and staying safe when doing so: www.fco.gov.uk/en/travel-and-living-abroad/staying-safe/. This contains a sub-section on health: http://www.fco.gov.uk/en/travel-and-living-abroad/staying-safe/health/.

www.lifelonglearningprogramme.org.uk/programme/erasmus. The website of the ELLP.

http://bit.ly/YIBzUC. Information on the European Health Insurance Card (EHIC).

https://estaapply.net/uk. Information on ESTA US business travel visa applications.

http://www.fnif.org/index.html. The International Council of Nurses (ICN).

http://bit.ly/Yfj25X. The National Union of Students (NUS).

www.oxfam.org.uk/education/gc/Oxfam. Information on global citizenship.

http://bit.ly/XGS96Z. The Quality Assurance Agency for Higher Education (graduate attributes).

http://bit.ly/14vqI7O. The website for Robert Gordon University School of Nursing and Midwifery.

www.rcn.org.uk/support/legal/indemnityscheme. Information from the RCN about professional indemnity exclusions (i.e. USA and Canada).

http://travel.state.gov/visa/visa_1750.html. Information from the United States Department of State (USDS) on US visa applications.

References

Bologna Process (European Higher Education Area) (2007) *European Higher Education in a Global Setting: A Strategy for the External Dimension of the Bologna Process*, available at: http://bit.ly/ZpRG8D.

British Council (2012) *Erasmus Programmes*, available at: http://www.britishcouncil.org/erasmus-programmes-content.htm.

CRE (Confederation of European Union Rectors' Conferences and the Association of European Universities) (2000) *The Bologna Declaration on the European Space for Higher Education: An Explanation*, available at: http://ec.europa.eu/education/policies/educ/bologna/bologna.pdf.

Diamond, A., Walkley, L., Forbes, P., Hughes, T. and Sheen, J. (2011a) *Global Graduated to Global Leaders*. London: The Council for Industry and Higher Education.

Diamond, A., Walkley, L. and Scott-Davies, S. (2011b) *Global Graduated to Global Leaders. Executive Summary*. London: The Council for Industry and Higher Education.

European Commission (2005) *Directive of the European Parliament and of the Council on the Recognition of Professional Qualifications*, available at: http://bit.ly/WW7bIN.

European Commission (2009a) *Green Paper: Promoting the Learning Mobility of Young People*, available at: http://bit.ly/YErr2k.

European Commission (2009b) *Standards and Guidelines for Quality Assurance in the European Higher Education Area*, 3rd edn, available at: http://bit.ly/11MzkCs.

European Commission (2010) *The Erasmus Programme: Studying in Europe and More*, available at: http://ec.europa.eu/education/lifelong-learning-programme/doc80_en.htm.

European Commission (2011a) *The Bologna Process: Towards the European Higher Education Area*, available at: http://ec.europa.eu/education/higher-education/doc1290_en.htm.

European Commission (2011b) *European Credit Transfer and Accumulation System (ECTS)*, available at: http://www.ec.europa.eu/education/lifelong-learning-policy/doc48_en.htm.

Fielden, J., Middlehurst, R. and Woodfield, S. (2007) *Global Horizons for UK Students: A Guide for Universities*. London: The Council for Industry and Higher Education.

GANES (Global Alliance for Leadership in Nursing Education and Science) (2011) *Investing in Nursing Education to Advance Global Health: A Position of the Global Alliance for Leadership in Nursing Education and Science*, available at: www.ganes.info/documents/GANESPositionFinal5.26.11.pdf.

Gobbi, M.(2005) *Tuning Educational Structures in Europe: Summary of Outcomes – Nursing*, available at: http://bit.ly/11M7mdL.

Greatrex-White, S. (2008) Uncovering study abroad: foreignness and its relevance to nurse education and cultural competence, *Nurse Education Today*, 28: 530–8.

Hounsell, D. (2011) *Graduates for the 21st Century: Integrating the Enhancement Themes. Institutional Activities*. Glasgow: The Quality Assurance Agency for Higher Education.

Kokko, R. (2011) Future nurses' cultural competencies: what are their learning experiences during exchange and studies abroad? A systematic literature review, *Journal of Nursing Management,* 19: 673–82.

Lee, N.J. (2004) The impact of international experience on student nurses' personal and professional development, *International Nursing Review*, 51: 113–22.

Lee, R.L.T., Pang, S.M.C., Wong, T.K.S. and Chan, M.F. (2007) Evaluation of an innovative nursing exchange programme: health counseling skills and cultural awareness, *Nurse Education Today*, 27: 868–77.

Leininger, M. (2002) Cultural care theory: a major contribution to advance transcultural nursing knowledge and practices, *Journal of Transcultural Nursing*, 13: 189–92.

NMC (Nursing and Midwifery Council) (2010) *Standards for Pre-registration Nursing Education*. London: NMC.

Oxfam (2006) *Education for Global Citizenship: A Guide for Schools.* London: Oxfam Development Education Programme.

Papadopoulos, I., Tilki, M. and Lees, S. (2004) Promoting cultural competence in healthcare through a research-based intervention in the UK, *Diversity in Health and Social Care*, 1: 107–15.

RCN (Royal College of Nursing) (2012) Student membership, available at: www.rcn.org.uk/membership/student_member.

Scottish Government (2011) Protecting Vulnerable Groups Scheme, available at: http://www.scotland.gov.uk/Topics/People/Young-People/children-families/pvglegislation.

Siantz, M.L.D. and Meleis, A.F. (2007) Integrating cultural competence into nursing education and practice: 21st century action steps, *Journal of Transcultural Nursing*, 18: S86–90.

Wimpenny, P., Gault, B., MacLennan, V., Boast-Bowen, L. and Shepherd, P. (2005) Teaching and learning about culture: a European journey, *Nurse Education Today*, 25: 398–404.

WHO (World Health Organization) (2009) *Global Standards for the Initial Education of Professional Nurses and Midwives*. Geneva: WHO, available at: http://bit.ly/15UAooh.

Domains Appendix

NMC Competencies for entry to the register: Adult nursing

Domain 1: Professional values

Generic standard for competence

All nurses must act first and foremost to care for and safeguard the public. They must practise autonomously and be responsible and accountable for safe, compassionate, person-centred, evidence-based nursing that respects and maintains dignity and human rights. They must show professionalism and integrity and work within recognised professional, ethical and legal frameworks. They must work in partnership with other health and social care professionals and agencies, service users, their carers and families in all settings, including the community, ensuring that decisions about care are shared.

Field standard for competence

Adult nurses must also be able at all times to promote the rights, choices and wishes of all adults and, where appropriate, children and young people, paying particular attention to equality, diversity and the needs of an ageing population. They must be able to work in partnership to address people's needs in all healthcare settings.

Competencies

1 All nurses must practise with confidence according to *The code: Standards of conduct, performance and ethics for nurses and midwives* (NMC 2008), and within other recognised ethical and legal frameworks. They must be able to recognize and address ethical challenges relating to people's choices and decision-making about their care, and act within the law to help them and their families and carers find acceptable solutions.

    1.1 **Adult nurses** must understand and apply current legislation to all service users, paying special attention to the protection of vulnerable people, including those with complex needs arising from ageing, cognitive impairment, long-term conditions and those approaching the end of life.

2 All nurses must practise in a holistic, non-judgmental, caring and sensitive manner that avoids assumptions, supports social inclusion; recognises and respects individual choice; and acknowledges diversity. Where necessary, they must challenge inequality, discrimination and exclusion from access to care.

3 All nurses must support and promote the health, wellbeing, rights and dignity of people, groups, communities and populations. These include people whose lives are affected by ill health, disability, ageing, death and dying. Nurses must understand how these activities influence public health.

4 All nurses must work in partnership with service users, carers, families, groups, communities and organisations. They must manage risk, and promote health and wellbeing while aiming to empower choices that promote self-care and safety.

5 All nurses must fully understand the nurse's various roles, responsibilities and functions, and adapt their practice to meet the changing needs of people, groups, communities and populations.

6 All nurses must understand the roles and responsibilities of other health and social care professionals, and seek to work with them collaboratively for the benefit of all who need care.

7 All nurses must be responsible and accountable for keeping their knowledge and skills up to date through continuing professional development. They must aim to improve their performance and enhance the safety and quality of care through evaluation, supervision and appraisal.

8 All nurses must practise independently, recognising the limits of their competence and knowledge. They must reflect on these limits and seek advice from, or refer to, other professionals where necessary.

9 All nurses must appreciate the value of evidence in practice, be able to understand and appraise research, apply relevant theory and research findings to their work, and identify areas for further investigation.

 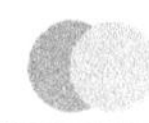

Domain 2: Communication and interpersonal skills

Generic standard for competence

All nurses must use excellent communication and interpersonal skills. Their communications must always be safe, effective, compassionate and respectful. They must communicate effectively using a wide range of strategies and interventions including the effective use of communication technologies. Where people have a disability, nurses must be able to work with service users and others to obtain the information needed to make reasonable adjustments that promote optimum health and enable equal access to services.

Field standard for competence

Adult nurses must demonstrate the ability to listen with empathy. They must be able to respond warmly and positively to people of all ages who may be anxious, distressed, or facing problems with their health and wellbeing.

Competencies

1 All nurses must build partnerships and therapeutic relationships through safe, effective and non-discriminatory communication. They must take account of individual differences, capabilities and needs.

2 All nurses must use a range of communication skills and technologies to support person-centred care and enhance quality and safety. They must ensure people receive all the information they need in a language and manner that allows them to make informed choices and share decision making. They must recognise when language interpretation or other communication support is needed and know how to obtain it.

3 All nurses must use the full range of communication methods, including verbal, non-verbal and written, to acquire, interpret and record their knowledge and understanding of people's needs. They must be aware of their own values and beliefs and the impact this may have on their communication with others. They must take account of the many different ways in which people communicate and how these may be influenced by ill health, disability and other factors, and be able to recognise and respond effectively when a person finds it hard to communicate.

 3.1 **Adult nurses** must promote the concept, knowledge and practice of self-care with people with acute and long-term conditions, using a range of communication skills and strategies.

4 All nurses must recognise when people are anxious or in distress and respond effectively, using therapeutic principles, to promote their wellbeing, manage personal safety and resolve conflict. They must use effective communication strategies and negotiation techniques to achieve best outcomes, respecting the dignity and human rights of all concerned. They must know when to consult a third party and how to make referrals for advocacy, mediation or arbitration.

5 All nurses must use therapeutic principles to engage, maintain and, where appropriate, disengage from professional caring relationships, and must always respect professional boundaries.

6 All nurses must take every opportunity to encourage health-promoting behaviour through education, role modelling and effective communication.

7 All nurses must maintain accurate, clear and complete records, including the use of electronic formats, using appropriate and plain language.

8 All nurses must respect individual rights to confidentiality and keep information secure and confidential in accordance with the law and relevant ethical and regulatory frameworks, taking account of local protocols. They must also actively share personal information with others when the interests of safety and protection override the need for confidentiality.

 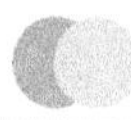

Domain 3: Nursing practice and decision-making

Generic standard for competence

All nurses must practise autonomously, compassionately, skilfully and safely, and must maintain dignity and promote health and wellbeing. They must assess and meet the full range of essential physical and mental health needs of people of all ages who come into their care. Where necessary they must be able to provide safe and effective immediate care to all people prior to accessing or referring to specialist services irrespective of their field of practice. All nurses must also meet more complex and coexisting needs for people in their own nursing field of practice, in any setting including hospital, community and at home. All practice should be informed by the best available evidence and comply with local and national guidelines. Decision-making must be shared with service users, carers and families and informed by critical analysis of a full range of possible interventions, including the use of up-to-date technology. All nurses must also understand how behaviour, culture, socioeconomic and other factors, in the care environment and its location, can affect health, illness, health outcomes and public health priorities and take this into account in planning and delivering care.

Field standard for competence

Adult nurses must be able to carry out accurate assessment of people of all ages using appropriate diagnostic and decision-making skills. They must be able to provide effective care for service users and others in all settings. They must have in-depth understanding of and competence in medical and surgical nursing to respond to adults' full range of health and dependency needs. They must be able to deliver care to meet essential and complex physical and mental health needs.

Competencies

1 All nurses must use up-to-date knowledge and evidence to assess, plan, deliver and evaluate care, communicate findings, influence change and promote health and best practice. They must make person-centred, evidence-based judgments and decisions, in partnership with others involved in the care process, to ensure high quality care. They must be able to recognise when the complexity of clinical decisions requires specialist knowledge and expertise, and consult or refer accordingly.

1.1 **Adult nurses** must be able to recognise and respond to the needs of all people who come into their care including babies, children and young people, pregnant and postnatal women, people with mental health problems, people with physical disabilities, people with learning disabilities, older people, and people with long term problems such as cognitive impairment.

2 All nurses must possess a broad knowledge of the structure and functions of the human body, and other relevant knowledge from the life, behavioural and social sciences as applied to health, ill health, disability, ageing and death. They must have an in-depth knowledge of common physical and mental health problems and treatments in their own field of practice, including co-morbidity and physiological and psychological vulnerability.

3 All nurses must carry out comprehensive, systematic nursing assessments that take account of relevant physical, social, cultural, psychological, spiritual, genetic and environmental factors, in partnership with service users and others through interaction, observation and measurement.

3.1 **Adult nurses** must safely use a range of diagnostic skills, employing appropriate technology, to assess the needs of service users.

4 All nurses must ascertain and respond to the physical, social and psychological needs of people, groups and communities. They must then plan, deliver and evaluate safe, competent, person-centred care in partnership with them, paying special attention to changing health needs during different life stages, including progressive illness and death, loss and bereavement.

4.1 **Adult nurses** must safely use invasive and non-invasive procedures, medical devices, and current technological and pharmacological interventions, where relevant, in medical and surgical nursing practice, providing information and taking account of individual needs and preferences.

4.2 **Adult nurses** must recognise and respond to the changing needs of adults, families and carers during terminal illness. They must be aware of how treatment goals and service users' choices may change at different stages of progressive illness, loss and bereavement.

5 All nurses must understand public health principles, priorities and practice in order to recognise and respond to the major causes and social determinants of health, illness and health inequalities. They must use a range of information and data to assess the needs of people, groups, communities and populations, and work to improve health, wellbeing and experiences of healthcare; secure equal access to health screening, health promotion and healthcare; and promote social inclusion.

6 All nurses must practise safely by being aware of the correct use, limitations and hazards of common interventions, including nursing activities, treatments, and the use of medical devices and equipment. The nurse must be able to evaluate their use, report any concerns promptly through appropriate channels and modify care where necessary to maintain safety. They must contribute to the collection of local and national data and formulation of policy on risks, hazards and adverse outcomes.

7 All nurses must be able to recognise and interpret signs of normal and deteriorating mental and physical health and respond promptly to maintain or improve the health and comfort of the service user, acting to keep them and others safe.

7.1 **Adult nurses** must recognise the early signs of illness in people of all ages. They must make accurate assessments and start appropriate and timely management of those who are acutely ill, at risk of clinical deterioration, or require emergency care.

7.2 **Adult nurses** must understand the normal physiological and psychological processes of pregnancy and childbirth. They must work with the midwife and other professionals and agencies to provide basic nursing care to pregnant women and families during pregnancy and after childbirth. They must be able to respond safely and effectively in an emergency to safeguard the health of mother and baby.

8 All nurses must provide educational support, facilitation skills and therapeutic nursing interventions to optimise health and wellbeing. They must promote self-care and management whenever possible, helping people to make choices about their healthcare needs, involving families and carers where appropriate, to maximise their ability to care for themselves.

8.1 **Adult nurses** must work in partnership with people who have long-term conditions that require medical or surgical nursing, and their families and carers, to provide therapeutic nursing interventions, optimise health and wellbeing, facilitate choice and maximise self-care and self-management.

9 All nurses must be able to recognise when a person is at risk and in need of extra support and protection and take reasonable steps to protect them from abuse.

10 All nurses must evaluate their care to improve clinical decision-making, quality and outcomes, using a range of methods, amending the plan of care, where necessary, and communicating changes to others.

Domain 4: Leadership, management and team working

Generic standard for competence

All nurses must be professionally accountable and use clinical governance processes to maintain and improve nursing practice and standards of healthcare. They must be able to respond autonomously and confidently to planned and uncertain situations, managing themselves and others effectively. They must create and maximise opportunities to improve services. They must also demonstrate the potential to develop further management and leadership skills during their period of preceptorship and beyond.

Field standard for competence

Adult nurses must be able to provide leadership in managing adult nursing care, understand and coordinate interprofessional care when needed, and liaise with specialist teams. They must be adaptable and flexible, and able to take the lead in responding to the needs of people of all ages in a variety of circumstances, including situations where immediate or urgent care is needed. They must recognise their leadership role in disaster management, major incidents and public health emergencies, and respond appropriately according to their levels of competence.

Competencies

1 All nurses must act as change agents and provide leadership through quality improvement and service development to enhance people's wellbeing and experiences of healthcare.

2 All nurses must systematically evaluate care and ensure that they and others use the findings to help improve people's experience and care outcomes and to shape future services.

3 All nurses must be able to identify priorities and manage time and resources effectively to ensure the quality of care is maintained or enhanced.

4 All nurses must be self-aware and recognise how their own values, principles and assumptions may affect their practice. They must maintain their own personal and professional development, learning from experience, through supervision, feedback, reflection and evaluation.

5 All nurses must facilitate nursing students and others to develop their competence, using a range of professional and personal development skills.

6 All nurses must work independently as well as in teams. They must be able to take the lead in coordinating, delegating and supervising care safely, managing risk and remaining accountable for the care given.

7 All nurses must work effectively across professional and agency boundaries, actively involving and respecting others' contributions to integrated person-centred care. They must know when and how to communicate with and refer to other professionals and agencies in order to respect the choices of service users and others, promoting shared decision making, to deliver positive outcomes and to coordinate smooth, effective transition within and between services and agencies.

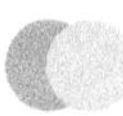

Competencies for entry to the register: Mental health nursing

Domain 1: Professional values

Generic standard for competence

All nurses must act first and foremost to care for and safeguard the public. They must practise autonomously and be responsible and accountable for safe, compassionate, person-centred, evidence-based nursing that respects and maintains dignity and human rights. They must show professionalism and integrity and work within recognised professional, ethical and legal frameworks. They must work in partnership with other health and social care professionals and agencies, service users, their carers and families in all settings, including the community, ensuring that decisions about care are shared.

Field standard for competence

Mental health nurses must work with people of all ages using values-based mental health frameworks. They must use different methods of engaging people, and work in a way that promotes positive relationships focused on social inclusion, human rights and recovery, that is, a person's ability to live a self-directed life, with or without symptoms, that they believe is meaningful and satisfying.

Competencies

1 All nurses must practise with confidence according to *The code: Standards of conduct, performance and ethics for nurses and midwives* (NMC 2008), and within other recognised ethical and legal frameworks. They must be able to recognize and address ethical challenges relating to people's choices and decision-making about their care, and act within the law to help them and their families and carers find acceptable solutions.

1.1 **Mental health nurses** must understand and apply current legislation to all service users, paying special attention to the protection of vulnerable people, including those with complex needs arising from ageing, cognitive impairment, long-term conditions and those approaching the end of life.

2 All nurses must practise in a holistic, non-judgmental, caring and sensitive manner that avoids assumptions, supports social inclusion; recognises and respects individual choice; and acknowledges diversity. Where necessary, they must challenge inequality, discrimination and exclusion from access to care.

2.1 **Mental health nurses** must practise in a way that addresses the potential power imbalances between professionals and people experiencing mental health problems, including situations when compulsory measures are used, by helping people exercise their rights, upholding safeguards and ensuring minimal restrictions on their lives. They must have an in depth understanding of mental health legislation and how it relates to care and treatment of people with mental health problems.

3 All nurses must support and promote the health, wellbeing, rights and dignity of people, groups, communities and populations. These include people whose lives are affected by ill health, disability, inability to engage, ageing or death. Nurses must act on their understanding of how these conditions influence public health.

3.1 **Mental health nurses** must promote mental health and wellbeing, while challenging the inequalities and discrimination that may arise from or contribute to mental health problems.

4 All nurses must work in partnership with service users, carers, groups, communities and organisations. They must manage risk, and promote health and wellbeing while aiming to empower choices that promote self-care and safety.

4.1 **Mental health nurses** must work with people in a way that values, respects and explores the meaning of their individual lived experiences of mental health problems, to provide person-centred and recovery-focused practice.

5 All nurses must fully understand the nurse's various roles, responsibilities and functions, and adapt their practice to meet the changing needs of people, groups, communities and populations.

6 All nurses must understand the roles and responsibilities of other health and social care professionals, and seek to work with them collaboratively for the benefit of all who need care.

7 All nurses must be responsible and accountable for keeping their knowledge and skills up to date through continuing professional development. They must aim to improve their performance and enhance the safety and quality of care through evaluation, supervision and appraisal.

8 All nurses must practise independently, recognising the limits of their competence and knowledge. They must reflect on these limits and seek advice from, or refer to, other professionals where necessary.

8.1 **Mental health nurses** must have and value an awareness of their own mental health and wellbeing. They must also engage in reflection and supervision to explore the emotional impact on self of working in mental health; how personal values, beliefs and emotions impact on practice, and how their own practice aligns with mental health legislation, policy and values-based frameworks.

9 All nurses must appreciate the value of evidence in practice, be able to understand and appraise research, apply relevant theory and research findings to their work, and identify areas for further investigation.

 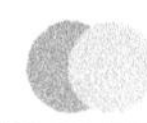

Domain 2: Communication and interpersonal skills

Generic standard for competence

All nurses must use excellent communication and interpersonal skills. Their communications must always be safe, effective, compassionate and respectful. They must communicate effectively using a wide range of strategies and interventions including the effective use of communication technologies. Where people have a disability, nurses must be able to work with service users and others to obtain the information needed to make reasonable adjustments that promote optimum health and enable equal access to services,

Field standard for competence

Mental health nurses must practise in a way that focuses on the therapeutic use of self. They must draw on a range of methods of engaging with people of all ages experiencing mental health problems, and those important to them, to develop and maintain therapeutic relationships. They must work alongside people, using a range of interpersonal approaches and skills to help them explore and make sense of their experiences in a way that promotes recovery.

Competencies

1 All nurses must build partnerships and therapeutic relationships through safe, effective and non-discriminatory communication. They must take account of individual differences, capabilities and needs.

    1.1 **Mental health nurses** must use skills of relationship-building and communication to engage with and support people distressed by hearing voices, experiencing distressing thoughts or experiencing other perceptual problems.

    1.2 **Mental health nurses** must use skills and knowledge to facilitate therapeutic groups with people experiencing mental health problems and their families and carers.

2 All nurses must use a range of communication skills and technologies to support person-centred care and enhance quality and safety. They must ensure people receive all the information they need in a language and manner that allows them to make informed choices and share decision making. They must recognise when language interpretation or other communication support is needed and know how to obtain it.

3 All nurses must use the full range of communication methods, including verbal, non-verbal and written, to acquire, interpret and record their knowledge and understanding of people's needs. They must be aware of their own values and beliefs and the impact this may have on their communication with others. They must take account of the many different ways in which people communicate and how these may be influenced by ill health, disability and other factors, and be able to recognise and respond effectively when a person finds it hard to communicate.

4 All nurses must recognise when people are anxious or in distress and respond effectively, using therapeutic principles, to promote their wellbeing, manage personal safety and resolve conflict. They must use effective communication strategies and negotiation techniques to achieve best outcomes, respecting the dignity and human rights of all concerned. They must know when to consult a third party and how to make referrals for advocacy, mediation or arbitration.

    4.1 **Mental health nurses** must be sensitive to, and take account of, the impact of abuse and trauma on people's wellbeing and the development of mental health problems. They must use interpersonal skills and make interventions that help people disclose and discuss their experiences as part of their recovery.

5 All nurses must use therapeutic principles to engage, maintain and, where appropriate, disengage from professional caring relationships, and must always respect professional boundaries.

5.1 **Mental health nurses** must use their personal qualities, experiences and interpersonal skills to develop and maintain therapeutic, recovery-focused relationships with people and therapeutic groups. They must be aware of their own mental health, and know when to share aspects of their own life to inspire hope while maintaining professional boundaries.

6 All nurses must take every opportunity to encourage health-promoting behaviour through education, role modelling and effective communication.

6.1 **Mental health nurses** must foster helpful and enabling relationships with families, carers and other people important to the person experiencing mental health problems. They must use communication skills that enable psychosocial education, problem-solving and other interventions to help people cope and to safeguard those who are vulnerable.

7 All nurses must maintain accurate, clear and complete records, including the use of electronic formats, using appropriate and plain language.

8 All nurses must respect individual rights to confidentiality and keep information secure and confidential in accordance with the law and relevant ethical and regulatory frameworks, taking account of local protocols. They must also actively share personal information with others when the interests of safety and protection override the need for confidentiality.

Domain 3: Nursing practice and decision-making

Generic standard for competence

All nurses must practise autonomously, compassionately, skilfully and safely, and must maintain dignity and promote health and wellbeing. They must assess and meet the full range of essential physical and mental health needs of people of all ages who come into their care. Where necessary they must be able to provide safe and effective immediate care to all people prior to accessing or referring to specialist services irrespective of their field of practice. All nurses must also meet more complex and coexisting needs for people in their own nursing field of practice, in any setting including hospital, community and at home. All practice should be informed by the best available evidence and comply with local and national guidelines. Decision-making must be shared with service users, carers and families and informed by critical analysis of a full range of possible interventions, including the use of up-to-date technology. All nurses must also understand how behaviour, culture, socioeconomic and other factors, in the care environment and its location, can affect health, illness, health outcomes and public health priorities and take this into account in planning and delivering care.

Field standard for competence

Mental health nurses must draw on a range of evidence-based psychological, psychosocial and other complex therapeutic skills and interventions to provide person-centred support and care across all ages, in a way that supports self-determination and aids recovery. They must also promote improvements in physical and mental health and wellbeing and provide direct care to meet both the essential and complex physical and mental health needs of people with mental health problems.

Competencies

1 All nurses must use up-to-date knowledge and evidence to assess, plan, deliver and evaluate care, communicate findings, influence change and promote health and best practice. They must make person-centred, evidence-based judgments and decisions, in partnership with others involved in the care process, to ensure high quality care. They must be able to recognise when the complexity of clinical decisions requires specialist knowledge and expertise, and consult or refer accordingly.

1.1 **Mental health nurses** must be able to recognise and respond to the needs of all people who come into their care including babies, children and young people, pregnant and postnatal women, people with physical health problems, people with physical disabilities, people with learning disabilities, older people, and people with long term problems such as cognitive impairment.

2 All nurses must possess a broad knowledge of the structure and functions of the human body, and other relevant knowledge from the life, behavioral and social sciences as applied to health, ill health, disability, ageing and death. They must have an in-depth knowledge of common physical and mental health problems and treatments in their own field of practice, including co-morbidity and physiological and psychological vulnerability.

3 All nurses must carry out comprehensive, systematic nursing assessments that take account of relevant physical, social, cultural, psychological, spiritual, genetic and environmental factors, in partnership with service users and others through interaction, observation and measurement.

3.1 **Mental health nurses** must be able to apply their knowledge and skills in a range of evidence-based individual and group psychological and psychosocial interventions, to carry out systematic needs assessments, develop case formulations and negotiate goals.

4 All nurses must ascertain and respond to the physical, social and psychological needs of people, groups and communities. They must then plan, deliver and evaluate safe, competent, person-centred care in partnership with them, paying special attention to changing health needs during different life stages, including progressive illness and death, loss and bereavement.

4.1 **Mental health nurses** must be able to apply their knowledge and skills in a range of evidence-based psychological and psychosocial individual and group interventions to develop and implement care plans and evaluate outcomes, in partnership with service users and others.

5 All nurses must understand public health principles, priorities and practice in order to recognise and respond to the major causes and social determinants of health, illness and health inequalities. They must use a range of information and data to assess the needs of people, groups, communities and populations, and work to improve health, wellbeing and experiences of healthcare; secure equal access to health screening, health promotion and healthcare; and promote social inclusion.

5.1 **Mental health nurses** must work to promote mental health, help prevent mental health problems in at-risk groups, and enhance the health and wellbeing of people with mental health problems.

6 All nurses must practise safely by being aware of the correct use, limitations and hazards of common interventions, including nursing activities, treatments, and the use of medical devices and equipment. The nurse must be able to evaluate their use, report any concerns promptly through appropriate channels and modify care where necessary to maintain safety. They must contribute to the collection of local and national data and formulation of policy on risks, hazards and adverse outcomes.

6.1 **Mental health nurses** must help people experiencing mental health problems to make informed choices about pharmacological and physical treatments, by providing education and information on the benefits and unwanted effects, choices and alternatives. They must support people to identify actions that promote health and help to balance benefits and unwanted effects.

7 All nurses must be able to recognise and interpret signs of normal and deteriorating mental and physical health and respond promptly to maintain or improve the health and comfort of the service user, acting to keep them and others safe.

7.1 **Mental health nurses** must provide support and therapeutic interventions for people experiencing critical and acute mental health problems. They must recognise the health and social factors that can contribute to crisis and relapse and use skills in early intervention, crisis resolution and relapse management in a way that ensures safety and security and promotes recovery.

7.2 **Mental health nurses** must work positively and proactively with people who are at risk of suicide or self-harm, and use evidence-based models of suicide prevention, intervention and harm reduction to minimise risk.

8 All nurses must provide educational support, facilitation skills and therapeutic nursing interventions to optimise health and wellbeing. They must promote self-care and management whenever possible, helping people to make choices about their healthcare needs, involving families and carers where appropriate, to maximise their ability to care for themselves.

8.1 **Mental health nurses** must practise in a way that promotes the self-determination and expertise of people with mental health problems, using a range of approaches and tools that aid wellness and recovery and enable self-care and self-management.

9 All nurses must be able to recognise when a person is at risk and in need of extra support and protection and take reasonable steps to protect them from abuse.

9.1 **Mental health nurses** must use recovery-focused approaches to care in situations that are potentially challenging, such as times of acute distress; when compulsory measures are used; and in forensic mental health settings. They must seek to maximise service user involvement and therapeutic engagement, using interventions that balance the need for safety with positive risk-taking.

10 All nurses must evaluate their care to improve clinical decision-making, quality and outcomes, using a range of methods, amending the plan of care, where necessary, and communicating changes to others.

Domain 4: Leadership, management and team working

Generic standard for competence

All nurses must be professionally accountable and use clinical governance processes to maintain and improve nursing practice and standards of healthcare. They must be able to respond autonomously and confidently to planned and uncertain situations, managing themselves and others effectively. They must create and maximise opportunities to improve services. They must also demonstrate the potential to develop further management and leadership skills during their period of preceptorship and beyond.

Field standard for competence

Mental health nurses must contribute to the leadership, management and design of mental health services. They must work with service users, carers, other professionals and agencies to shape future services, aid recovery and challenge discrimination and inequality.

Competencies

1 All nurses must act as change agents and provide leadership through quality improvement and service development to enhance people's wellbeing and experiences of healthcare.

2 All nurses must systematically evaluate care and ensure that they and others use the findings to help improve people's experience and care outcomes and to shape future services.

3 All nurses must be able to identify priorities and manage time and resources effectively to ensure the quality of care is maintained or enhanced.

4 All nurses must be self-aware and recognise how their own values, principles and assumptions may affect their practice. They must maintain their own personal and professional development, learning from experience, through supervision, feedback, reflection and evaluation.

4.1 **Mental health nurses** must actively promote and participate in clinical supervision and reflection, within a values-based mental health framework, to explore how their values, beliefs and emotions affect their leadership, management and practice.

5 All nurses must facilitate nursing students and others to develop their competence, using a range of professional and personal development skills.

5.1 **Mental health nurses** must help raise awareness of mental health, and provide advice and support in best practice in mental health care and treatment to members of the multiprofessional team and others working in health, social care and other services and settings.

6 All nurses must work independently as well as in teams. They must be able to take the lead in coordinating, delegating and supervising care safely, managing risk and remaining accountable for the care given.

6.1 **Mental health nurses** must contribute to the management of mental health care environments by giving priority to actions that enhance people's safety, psychological security and therapeutic outcomes, and by ensuring effective communication, positive risk management and continuity of care across service boundaries.

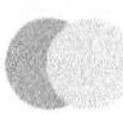

7 All nurses must work effectively across professional and agency boundaries, actively involving and respecting others' contributions to integrated person-centred care. They must know when and how to communicate with and refer to other professionals and agencies in order to respect the choices of service users and others, promoting shared decision making, to deliver positive outcomes and to coordinate smooth, effective transition within and between services and agencies.

Competencies for entry to the register: Learning disabilities nursing

Domain 1: Professional values

Generic standard for competence

All nurses must act first and foremost to care for and safeguard the public. They must practise autonomously and be responsible and accountable for safe, compassionate, person-centred, evidence-based nursing that respects and maintains dignity and human rights. They must show professionalism and integrity and work within recognised professional, ethical and legal frameworks. They must work in partnership with other health and social care professionals and agencies, service users, their carers and families in all settings, including the community, ensuring that decisions about care are shared.

Field standard for competence

Learning disabilities nurses must promote the individuality, independence, rights, choice and social inclusion of people with learning disabilities and highlight their strengths and abilities at all times while encouraging others do the same. They must facilitate the active participation of families and carers.

Competencies

1 All nurses must practise with confidence according to *The code: Standards of conduct, performance and ethics for nurses and midwives* (NMC 2008), and within other recognised ethical and legal frameworks. They must be able to recognize and address ethical challenges relating to people's choices and decision-making about their care, and act within the law to help them and their families and carers find acceptable solutions.

1.1 **Learning disabilities nurses** must understand and apply current legislation to all service users, paying special attention to the protection of vulnerable people, including those with complex needs arising from ageing, cognitive impairment, long-term conditions and those approaching the end of life.

2 All nurses must practise in a holistic, non-judgmental, caring and sensitive manner that avoids assumptions, supports social inclusion; recognises and respects individual choice; and acknowledges diversity. Where necessary, they must challenge inequality, discrimination and exclusion from access to care.

2.1 **Learning disabilities nurses** must always promote the autonomy, rights and choices of people with learning disabilities and support and involve their families and carers, ensuring that each person's rights are upheld according to policy and the law.

3 All nurses must support and promote the health, wellbeing, rights and dignity of people, groups, communities and populations. These include people whose lives are affected by ill health, disability, inability to engage, ageing or death. Nurses must act on their understanding of how these conditions influence public health.

3.1 **Learning disabilities nurses** must use their knowledge and skills to exercise professional advocacy, and recognise when it is appropriate to refer to independent advocacy services to safeguard dignity and human rights.

4 All nurses must work in partnership with service users, carers, groups, communities and organisations. They must manage risk, and promote health and wellbeing while aiming to empower choices that promote self-care and safety.

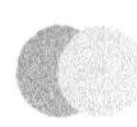

4.1 **Learning disabilities nurses** must recognise that people with learning disabilities are full and equal citizens, and must promote their health and wellbeing by focusing on and developing their strengths and abilities.

5 All nurses must fully understand the nurse's various roles, responsibilities and functions, and adapt their practice to meet the changing needs of people, groups, communities and populations.

6 All nurses must understand the roles and responsibilities of other health and social care professionals, and seek to work with them collaboratively for the benefit of all who need care.

7 All nurses must be responsible and accountable for keeping their knowledge and skills up to date through continuing professional development. They must aim to improve their performance and enhance the safety and quality of care through evaluation, supervision and appraisal.

8 All nurses must practise independently, recognising the limits of their competence and knowledge. They must reflect on these limits and seek advice from, or refer to, other professionals where necessary.

9 All nurses must appreciate the value of evidence in practice, be able to understand and appraise research, apply relevant theory and research findings to their work, and identify areas for further investigation.

Domain 2: Communication and interpersonal skills

Generic standard for competence
All nurses must use excellent communication and interpersonal skills. Their communications must always be safe, effective, compassionate and respectful. They must communicate effectively using a wide range of strategies and interventions including the effective use of communication technologies. Where people have a disability, nurses must be able to work with service users and others to obtain the information needed to make reasonable adjustments that promote optimum health and enable equal access to services,

Field standard for competence
Learning disabilities nurses must use complex communication and interpersonal skills and strategies to work with people of all ages who have learning disabilities and help them to express themselves. They must also be able to communicate and negotiate effectively with other professionals, services and agencies, and ensure that people with learning disabilities, their families and carers, are fully involved in decision-making.

Competencies

1 All nurses must build partnerships and therapeutic relationships through safe, effective and non-discriminatory communication. They must take account of individual differences, capabilities and needs.

1.1 **Learning disabilities nurses** must use the full range of person-centred alternative and augmentative communication strategies and skills to build partnerships and therapeutic relationships with people with learning disabilities.

2 All nurses must use a range of communication skills and technologies to support person-centred care and enhance quality and safety. They must ensure people receive all the information they need in a language and manner that allows them to make informed choices and share decision making. They must recognise when language interpretation or other communication support is needed and know how to obtain it.

2.1 **Learning disabilities nurses** must be able to make all relevant information accessible to and understandable by people with learning disabilities, including adaptation of format, presentation and delivery.

3 All nurses must use the full range of communication methods, including verbal, non-verbal and written, to acquire, interpret and record their knowledge and understanding of people's needs. They must be aware of their own values and beliefs and the impact this may have on their communication with others. They must take account of the many different ways in which people communicate and how these may be influenced by ill health, disability and other factors, and be able to recognise and respond effectively when a person finds it hard to communicate.

3.1 **Learning disabilities nurses** must use a structured approach to assess, communicate with, interpret and respond therapeutically to people with learning disabilities who have complex physical and psychological health needs or those in behavioural distress.

4 All nurses must recognise when people are anxious or in distress and respond effectively, using therapeutic principles, to promote their wellbeing, manage personal safety and resolve conflict. They must use effective communication strategies and negotiation techniques to achieve best

outcomes, respecting the dignity and human rights of all concerned. They must know when to consult a third party and how to make referrals for advocacy, mediation or arbitration.

4.1 **Learning disabilities nurses** must recognise and respond therapeutically to the complex behaviour that people with learning disabilities may use as a means of communication.

5 All nurses must use therapeutic principles to engage, maintain and, where appropriate, disengage from professional caring relationships, and must always respect professional boundaries.

6 All nurses must take every opportunity to encourage health-promoting behaviour through education, role modelling and effective communication.

7 All nurses must maintain accurate, clear and complete records, including the use of electronic formats, using appropriate and plain language.

8 All nurses must respect individual rights to confidentiality and keep information secure and confidential in accordance with the law and relevant ethical and regulatory frameworks, taking account of local protocols. They must also actively share personal information with others when the interests of safety and protection override the need for confidentiality.

Domain 3: Nursing practice and decision-making

Generic standard for competence

All nurses must practise autonomously, compassionately, skilfully and safely, and must maintain dignity and promote health and wellbeing. They must assess and meet the full range of essential physical and mental health needs of people of all ages who come into their care. Where necessary they must be able to provide safe and effective immediate care to all people prior to accessing or referring to specialist services irrespective of their field of practice. All nurses must also meet more complex and coexisting needs for people in their own nursing field of practice, in any setting including hospital, community and at home. All practice should be informed by the best available evidence and comply with local and national guidelines. Decision-making must be shared with service users, carers and families and informed by critical analysis of a full range of possible interventions, including the use of up-to-date technology. All nurses must also understand how behaviour, culture, socioeconomic and other factors, in the care environment and its location, can affect health, illness, health outcomes and public health priorities and take this into account in planning and delivering care.

Field standard for competence

Learning disabilities nurses must have an enhanced knowledge of the health and developmental needs of all people with learning disabilities, and the factors that might influence them. They must aim to improve and maintain their health and independence through skilled direct and indirect nursing care. They must also be able to provide direct care to meet the essential and complex physical and mental health needs of people with learning disabilities.

Competencies

1 All nurses must use up-to-date knowledge and evidence to assess, plan, deliver and evaluate care, communicate findings, influence change and promote health and best practice. They must make person-centred, evidence-based judgments and decisions, in partnership with others involved in the care process, to ensure high quality care. They must be able to recognise when the complexity of clinical decisions requires specialist knowledge and expertise, and consult or refer accordingly.

1.1 **Learning disabilities nurses** must be able to recognise and respond to the needs of all people who come into their care including babies, children and young people, pregnant and postnatal women, people with mental health, people with physical health problems and disabilities, older people, and people with long term problems such as cognitive impairment.

2 All nurses must possess a broad knowledge of the structure and functions of the human body, and other relevant knowledge from the life, behavioural and social sciences as applied to health, ill health, disability, ageing and death. They must have an in-depth knowledge of common physical and mental health problems and treatments in their own field of practice, including co-morbidity and physiological and psychological vulnerability.

3 All nurses must carry out comprehensive, systematic nursing assessments that take account of relevant physical, social, cultural, psychological, spiritual, genetic and environmental factors, in partnership with service users and others through interaction, observation and measurement.

3.1 **Learning disabilities nurses** must use a structured, person-centred approach to assess, interpret and respond therapeutically to people with learning disabilities, and their often

complex, pre-existing physical and psychological health needs. They must work in partnership with service users, carers and other professionals, services and agencies to agree and implement individual care plans and ensure continuity of care.

4 All nurses must ascertain and respond to the physical, social and psychological needs of people, groups and communities. They must then plan, deliver and evaluate safe, competent, person-centred care in partnership with them, paying special attention to changing health needs during different life stages, including progressive illness and death, loss and bereavement.

5 All nurses must understand public health principles, priorities and practice in order to recognise and respond to the major causes and social determinants of health, illness and health inequalities. They must use a range of information and data to assess the needs of people, groups, communities and populations, and work to improve health, wellbeing and experiences of healthcare; secure equal access to health screening, health promotion and healthcare; and promote social inclusion.

5.1 **Learning disabilities nurses** must lead the development, implementation and review of individual plans for all people with learning disabilities, to promote their optimum health and wellbeing and facilitate their equal access to all health, social care and specialist services.

6 All nurses must practise safely by being aware of the correct use, limitations and hazards of common interventions, including nursing activities, treatments, and the use of medical devices and equipment. The nurse must be able to evaluate their use, report any concerns promptly through appropriate channels and modify care where necessary to maintain safety. They must contribute to the collection of local and national data and formulation of policy on risks, hazards and adverse outcomes.

7 All nurses must be able to recognise and interpret signs of normal and deteriorating mental and physical health and respond promptly to maintain or improve the health and comfort of the service user, acting to keep them and others safe.

8 All nurses must provide educational support, facilitation skills and therapeutic nursing interventions to optimise health and wellbeing. They must promote self-care and management whenever possible, helping people to make choices about their healthcare needs, involving families and carers where appropriate, to maximise their ability to care for themselves.

8.1 **Learning disabilities nurses** must work in partnership with people with learning disabilities and their families and carers to facilitate choice and maximise self-care and self-management and co-ordinate the transition between different services and agencies.

9 All nurses must be able to recognise when a person is at risk and in need of extra support and protection and take reasonable steps to protect them from abuse.

10 All nurses must evaluate their care to improve clinical decision-making, quality and outcomes, using a range of methods, amending the plan of care, where necessary, and communicating changes to others.

Domain 4: Leadership, management and team working

Generic standard for competence

All nurses must be professionally accountable and use clinical governance processes to maintain and improve nursing practice and standards of healthcare. They must be able to respond autonomously and confidently to planned and uncertain situations, managing themselves and others effectively. They must create and maximise opportunities to improve services. They must also demonstrate the potential to develop further management and leadership skills during their period of preceptorship and beyond.

Field standard for competence

Learning disabilities nurses must exercise collaborative management, delegation and supervision skills to create, manage and support therapeutic environments for people with learning disabilities.

Competencies

1 All nurses must act as change agents and provide leadership through quality improvement and service development to enhance people's wellbeing and experiences of healthcare.

 1.1 **Learning disabilities nurses** must take the lead in ensuring that people with learning disabilities receive support that creatively addresses their physical, social, economic, psychological, spiritual and other needs, when assessing, planning and delivering care.

 1.2 **Learning disabilities nurses** must provide direction through leadership and education to ensure that their unique contribution is recognised in service design and provision.

2 All nurses must systematically evaluate care and ensure that they and others use the findings to help improve people's experience and care outcomes and to shape future services.

 2.1 **Learning disabilities nurses** must use data and research findings on the health of people with learning disabilities to help improve people's experiences and care outcomes, and shape of future services.

3 All nurses must be able to identify priorities and manage time and resources effectively to ensure the quality of care is maintained or enhanced.

4 All nurses must be self-aware and recognise how their own values, principles and assumptions may affect their practice. They must maintain their own personal and professional development, learning from experience, through supervision, feedback, reflection and evaluation.

5 All nurses must facilitate nursing students and others to develop their competence, using a range of professional and personal development skills.

6 All nurses must work independently as well as in teams. They must be able to take the lead in coordinating, delegating and supervising care safely, managing risk and remaining accountable for the care given.

 6.1 **Learning disabilities nurses** must use leadership, influencing and decision-making skills to engage effectively with a range of agencies and professionals. They must also be able, when needed, to represent the health needs and protect the rights of people with learning disabilities and challenge negative stereotypes.

 6.2 **Learning disabilities nurses** must work closely with stakeholders to enable people with learning disabilities to exercise choice and challenge discrimination.

7 All nurses must work effectively across professional and agency boundaries, actively involving and respecting others' contributions to integrated person-centred care. They must know when and how to communicate with and refer to other professionals and agencies in order to respect the choices of service users and others, promoting shared decision making, to deliver positive outcomes and to coordinate smooth, effective transition within and between services and agencies.

Competencies for entry to the register: Children's nursing

Domain 1: Professional values

Generic standard for competence

All nurses must act first and foremost to care for and safeguard the public. They must practise autonomously and be responsible and accountable for safe, compassionate, person-centred, evidence-based nursing that respects and maintains dignity and human rights. They must show professionalism and integrity and work within recognised professional, ethical and legal frameworks. They must work in partnership with other health and social care professionals and agencies, service users, their carers and families in all settings, including the community, ensuring that decisions about care are shared.

Field standard for competence

Children's nurses must understand their role as an advocate for children, young people and their families, and work in partnership with them. They must deliver child and family-centred care; empower children and young people to express their views and preferences; and maintain and recognise their rights and best interests.

Competencies

1 All nurses must practise with confidence according to *The code: Standards of conduct, performance and ethics for nurses and midwives* (NMC 2008), and within other recognised ethical and legal frameworks. They must be able to recognize and address ethical challenges relating to people's choices and decision-making about their care, and act within the law to help them and their families and carers find acceptable solutions.

1.1 **Children's nurses** must understand the laws relating to child and parental consent, including giving and refusing consent, withdrawal of treatment and legal capacity.

2 All nurses must practise in a holistic, non-judgmental, caring and sensitive manner that avoids assumptions, supports social inclusion; recognises and respects individual choice; and acknowledges diversity. Where necessary, they must challenge inequality, discrimination and exclusion from access to care.

2.1 **Children's nurses** must recognise that all children and young people have the right to be safe, enjoy life and reach their potential. They must practice in a way that recognises, respects and responds to the individuality of every child and young person.

3 All nurses must support and promote the health, wellbeing, rights and dignity of people, groups, communities and populations. These include people whose lives are affected by ill health, disability, inability to engage, ageing or death. Nurses must act on their understanding of how these conditions influence public health.

3.1 **Children's nurses** must act as advocates for the right of all children and young people to lead full and independent lives.

4 All nurses must work in partnership with service users, carers, groups, communities and organisations. They must manage risk, and promote health and wellbeing while aiming to empower choices that promote self-care and safety.

4.1 **Children's nurses** must work in partnership with children, young people and their families to negotiate, plan and deliver child and family-centred care, education and support. They must recognise the parent's or carer's primary role in achieving and maintaining the child's or young person's health and wellbeing, and offer advice and support on parenting in health and illness.

5 All nurses must fully understand the nurse's various roles, responsibilities and functions, and adapt their practice to meet the changing needs of people, groups, communities and populations.

6 All nurses must understand the roles and responsibilities of other health and social care professionals, and seek to work with them collaboratively for the benefit of all who need care.

7 All nurses must be responsible and accountable for keeping their knowledge and skills up to date through continuing professional development. They must aim to improve their performance and enhance the safety and quality of care through evaluation, supervision and appraisal.

8 All nurses must practise independently, recognising the limits of their competence and knowledge. They must reflect on these limits and seek advice from, or refer to, other professionals where necessary.

9 All nurses must appreciate the value of evidence in practice, be able to understand and appraise research, apply relevant theory and research findings to their work, and identify areas for further investigation.

Domain 2: Communication and interpersonal skills

Generic standard for competence

All nurses must use excellent communication and interpersonal skills. Their communications must always be safe, effective, compassionate and respectful. They must communicate effectively using a wide range of strategies and interventions including the effective use of communication technologies. Where people have a disability, nurses must be able to work with service users and others to obtain the information needed to make reasonable adjustments that promote optimum health and enable equal access to services.

Field standard for competence

Children's nurses must take account of each child and young person's individuality, including their stage of development, ability to understand, culture, learning or communication difficulties and health status. They must communicate effectively with them and with parents and carers.

Competencies

1 All nurses must build partnerships and therapeutic relationships through safe, effective and non-discriminatory communication. They must take account of individual differences, capabilities and needs.

1.1 **Children's nurses** must work with the child, young person and others to ensure that they are actively involved in decision-making, in order to maintain their independence and take account of their ongoing intellectual, physical and emotional needs.

2 All nurses must use a range of communication skills and technologies to support person-centred care and enhance quality and safety. They must ensure people receive all the information they need in a language and manner that allows them to make informed choices and share decision making. They must recognise when language interpretation or other communication support is needed and know how to obtain it.

2.1 **Children's nurses** must understand all aspects of development from infancy to young adulthood, and identify each child or young person's developmental stage, in order to communicate effectively with them. They must use play, distraction and communication tools appropriate to the child's or young person's stage of development, including for those with sensory or cognitive impairment.

3 All nurses must use the full range of communication methods, including verbal, non-verbal and written, to acquire, interpret and record their knowledge and understanding of people's needs. They must be aware of their own values and beliefs and the impact this may have on their communication with others. They must take account of the many different ways in which people communicate and how these may be influenced by ill health, disability and other factors, and be able to recognise and respond effectively when a person finds it hard to communicate.

3.1 Children's nurses must ensure that, where possible, children and young people understand their healthcare needs and can make or contribute to informed choices about all aspects of their care.

4 All nurses must recognise when people are anxious or in distress and respond effectively, using therapeutic principles, to promote their wellbeing, manage personal safety and resolve conflict. They must use effective communication strategies and negotiation techniques to achieve best

outcomes, respecting the dignity and human rights of all concerned. They must know when to consult a third party and how to make referrals for advocacy, mediation or arbitration.

5 All nurses must use therapeutic principles to engage, maintain and, where appropriate, disengage from professional caring relationships, and must always respect professional boundaries.

6 All nurses must take every opportunity to encourage health-promoting behaviour through education, role modelling and effective communication.

7 All nurses must maintain accurate, clear and complete records, including the use of electronic formats, using appropriate and plain language.

8 All nurses must respect individual rights to confidentiality and keep information secure and confidential in accordance with the law and relevant ethical and regulatory frameworks, taking account of local protocols. They must also actively share personal information with others when the interests of safety and protection override the need for confidentiality.

Domain 3: Nursing practice and decision-making

Generic standard for competence

All nurses must practise autonomously, compassionately, skilfully and safely, and must maintain dignity and promote health and wellbeing. They must assess and meet the full range of essential physical and mental health needs of people of all ages who come into their care. Where necessary they must be able to provide safe and effective immediate care to all people prior to accessing or referring to specialist services irrespective of their field of practice. All nurses must also meet more complex and coexisting needs for people in their own nursing field of practice, in any setting including hospital, community and at home. All practice should be informed by the best available evidence and comply with local and national guidelines. Decision-making must be shared with service users, carers and families and informed by critical analysis of a full range of possible interventions, including the use of up-to-date technology. All nurses must also understand how behaviour, culture, socioeconomic and other factors, in the care environment and its location, can affect health, illness, health outcomes and public health priorities and take this into account in planning and delivering care.

Field standard for competence

Children's nurses must be able to care safely and effectively for children and young people in all settings, and recognise their responsibility for safeguarding them. They must be able to deliver care to meet essential and complex physical and mental health needs informed by deep understanding of biological, psychological and social factors throughout infancy, childhood and adolescence.

Competencies

1 All nurses must use up-to-date knowledge and evidence to assess, plan, deliver and evaluate care, communicate findings, influence change and promote health and best practice. They must make person-centred, evidence-based judgments and decisions, in partnership with others involved in the care process, to ensure high quality care. They must be able to recognise when the complexity of clinical decisions requires specialist knowledge and expertise, and consult or refer accordingly.

1.1 **Children's nurses** must be able to recognise and respond to the essential needs of all people who come into their care including babies, pregnant and postnatal women, adults, people with mental health problems, people with physical disabilities, people with learning disabilities, and people with long term problems such as cognitive impairment.

1.2 **Children's nurses** must use recognised, evidence-based, child-centred frameworks to assess, plan, implement, evaluate and record care, and to underpin clinical judgments and decision-making. Care planning and delivery must be informed by knowledge of pharmacology, anatomy and physiology, pathology, psychology and sociology, from infancy to young adulthood.

2 All nurses must possess a broad knowledge of the structure and functions of the-human body, and other relevant knowledge from the life, behavioural and social sciences as applied to health, ill health, disability, ageing and death. They must have an in-depth knowledge of common physical and mental health problems and treatments in their own field of practice, including co-morbidity and physiological and psychological vulnerability.

3 All nurses must carry out comprehensive, systematic nursing assessments that take account of relevant physical, social, cultural, psychological, spiritual, genetic and environmental

factors, in partnership with service users and others through interaction, observation and measurement.

3.1 **Children's nurses** must carry out comprehensive nursing assessments of children and young people, recognising the particular vulnerability of infants and young children to rapid physiological deterioration.

4 All nurses must ascertain and respond to the physical, social and psychological needs of people, groups and communities. They must then plan, deliver and evaluate safe, competent, person-centred care in partnership with them, paying special attention to changing health needs during different life stages, including progressive illness and death, loss and bereavement.

5 All nurses must understand public health principles, priorities and practice in order to recognise and respond to the major causes and social determinants of health, illness and health inequalities. They must use a range of information and data to assess the needs of people, groups, communities and populations, and work to improve health, wellbeing and experiences of healthcare; secure equal access to health screening, health promotion and healthcare; and promote social inclusion.

5.1 **Children's nurses** must include health promotion, and illness and injury prevention, in their nursing practice. They must promote early intervention to address the links between early life adversity and adult ill health, and the risks to the current and future physical, mental, emotional and sexual health of children and young people.

6 All nurses must practise safely by being aware of the correct use, limitations and hazards of common interventions, including nursing activities, treatments, the calculation and administration of medicines, and the use of medical devices and equipment. The nurse must be able to evaluate their use, report any concerns promptly through appropriate channels and modify care where necessary to maintain safety. They must contribute to the collection of local and national data and formulation of policy on risks, hazards and adverse outcomes.

6.1 **Children's nurses** must have numeracy skills for medicines management, assessment, measuring, monitoring and recording which recognise the particular vulnerability of infants and young children in relation accurate medicines calculation.

7 All nurses must be able to recognise and interpret signs of normal and deteriorating mental and physical health and respond promptly to maintain or improve the health and comfort of the service user, acting to keep them and others safe.

8 All nurses must provide educational support, facilitation skills and therapeutic nursing interventions to optimise health and wellbeing. They must promote self-care and management whenever possible, helping people to make choices about their healthcare needs, involving families and carers where appropriate, to maximise their ability to care for themselves.

8.1 **Children's nurses** must use negotiation skills to ensure the best interests of children and young people in all decisions, including the continuation or withdrawal of care. Negotiation must include the child or young person, their family and members of the multidisciplinary and interagency team where appropriate.

9 All nurses must be able to recognise when a person is at risk and in need of extra support and protection and take reasonable steps to safeguard them against abuse.

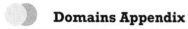

9.1 **Children's nurses** must understand their central role in preventing maltreatment, and safeguarding children and young people. They must work closely with relevant agencies and professionals, and know when and how to identify and refer those at risk or experiencing harm.

10 All nurses must evaluate their care to improve clinical decision-making, quality and outcomes, using a range of methods, amending the plan of care, where necessary, and communicating changes to others.

 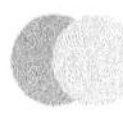

Domain 4: Leadership, management and team working

Generic standard for competence

All nurses must be professionally accountable and use clinical governance processes to maintain and improve nursing practice and standards of healthcare. They must be able to respond autonomously and confidently to planned and uncertain situations, managing themselves and others effectively. They must create and maximise opportunities to improve services. They must also demonstrate the potential to develop further management and leadership skills during their period of preceptorship and beyond.

Field standard for competence

Children's nurses must listen and respond to the wishes of children and young people. They must influence the delivery of health and social care services to optimise the care of children and young people. They must work closely with other agencies and services to ensure seamless and well-supported transition to adult services.

Competencies

1 All nurses must act as change agents and provide leadership through quality improvement and service development to enhance people's wellbeing and experiences of healthcare.

   1.1 **Children's nurses** must understand health and social care policies relating to the health and wellbeing of children and young people. They must, where possible, empower and enable children, young people, parents and carers to influence the quality of care and develop future policies and strategies.

   1.2 **Children's nurses** must ensure that, wherever possible, care is delivered in the child or young person's home, or in another environment that suits their age, needs and preferences.

2 All nurses must systematically evaluate care and ensure that they and others use the findings to help improve people's experience and care outcomes and to shape future services.

3 All nurses must be able to identify priorities and manage time and resources effectively to ensure the quality of care is maintained or enhanced.

4 All nurses must be self-aware and recognise how their own values, principles and assumptions may affect their practice. They must maintain their own personal and professional development, learning from experience, through supervision, feedback, reflection and evaluation.

5 All nurses must facilitate nursing students and others to develop their competence, using a range of professional and personal development skills.

6 All nurses must work independently as well as in teams. They must be able to take the lead in coordinating, delegating and supervising care safely, managing risk and remaining accountable for the care given.

   6.1 **Children's nurses** must use effective clinical decision-making skills when managing complex and unpredictable situations, especially where the views of children or young people and their parents and carers differ. They must recognise when to seek extra help or advice to manage the situation safely.

7 All nurses must work effectively across professional and agency boundaries, actively involving and respecting others' contributions to integrated person-centred care. They must know when and how to communicate with and refer to other professionals and agencies in order to respect

the choices of service users and others, promoting shared decision making, to deliver positive outcomes and to coordinate smooth, effective transition within and between services and agencies.

7.1 **Children's nurses** must work effectively with young people who have continuing health needs, their families, the multidisciplinary team and other agencies to manage smooth and effective transition from children's services to adult services, taking account of individual needs and preferences.

Index

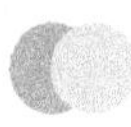

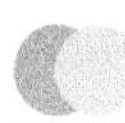

 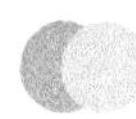

 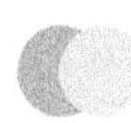

 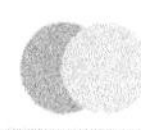

 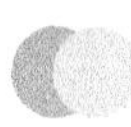